EFFECTIVE LEADERSHIP & MANAGEMENT

in Nutrition & Dietetics

EDITORS

Julie Grim, MPH, RDN, LD

Susan Renee Roberts, DCN, RDN, LDN, CNSC, FAND

eat right.® Academy of Nutrition and Dietetics

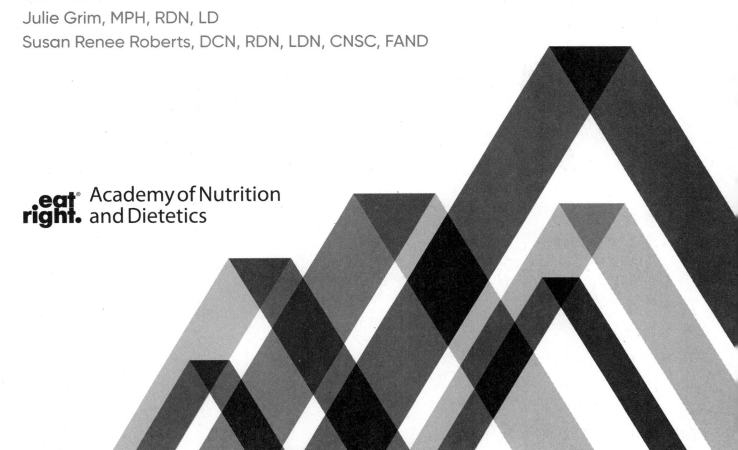

eat right. Academy of Nutrition and Dietetics

Academy of Nutrition and Dietetics
120 S. Riverside Plaza, Suite 2190
Chicago, IL 60606

Effective Leadership & Management in Nutrition & Dietetics

ISBN 978-0-88091-202-0 (print)
ISBN 978-0-88091-211-2 (eBook)
Catalog Number 202023 (print)
Catalog Number 202023e (eBook)

10   9   8   7   6   5   4   3   2   1

For more information on the Academy of Nutrition and Dietetics, visit www.eatright.org.

Library of Congress Cataloging-in-Publication Data
Names: Grim, Julie A., editor. | Roberts, Susan Renee, editor.
Title: Effective leadership & management in nutrition & dietetics / editors
   Julie Grim, MPH, RDN, LD, Susan Renee Roberts, DCN, RDN, LD, CNSC, FAND.

Other titles: Effective leadership and management in nutrition and
   dietetics
Description: Chicago, IL : Academy of Nutrition and Dietetics, [2023] |
   Includes bibliographical references and index.
Identifiers: LCCN 2022060612 (print) | LCCN 2022060613 (ebook) | ISBN
   9780880912020 (paperback) | ISBN 9780880912112 (ebook)
Subjects: LCSH: Dietetics--Vocational guidance. | Nutrition
   counseling--Vocational guidance.
Classification: LCC RM218.5 .E34 2023 (print) | LCC RM218.5 (ebook) | DDC
   613.2023--dc23/eng/20230314
LC record available at https://lccn.loc.gov/2022060612
LC ebook record available at https://lccn.loc.gov/2022060613

CONTENTS

CONTRIBUTORS

Kim Brenkus, MBA, RDN, LD, FAND
Director of Learning and Development, Metz Culinary Management
Auburn, AL

Pamela Charney, PhD, MS, RDN, LDN, FAND
Clinical Dietitian, Geisinger
Wilkes-Barre, PA

Mandy L. Corrigan, MPH, RD, CNSC, FAND, FASPEN
Nutrition Manager, Cleveland Clinic
Cleveland, OH

Julie Grim, MPH, RDN, LD
National Nutrition Director, American Diabetes Association
Plano, TX

Janelle Gunn, MPH, RD
Associate Director for Policy, Partnerships and Communications, Division of Nutrition, Physical Activity and Obesity, Centers for Disease Control and Prevention

Samia Hamdan, MPH, RDN
Division Director, USDA Food and Nutrition Service Agency
Chicago, IL

Cindy Hamilton, MS, RD, LD, FAND
Senior Director (Retired), Nutrition, Center for Human Nutrition, Cleveland Clinic
Cleveland, OH

Bonnie Javurek, MEd, RDN, LD
Clinical Nutrition Manager (Retired), Cleveland Clinic
Cleveland, OH

Deanna Belleny Lewis, MPH, RDN
Co-Founder, Diversify Dietetics
Atlanta, GA

Claire Loose, MA, RD, LD
Manager, Clinical Nutrition, Cleveland Clinic Akron General: Lodi and Union Hospitals
Akron, OH

Julie O'Sullivan-Maillet, PhD, RDN, FADA, FAND
Professor, Rutgers School of Health Professions
Newark, NJ

Ashley Mullins, MS, RDN, LD, CNSC
Dietetic Internship Director, Aramark Healthcare+ at Baylor University Medical Center
Dallas, TX

John A. Papazoglou, MPA/HCA
Associate Vice President, The Pennsylvania State University
State College, PA

Wendy Phillips, MS, RD, CLE, NWCC, FAND
Regional Vice President, Morrison Healthcare
Cleveland, OH

Camille Range, MPH, RDN
Doctoral Candidate, University of the District of Columbia
Washington, DC

Kristin Ringo, RDN, LD, CNSC
Consulting Dietitian, Baylor Health Care System/Aramark Healthcare
Dallas, TX

Susan Renee Roberts, DCN, RDN, LDN, CNSC, FAND
Director, Dietetics and Nutrition Coordinated Program, Keiser University
Melbourne, FL

Marsha Schofield, MS, RD, LD, FAND
Owner, Marsha Schofield & Associates LLC
Stow, OH

Agnieszka Sowa, MS, RD, LD
Clinical Nutrition Manager, Cleveland Clinic
Cleveland, OH

Janel Welch, MS, MPA, RDN, CDN, FAND, CPHQ, QCP, OHCC
Director of Quality & Risk Management/Corporate Compliance Officer, St Ann's Community
Rochester, NY

REVIEWERS

Deanne Brandstetter, MBA, RDN, CDN, FAND
Vice President, Nutrition & Wellness, Compass Group
Rye Brook, NY

Ann F. Childers, MS, MHA, RDN, LD
Manager (Retired), Clinical Nutrition and Informatics, Prisma Health Richland Hospital
Columbia, SC

Mary Lee Chin, MS, RDN
Nutrition Communications Consultant, Nutrition Edge Communications
Denver, CO

Kathleen M. Cullinen, PhD, MS, RDN
Program Manager, Disease Prevention & Control, New Jersey Department of Health, Division of Community Health Services, Community Health and Wellness Unit
Newark, NJ

Jennifer Doley, MBA, RD, CNSC, FAND
Malnutrition Program Manager, Morrison Healthcare
Tucson, AZ

Laura Feldman, MS, RDN, CDN, CDCES
Assistant Professor and Director of Didactic Program in Dietetics, Long Island University Post
Greenvale, NY

Cecilia Pozo Fileti, MS, RDN, FADA
President, Latino Health Communications, Inc. Palm Beach Gardens, FL

Sharon Foley, PhD, RDN
Associate Professor, Rush University
Chicago, IL

Rosa K. Hand, PhD, RDN, LD, FAND
Assistant Professor, Department of Nutrition, Case Western Reserve University
Cleveland, OH

Gisele Leger, MS, RDN, LDN, CNSC, FAND
National Director, Clinical Nutrition, Morrison Healthcare
Atlanta, GA

Paul Moore, PhD, MBA, RD, CSSD, LDN, CSCS, NSCA-CPT
Senior Lecturer
Appalachian State University
Boone, NC

Caroline W. Passerrello, MS, RDN, LDN
Instructor, University of Pittsburgh
Pittsburgh, PA

Kathleen M. Pellechia, MS, RDN, PMP
Associate Director, Projects and Programs, FHI 360
Washington, DC

Wendy Phillips, MS, RD, CLE, NWCC, FAND
Regional Vice President, Morrison Healthcare
Cleveland, OH

Judith Rodriguez , PhD, RDN
Professor Emeritus, University of North Florida
Jacksonville, FL

Shaynee Roper, DCN, MEd, RD, LDN, FAND
Corporate Dietitian, Home Health and Hospice
Oxford, NC

Kevin L. Sauer, PhD, RDN, LD, FAND
Professor, Kansas State University
Manhattan, KS

Shey L. Schnell, MHA, RD
Regional Director, Performance Improvement, University of Vermont Health Network, Champlain Valley Physicians Hospital
Plattsburgh, NY

Aaron Schwartz, MBA, MS, RD, LD
Lecturer, Dietetic Internship Director, Director of Undergraduate Studies, University of Kentucky
Lexington, KY

Amber Smith, MBA, RD, ACC, TMP, PMP
Director, Leader Development, Advisory Board
Washington DC

Paula Milas Sochacki, EdD, MPH, RDN, LDN
Assistant Professor/DPD Program Director, Benedictine University
Lisle, IL

Liset L. Vasquez, PhD, RDN, LD, CHES
Dietetic Director/Assistant Professor in Practice, University of Texas at San Antonio
San Antonio, TX

Kate Willcutts, DCN, RDN, CNSC, FASPEN
VA Western Colorado Health Care System
Grand Junction, CO

Mary K. Young, MS, RD
Principal, MKYoung Food & Nutrition Strategies
Franktown, CO

FOREWORD

Leadership occurs when people reach goals together, and then instinctively gain momentum and continue forward because they are inspired to do so. So get ready to be inspired by this book—it certainly motivated me!

Though we cannot predict the future, we can cocreate it through the continual reflection and development of our own management and leadership skills. Said professional development will be paramount to move the dietetics profession forward through the 21st century.

Appropriate and effective nutrition care does not occur by accident nor by technical abilities alone: it is only possible through financial resource managament, effective leadership and communication, workforce diversity, appropriate use of technology, quality improvement, strategic planning, and more—all key topics that mirror well throughout the chapters in this book. Drawing upon the experiences of distinguished practicing managers and leaders in the nutrition field, this book aims to provide the important whats and whys of applicable leadership and management. Key principles and moments of sage advice are shared through the lenses of those with substantial experience and will offer new perspectives to inspire both current and potential leaders. The book is designed to inform practitioners across a variety of practice settings and organizational structures and will be especially helpful to registered dietitian nutritionists and nutrition and dietetics technicians, registered, at various career stages and transitions. Indeed, this resource is applicable anywhere there are groups of people working hard toward a common cause to improve the human condition through nutrition and care.

I know that you will find *Effective Leadership & Management in Nutrition & Dietetics* to be immediately useful and a source of reference for a successful future. Clearly, this book was written *by leaders for leaders*.

Kevin L. Sauer, PhD, RDN, LD, FAND
Professor, Dietetics
Co-Director, Center for Food Safety in Child Nutrition Programs
Department of Food, Nutrition, Dietetics, and Health
Kansas State University, College of Health and Human Sciences
Past President, Academy of Nutrition and Dietetics

When we go through training to become registered dietitian nutritionists (RDNs) or nutrition and dietetics technicians, registered (NDTRs), our exposure to leadership and management principles and skills is often limited. When we then find ourselves in a role that requires these skills, it is not always easy to find practical resources to hasten the learning curve. The impact of the COVID-19 pandemic and resulting challenges in delivering food and nutrition services in dramatically different environments, embracing new technologies, and managing through substantial staffing challenges made the need for effective leaders in our profession even more evident.

Following the success of *The Clinical Nutrition Manager's Handbook: Solutions for the Busy Professional*, we were asked to consider leading a new edition but with a broader focus on management in other settings. This led to discussion of how leadership is critical in all aspects of the profession, including in management roles, and the concept for this book was established. During development, it became clear that an expanded focus on diversity was also essential for nutrition managers and leaders, and an excellent chapter devoted to embracing diversity and embodying inclusive leadership is now included.

Whether you have a formal or informal leadership role, are experienced or early in your career, all dietetics professionals can benefit from useful, applicable information. Leaders can emerge in any environment and work to inspire people. Managers inhabit formal roles within an organization and supervise staff and activities. The two are separate yet complementary. This book is designed to build management and leadership knowledge and skills in key areasincluding negotiation, staff development, budgeting, strategic planning, quality improvement, and regulatory compliance, among others. We hope that it will help you navigate your own distinct career path and assist you with solving common problems you may encounter along the way. In addition, the book features many practical ideas and best practices from a distinguished group of RDN leaders in a variety of professional roles and practice areas.

There are many ways to use this book. You may wish to start at the beginning and read cover to cover. Alternatively, we encourage you to turn to the chapters that are most relevant to your current or desired role or begin with the topics that are least familiar to you. Our hope is that the information in this book will make you more knowledgeable, successful, and effective in your role as a food and nutrition leader.

Julie Grim, MPH, RDN, LD
Susan Renee Roberts, DCN, RDN, LDN, CNSC, FAND

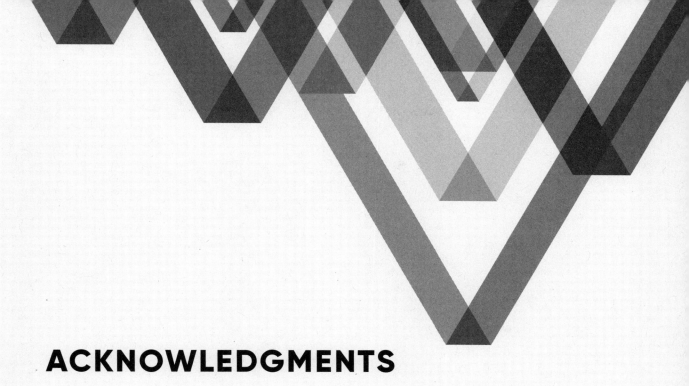

ACKNOWLEDGMENTS

This book is dedicated to our families who provided unending love and support. We want to express our appreciation to the authors and reviewers for their willingness to give back to their profession by sharing their time and expertise. And finally, we would like to thank the many registered dietitians and other health care professionals who have mentored and encouraged us over the years.

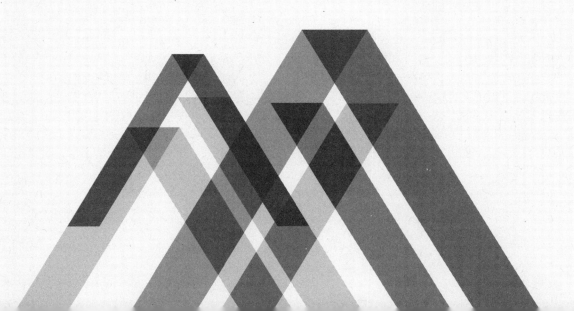

Julie Grim, MPH, RDN, LD, is a registered dietitian and licensed dietitian/nutritionist with a master's degree in public health and a passion for the role of nutrition in the prevention and management of chronic disease. She has more than 25 years of experience in food and nutrition leadership and health care administration as well as teaching experience at the graduate level. Julie is currently the director of nutrition for the American Diabetes Association. She has served in many national leadership roles for the Academy of Nutrition and Dietetics, including the Accreditation Council for Education in Nutrition and Dietetics (ACEND), the Nutrition Care Process Committee, and the Nominating Committee. Julie is the coeditor of the *Clinical Nutrition Manager's Handbook: Solutions for the Busy Professional*. She speaks nationally on leadership development and the role of nutrition in chronic disease prevention. In her spare time, Julie is an organic gardener and an artist. She lives in North Texas and is married with two grown children and one grandson.

Susan Renee Roberts, DCN, RDN, LDN, CNSC, FAND, is a registered and licensed dietitian/nutritionist with a doctorate in clinical nutrition from Rutgers University, and master's and bachelor's degrees from Texas A&M University. She has more than 30 years of experience in the field of dietetics with expertise in oncology, critical care, clinical research, clinical nutrition management, and dietetics education. Susan has served as an educator to graduate, undergraduate, and dietetic internship students and is currently program director for the Coordinated Program in Dietetics at Keiser University in Melbourne, FL. She has held many different leadership roles within the Academy of Nutrition and Dietetics, including with the Dietitians in Nutrition Support dietetic practice group, the Nominating Committee, the Council on Future Practice, and the Board of Directors. She received the Medallion Award in 2018 and the Excellence in Clinical Practice Award in 2007. Throughout her career, Susan has presented on topics in her areas of expertise and has authored multiple peer-reviewed publications. When not engaged with work or professional activities, she enjoys pickleball and beach walks as well as trying out new recipes. She is married with two grown sons and two adorable dogs.

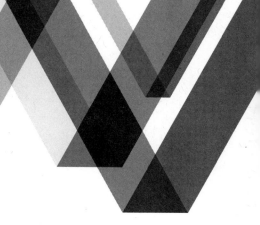

CHAPTER 1
Leadership Fundamentals

Julie Grim, MPH, RDN, LD

Introduction

Leadership in the dietetics profession (as well as in many professions), although widely discussed, is often poorly understood and not readily embraced. In spite of this, the need for effective leadership in dietetics has never been greater. According to Susan Calvert Finn, former president of the Academy of Nutrition and Dietetics, "Leadership skills are needed in all areas of dietetics to address the big issues of health care facing the world."[1] Changes in health care service and delivery, globalization, enhanced diversity in the work environment, and increases in both nutrition-related chronic disease and the need for sustainable food systems all present opportunities for food and nutrition professionals to step in and lead. Leadership skill and competency development can enable nutrition professionals to be ready when the opportunity arises.

The goal of this chapter is to discuss the core competencies to develop early in your career to maximize your current and future leadership abilities. There is a common misconception that leaders are born, not made. You may have been telling yourself that you don't have the personality for leadership. Or perhaps a negative early experience with an employee or a peer confrontation led you to feel discouraged about your ability to lead. Don't give up! Research shows—and leadership experts agree—that leadership is a set of competencies that can be learned through education, practice, experience, and coaching rather than innate talent.[2,3] In addition, leadership skills are transferable to other professions and can be utilized far beyond the work environment.

Why Leadership Skills and Competencies Are Essential

Leadership skills and competencies are necessary to be successful in life as well as work. The terms *skills* and *competencies* are often used interchangeably, but they are not the same. Skills are specific, learned activities that range widely in terms of complexity. Competencies are broader and define the knowledge, judgment, and required attitude in addition to skills.[4,5] Developing both skills and competencies enhances self-confidence and the ability to communicate and work effectively with others—critical in all aspects of life. Leadership training should start early in your career and combine knowledge and competency development through supervised practice. Although research indicates that experience, rather than formal training, may be the best way to develop leaders, educational training that replicates developmentally challenging experiences (such as simulations and case studies) can complement experience and enhance leadership competency.[3,6] This is accomplished by motivating people to think critically about situations, teaching them to analyze underlying causes and consequences of problems, and enabling them to develop new ways of working with others.[4] Some individuals may have particular character traits that make it easier to develop these skills, but the majority of competency development is the result of learning and actual experience.

Many opportunities to obtain leadership training exist. Options range from free online leadership courses and short seminars or webinars to certificate programs and advanced degrees. If your employer offers or subsidizes any of these types of opportunities, take advantage of them. Expanding your leadership skills will give you the confidence and visibility to take on expanded roles; seize opportunities; and gain insights into yourself, your supervisors, and your colleagues.

Leadership challenges and opportunities are not confined to the work environment. Many everyday activities (eg, serving on the board of a parent-teacher or homeowners association or volunteering as a committee member for a service, professional, or religious organization) present opportunities to lead. For example, serving on your homeowners association board can provide the opportunity to expand your negotiating and communication skills, both of which are essential for leadership in any setting.

Leadership Theory Overview

Theories on what makes a good leader have evolved over hundreds of years. These theories are often characterized by which aspect of leadership is thought to be most critical in defining the leader. One of the early widespread leadership theories, the great man theory, was based on the belief that only a "great" man could have the characteristics of a great leader. Many philosophers also thought that leadership traits were something an individual was born with, were intrinsic, and would emerge when confronted with the appropriate situation.[5,7] This trait-based thinking continued into the mid-1900s, when behavior-based theories began to emerge. Behavior-based theories reflected a new perspective that focused on the behaviors of the leaders instead of their mental, physical, or social characteristics. This resulted in a shift in belief that leadership was not innate but could be developed. The most salient leadership theories today build on this understanding and also begin to integrate followers' perspectives and the situations in which leaders and followers interact.[5,7]

As continued research in psychology and business practice provides new evidence on effective leadership strategies, many new theories have emerged. Examples from the last 50 years include the following[7,8]:

> Transactional leader theory, or the exchange leadership theory, describes a hierarchical form of leadership characterized by transactions made between the leader and the followers using a structure of rewards and consequences.

> Transformational leadership theory describes a system in which leaders encourage, inspire, and motivate employees to innovate and create change that will help grow the organization and shape its future success.

> Participative leadership theory suggests that the ideal leadership style considers multiple parties' input. Team members' involvement increases engagement and collaboration and results in improved decision making and business outcomes.

Additional resources on leadership theory are provided at the end of this chapter.

Management vs Leadership

Like *skills* and *competencies*, the terms *management* and *leadership* are often used interchangeably but are two separate and distinct entities. Management and leadership are necessary and complementary sets of competencies that add value in the workplace, and in many roles, you need both. Managers often possess a title (such as human resources manager or regional manager) or other designated position, whereas leaders can be found at all levels of an organization and in nonwork environments. Box 1.1 lists additional distinctions.[3,9,10]

BOX 1.1 Differences Between Leadership and Management[3,9,10]

Leadership	Management
Title, designation, seniority not required	Role formalized with title and delegated power within an organizational structure
Can be in any environment: work, school, community, etc	Workplace related
Supervisory authority can be formal or informal	Supervisory authority is formal
Emphasis on inspiring people	Emphasis on managing activities
Key functions: » selecting talent » motivating » coaching » building trust » inspiring » leading change	Key roles: » planning » budgeting » controlling » evaluating » communicating

Fundamental Leadership Competencies

Several core competencies can substantially impact the effectiveness of a new leader, regardless of the role. These include communication, self-awareness, empathy, influence, and learning agility.[3,10-13] These core competencies can enhance your effectiveness immediately and represent the building blocks for development of more advanced leadership skills and competencies. For example, the core competency of influence can lead to the ability to steer long-range objectives as well as set the stage for inspiring other individuals.[6-8,14]

Communication

Communication is an essential skill and a component in many other leadership competencies, such as negotiation or influence. According to the Center for Creative Leadership, "Communicating information and ideas is consistently rated among the most important skills for leaders to be successful."[11] Whether you manage employees in a child nutrition program, serve on a board, coordinate a team of volunteers, or organize your neighborhood carpool, your leadership skills are dependent on your ability to communicate effectively with others. The competency of effective communication can be broken down into three core components: active listening, speaking with clarity, and writing clearly.[3,10]

Active Listening

> *"Seek first to understand, then to be understood."* –Stephen R. Covey

Many experts think listening is the most important component of excellent communication skills and the most poorly executed.[3,10-13] The Sperry Corporation found that of our four basic workplace skills (listening, speaking, reading, and writing), listening is the most used but the least taught.[15] Studies show that the average listener retains only half of what is presented in a 10-minute presentation, and after 48 hours, retention drops by half again.[9] Managers, because they are in a position of power and usually short on time, are particularly vulnerable to poor listening behaviors. They tend to dominate the conversation, interrupt others to make their own points, ignore contributions of team members, and so on.[13]

Active listening involves fully concentrating on what is being said and listening for meaning. It represents a blend of skills that can be learned and begins with identifying your own personal barriers to listening. Signs that you might be a poor listener include getting impatient, jumping in with solutions, interrupting, planning your responses while the other person is still talking, not giving verbal cues that you are paying attention, and missing the meaning behind the conversation. The goal of listening should be to understand, not to formulate an answer.

Leadership experts recommend the following tactics to improve your listening skills[3,10,16]:

> Communicate your attention nonverbally by facing the speaker, nodding, smiling, and maintaining eye contact.

> Avoid distractions (for example, put your phone or watch on silent, turn it over, etc).

> Make listening your single focus. Don't multitask.

> Suspend judgment. Look for the worth of the content.

> Wait until the speaker is finished before formulating your response.

> After the speaker finishes speaking, pause for 3 to 5 seconds to formulate your response. By doing this, you avoid the risk of interrupting the speaker, who may just be taking a breath, and you show the speaker you are considering what they've said.

> Ask questions for clarification.

> Briefly summarize the message or information you have just heard. This can be a difficult practice to develop, but it is the most effective way to demonstrate that you have truly heard and understood the individual.

Even though active listening seems like a very basic skill, it has a substantial impact on leader effectiveness. Active listening allows you to gain insight into your managers and colleagues and helps you build trust, improve employee engagement, and avoid misunderstandings. An example of active listening in the workplace is described in the following Stories From the Field box.

STORIES FROM THE FIELD: Active Listening in the Workplace

A university nutrition department chairperson was preparing to meet with an upset faculty member regarding an issue of workload equity. Before the meeting, the chairperson reviewed faculty work-load assignments, forwarded their office phone calls, and put their cell phone on silent to ensure they would not be interrupted.

When the faculty member arrived, they immediately began sharing how frustrated they were that they taught more classes than their colleague and did much more work, even though they had less administrative time allocated. Even though the department chair had already researched the situation and thought the workloads were equitable, they let the faculty member air their grievance and then asked clarifying questions such as, "Can you tell me more about your current research obligations and any future research and grants that you have planned? You had three new course preps this year; how much time did you commit to that task? How do you handle a situation when a student comes to you rather than the other faculty member with issues related to the other faculty member or their class? What are your current service obligations at the university and with your profession?" The chairperson also made eye contact and nodded to indicate they were listening attentively and seeking to understand the source or sources of the faculty member's frustration. For example, was this truly a workload issue, or was it an issue of salary, lack of recognition, dissatisfaction with courses they were teaching, or something else?

Once the faculty member had finished sharing their issue, the chair summarized the issue to ensure they had heard the faculty member accurately. Then and only then, the chair shared their reasoning for the allocation of teaching and administrative responsibilities as well as factors that went into that allocation that the faculty member had not considered—for example, time that the other faculty member was spending administering a current grant and the additional grants and publications that the faculty member was preparing. In addition, the other faculty member was teaching several lab courses, so while the number of credits was lower, the time spent in the classroom actually exceeded the first faculty member's course load. By actively listening to the faculty member, the chairperson identified that a source of the faculty member's dissatisfaction was the number of new course preps they had done in the past year with little support in the classes from a teaching assistant. The faculty member was discouraged that much of the time dedicated to research was spent resubmitting publications, making the faculty member feel like no progress was being made on research. It also seemed unfair to the first faculty member that the other faculty member got administrative re-assigned time when they did not seem to enjoy working with and spending time with students.

By increasing teaching assistant support, the chairperson was able to ensure the faculty member felt valued and heard and was satisfied with the chairperson's response.

Speaking With Clarity

> *"To be clear, stop and think, and then proceed slowly."* –Brian Tracy[16]

Speaking with clarity is not just for public speaking. It is an essential skill if you will be directing the work of others, delegating, or leading in any way. When speaking with clarity, it is important to consider your audience. Unless you are speaking to a group of like-minded colleagues, keep your communications basic and clear. For example, nurses on a unit typically only have time for a 10-minute in-service meeting. If you speak much longer than that, you may be affecting breaks or contributing to staff members going into overtime. Worse yet, you might get cut off before you get to the most important information. In addition to being concise, avoid jargon or acronyms. Your audience may miss the key message if they are busy trying to decipher an unfamiliar word or acronym. Clarity is also essential when assigning or delegating a task or doing performance coaching. Keeping your communication simple and clear and asking for a recap from your audience can help ensure your message was received as intended. See Box 1.2 for an example of speaking with clarity.

> **BOX 1.2** Clarity in the Workplace
>
> **Original:** Pat, I know you have a lot on your plate, but it would be helpful if I could get a quick summary of our metrics in the next week or so. Nothing major, just the highlights. Thanks so much!
>
> **Better:** Pat, I need a presentation of five or six slides with graphs showing our quality and customer service metrics for the quarter ending June 30th by this Friday at 5:00 PM to present to senior leadership next week. Do you see any barriers to getting this report done by that deadline? Thanks so much!

Structured Communication Tools

The Situation, Background, Assessment, Recommendation (SBAR) technique and communication huddles are two structured communication tools adopted by many health care institutions that may be adapted to your environment to help improve communication with your team. Originally developed by the US military for use in the context of nuclear submarines, SBAR has been adopted in many health care settings to ensure prompt and appropriate communication. This tool can help your staff learn the key components needed to send a complete message. See Box 1.3 for an example of SBAR communication.[17,18]

> **BOX 1.3** Situation, Background, Assessment, Recommendation Technique Communication in the Workplace[17,18]

S = Situation (Describe what happened; be specific.)	**S:** At 8:30 AM, a customer fell in the Westside Cafe while carrying a tray to a table. The cashier helped the customer up and checked to see if they were okay. The customer reported they were fine and refused medical attention. The cashier called the supervisor, who got the customer another breakfast and filled out an incident report.
B = Background (Explain the circumstances leading to the situation.)	**B:** The Westside Cafe is typically crowded at that hour, so it is often difficult to navigate the seating area.
A = Assessment (Explain what you think the problem is, and what concerns you.)	**A:** The congestion may have contributed to the customer falling. I am concerned because this is the second time this quarter we have had a fall in the cafe.
R = Recommendation (Make a recommendation to correct the problem.)	**R:** I recommend we rearrange the tables to create a wider path through the seating areas, and remind the cashiers to offer assistance to unsteady or frail customers.

A second effective communication tool is communication huddles. Huddles are frequent, quick briefings to help the team stay informed. These quick check-ins focus on important issues the staff are dealing with on a daily basis, such as equipment failure, patient workload, staff coverage for a required training, and so on.[19,20] To make huddles successful, keep the focus on shift activities and problem solving, and actively and consistently include team members. Also, keep the meetings short—1 to 10 minutes is ideal.[15,16] The Institute for Healthcare Improvement (IHI) has good resources to assist with huddle implementation.[20] Nutrition-focused examples of the effective use of huddles are provided in Box 1.4.

BOX 1.4 Communication Huddles in Dietetics

Patient Meal Service: Nutrition and dietetics technicians, registered (NDTRs) huddle every morning to discuss patient food issues from the previous day, then attend the patient services huddle in the kitchen to share the identified issues with the kitchen team so they can quickly intervene.

Clinical Nutrition: Registered dietitian nutritionists (RDNs) (who do not attend multidisciplinary rounds on weekends) huddle to determine which patients do not get early enteral nutrition over the weekend. They then convene with all RDNs who work the weekend to set up a mechanism in the electronic health record to identify and prioritize intensive care unit patients ventilated in the last 24 to 48 hours to assess and start enteral nutrition, if appropriate.

Writing Clearly

An important skill of leaders at all levels is the ability to write clear, simple, direct messages. Be sure to use a professional, neutral tone in all written communication in the workplace. Written communication has advantages in many situations. It is especially valuable when giving instructions because the receiver can refer back to the instructions later. The two most common forms of written communication in the workplace are email and text communication, with texting rapidly overtaking email. According to Text Request, a company that works with organizations on managing text communication strategy, texting is the most common form of communication for US adults aged 50 years or less, with the average person sending 15 texts per day.[21] Business communication leaders recommend avoiding abbreviations that wouldn't be understood across all generations (such as ICYMI for "in case you missed it"), and avoiding emojis or using them sparingly, since both make texts informal. The focus of workplace text messages, especially to clients and managers, should remain centered on work at all times, unless the other party initiates a personal conversation about appropriate topics.[22]

The unprecedented increase in smartphone use and wearable devices, such as watches and trackers has made instant, discrete, and constant communication possible. Instant and spontaneous communication has benefits, but it also has detrimental, unintended consequences due to grammatical errors, autocorrect errors, and judgment errors due to lack of thought.[21,23] If you must respond immediately, pick up the phone or acknowledge receipt of the message via text or email to let the sender know you will get back to them within a stated time frame with more thorough information.

Despite the rise in texting, email is still used constantly in the workplace. It can be very useful for general, nonsensitive information when you don't need feedback or when you need to provide written instructions. Choose your communication method based on the type of information you are sending. Generally, the more impersonal the communication is, the less likely it is to be clear to everyone due to the inability to assess nonverbal cues, determine tone of voice, or ask clarifying questions. General tips for effective emails include the following:

> Don't overcommunicate by email, either in terms of frequency or content. Make good use of subject lines by keeping them brief and using key words, such as Action Required by (date), Vacation Request, and Update to draw attention to the email.[24,25] Keep messages clear and brief. Send information in discrete chunks by topic, using multiple emails if necessary. Make use of bullet points and numbered lists whenever possible.

> Be polite. Always be professional and respectful.

> Watch your tone. Choice of words, punctuation, capitalization, and sentence length can easily be misinterpreted without visual and verbal cues.

> Proofread. Typos and poor grammar reflect a lack of attention to detail.

> Use Reply All with care! Think carefully about who truly needs a response. Typically, that is someone who has been copied on the original email. You should avoid replying to all recipients if your response is not relevant to everyone, especially if your response relates to confidential or sensitive information.

> Indicate whether or not you expect a reply or other action to be taken as a result of the email.

Follow confidentiality guidelines with vigilance. Ensure that you and your team know which communication methods are approved and how to utilize encryption. Email encryption is the process of converting email messages and attachments into an unrecognizable form to protect the contents from being read by anyone other than the intended recipients. Encrypted email messages typically require authentication before they can be read. As you build relationships with your team, ask members how they prefer to communicate. For example, ask, "What's the best way for us to stay in touch on this project?"[26] Sensitive information, such as delivering bad news or addressing a performance issue, should never be communicated via email or text.[17,18] Communication of protected health information (PHI) via text may be allowed, but there are usually stringent requirements regarding its use. Finally, an unwritten but important rule is as follows: if email or text communication becomes volatile or contentious, the best recourse is to pick up the phone or arrange to discuss the matter face-to-face where there will be less chance of misinterpretation of intent or tone.

Self-Awareness

Self-awareness is the ability to monitor one's own emotions and reactions. Lack of self-awareness can easily derail a new leader. This can be one of the most challenging of the core skills to develop, but once developed, it can serve as the foundation for developing your other leadership skills.[3,11,27] According to Scisco et al, "We are the worst judges of our own strengths and weaknesses, so it's vitally important to have women and men whom we trust offer insights on what we're doing well and what we can do better."[27] The following actions are effective ways to increase your self-awareness[3,10,11,27]:

> Practice daily self-reflection through journaling, meditating, and thoughtfully considering feedback received. Block out time on your calendar to do this, so it will not be pushed aside as day-to-day business takes over.

> Know your emotional triggers, catch yourself reacting when your emotions are triggered, and consider what appropriate reactions should be.

> When listening, be sure to consider your attitudes, past history, and so on, and think about how they might affect your engagement. For example, if a particular nurse has complained to you about issues you felt were unimportant in the past, do not let that hinder your ability to pay attention in the future. Instead, consider that there may be a valid issue that needs addressing. In addition, do not let your body language reflect your emotions.

> Work with your supervisor, mentor, or a trusted colleague to obtain feedback. Listen and be open to receiving the feedback. See Box 1.5 for examples of creative ways to obtain feedback.[3,10,11,27]

BOX 1.5 Creative Ways to Obtain Feedback[3,10,11,27]

» **Ask, "What is one thing I did well and one thing I could improve on?"** This can be used equally effectively with your supervisor, colleagues, and students and with employees with whom you have a built a relationship of trust. If this is effective, you can expand it to ask for additional examples.

» **Be specific.** For example, rather than ask a general question ("Do you have any feedback for me?") try this: "When I reviewed the policy at the meeting, did I speak loudly enough and was my summary clear?"

» **If you plan to request feedback from a colleague or supervisor for your performance in a particular situation, notify them in advance so they can be watching for a particular behavior.** "When I present the protocol to the physicians, can you let me know if I use the word 'like' too often and if I answered their questions effectively?"

» **Use a mix of structured and open-ended questions in surveys and evaluation tools.** An example of an open-ended question is, "What is one thing you would change about your job?" An example of a structured question is, "On a scale of 1 to 5, how valued do you feel at work?"

» **When requesting feedback from others—especially subordinates—use methods that ensure anonymity** (such as SurveyMonkey and other online survey platforms).

» **Coach yourself: Pay attention to how others respond to your actions.** Assess how you respond in times of stress. Are you receptive? Do you lash out? Taking a good hard look at ourselves, particularly as we move into new roles that require new behaviors, can help us address issues early on when they are smaller and easier to fix.

Empathy

Empathy, as defined by the *Oxford English Dictionary*, is "the ability to understand and share the feelings of another."[28] An empathetic leader is able to utilize the awareness of another person's feelings to understand how those emotions influence the person's needs and perceptions.

Empathy is a core leadership skill because it enables you to build trust. You can't be an effective leader if your team doesn't trust you. Developing empathy can also make you more successful in understanding the motivations of others and gives you the ability to relate to different perspectives.

A survey conducted by the Center for Creative Leadership of more than 6,000 leaders in 38 countries found that empathy was positively related to job performance and that leaders who displayed more empathy toward their employees were viewed as better performers in their jobs by their bosses.[20] Empathy may seem like a character trait you either have or you don't, but empathy, like the other core leadership skills, can be developed with practice. The following tools and activities may help you strengthen your empathy skills, and thus help to build trust[10,11,27,29]:

> Practice active listening. If you have been working on this, you are on your way! The components of active listening—not interrupting, being fully present, asking clarifying questions, and displaying positive nonverbal behavior—all project empathy.

> Refer to people by name. Remember the names of people's spouses, children, and even pets, and refer to them by name. Recording this information may be helpful.

> Be cognizant of your own nonverbal communication. For example, smiling at others and making eye contact communicates your interest in what they are sharing.

> Tune into other people's nonverbal communication to identify whether your words, tone, or body language are having a negative impact or are unclear, and adjust accordingly.

> Encourage people when they speak up in meetings, particularly those who do not tend to do so. A nod or quick, affirming comment can help boost confidence.

> Take a personal interest in people. Ask them questions about their hobbies, their volunteer work, and their aspirations.

> Give praise that is genuine and specific.

Influence

Influence is the ability to impact the decisions, actions, opinions, or thinking of others. The core competency of influence enables you to get things done and achieve the outcomes you are working toward without coercion or individuals feeling they are being manipulated. If you do not have a formal leadership role, influence is about working effectively with coworkers over whom you have no managerial control. To effectively influence people, you need to be able to engage in give-and-take dialogues and present logical and compelling arguments to convince or persuade others to support an idea or a direction.[3,11,30]

The terms *influence* and *persuasion* are often used interchangeably, but they are two different strategies that may be utilized to achieve the same goal. Influence is about the messenger and involves feelings and values, and persuasion is more about the message. Persuading is more deliberate and obvious but also more short term. Influence is more art than science and, like the other key leadership skills, takes time and practice to master. The Stories From the Field box on the next page provides an example of developing influence.

STORIES FROM THE FIELD: Developing Influence in the Workplace

A registered dietitian nutritionist (RDN) volunteered to present the clinical nutrition department's volume-based tube feeding protocol to the Pharmacy and Therapeutics Committee for approval. The RDN knew that one of the physician committee members voiced skepticism of the potential effectiveness of the new protocol, so the RDN utilized the leadership competency of influence in the following ways:

» The RDN leveraged the literature to ensure that references were appropriately cited showing the positive impact of volume-based feeding and best practice examples from other hospitals of similar size, especially competitors.

» The RDN has a great relationship with the pharmacy director, so the RDN met with the director to share the initial idea and obtain support for it ahead of time.

» The RDN asked the pharmacy director about the skeptical physician and other key committee members' chief priorities for patient care (eg, decreased length of stay or patient safety), to tailor the presentation to show how volume-based feeding addresses those priorities.

» The RDN practiced answering potential questions from the committee members ahead of time with the clinical nutrition manager to help prepare for a successful presentation.

» The RDN identified one or two negotiable points, such as doing a shorter pilot program or restricting the protocol to a single unit initially if passage of the protocol did not appear likely.

Fortunately, there are multiple, practical strategies that can help you improve your influencing skills. If this is not a strength of yours, consider practicing this skill in low-risk situations or in one-on-one situations rather than trying to influence a larger group. Key strategies recommended by business leaders include the following[7,11,22]:

> Build rapport by remembering people's names, identifying common ground or shared experiences, listening actively, and asking questions to indicate genuine interest.

> Study and observe others to understand their personality style, what projects excite or frustrate them, how they prefer to work or solve problems, and so on.

> Establish trust by being respectful, transparent, and following through on commitments.

> Gather background information. Do your homework on topics you are trying to promote or influence. Have examples of actions and history to back up what you are saying.

> Know your desired outcome and what you are trying to achieve.

> Practice in front of a mirror until you like how you come across.

> Utilize active listening and pay attention to nonverbal and verbal cues. If you sense your approach is not working, try changing tone, asking questions, and so forth.

> Gain credibility by consistently working hard and getting good results.

> Take a training course specifically focused on building influence, such as those offered by Dale Carnegie, Learning Tree, and others.

Learning Agility

Learning agility is a set of skills that gives an individual the ability to learn something in one situation and apply that knowledge in a completely different situation.[11,31,32] Learning-agile individuals are highly skilled at learning from experience. They are often described by leadership experts as flexible, resourceful, adaptable, and thoughtful. Research conducted by Columbia University and the Center for Creative Leadership identified four behaviors that enable learning agility and one that derails it. The four enabling behaviors—innovating, performing, reflecting, and risking—were positively correlated with performance. *Innovating* is defined as being unafraid to challenge the status quo. *Performing* is used here to refer to the ability to remain calm in the face of stress or difficulty. *Reflecting* is taking the time to think back on one's experiences, and *risking* is intentionally putting oneself in challenging circumstances.[11,13]

Defending behavior was found to negatively impact learning agility or even derail it. Defensiveness has a negative impact on performance, particularly among leaders. The research team found that leaders who ranked high on the defending scale—those who remain closed or defensive when challenged or given critical feedback—tended to be lower in learning agility and were considered less effective.[31] Leaders at *Harvard Business Review* and *Forbes* suggest the following ways to develop learning agility[31,32]:

> **Innovating:** Seek out new solutions. Repeatedly ask yourself, "What else?" and "What are 10 more ways I could approach this?"

> **Performing:** Seek to identify patterns in complex situations. Find the similarities between current and past projects. Cultivate calm through meditation and other techniques. Enhance your listening skills, and learn to listen instead of simply (and immediately) reacting.

> **Reflecting:** Explore "what ifs" and alternative histories for projects you have been involved in. Regularly seek out honest input. Ask, "What are three or four things I or we could have done better here?"

> **Risking:** Look for "stretch assignments," where the success isn't a given. For example, implementing a farm-to-table program at your school's dining service or implementing the International Dysphagia Diet Standardization Initiative (IDDSI) at your extended care facility are challenging assignments that involve many stakeholders and require extensive coordination and oversight to implement effectively.

> **Avoid defending:** Acknowledge your failures (perhaps from those stretch assignments) and capture the lessons you've learned from them.

Emotional Intelligence

Emotional intelligence refers to the ability to understand and manage one's own emotions as well as recognize and influence other people's emotions.[3,10,33,34] Effective leadership competencies and emotional intelligence are closely related. In general, emotional intelligence consists of three skills: the ability to identify, name, and own your emotions; the ability to apply one's own emotions to tasks, such as problem solving; and the ability to help others manage their emotions.[3,33,34] Although there is limited evidence in the literature that emotional intelligence is directly linked to job performance, there is evidence that the characteristics of emotional intelligence such as empathy and influence have an impact.[7] Furthermore, since leadership is widely considered to be the ability to guide and influence others, the ability to successfully interact with others supports the need for emotional intelligence in leaders. Developing the five core leadership skills listed earlier in this chapter (communication, self-awareness, empathy, influence, and learning agility) will greatly assist you in improving your emotional intelligence, since these concepts are so closely aligned.

Common Mistakes New Leaders Make

New leaders may find themselves unprepared for their new roles. According to Daskal, "Everything you've done so far in your career has led you to this position. But the experiences and skills that landed you this new job will not be what allows you to succeed."[35] Research conducted by the Center for Creative Leadership shows that up to 40% of newly promoted managers and executives are no longer in their roles within 18 months of a promotion.[11] Business and leadership experts surmise that the most common and damaging mistakes made by new leaders typically involve communicating with people in the wrong way.[3,13,14,16] The following list details some of the most common mistakes new leaders make. These can be avoided or minimized with a focus on the core leadership competencies discussed earlier in this chapter.

Failing to develop trust with a new team Build trust through communication and empathy. New leaders need to listen to learn the environment and the people. Truly listening enables you to understand the content and the context of what your team member is saying. This can help you respond appropriately, avoid overreacting, and make better decisions. Getting to know your team members builds trust and enables you to gain an understanding of what motivates them. For example, it is a common mistake to assume lack of motivation is always tied to compensation; other factors that impact motivation include poor fit for the position, a perceived lack of fairness regarding workload or schedule, and frustration with underperforming coworkers. Another way to build trust is to obtain employee input before making any changes that impact them. It is also essential to explain clearly why you were unable to implement changes based on their feedback, if that is the situation. Being authentic, honest, sincere, and visible is key to building trust. Being visible can convey to your team that you are truly interested in resolving issues, care about their work load, and are willing to help when necessary.

Avoiding performance issues Leaders may avoid addressing team members' behavioral or performance problems due to fear of confrontation and lack of confidence in their ability to address the issues effectively. This can result in a lack of motivation in the employee and escalation of the issue, and it can also negatively impact other team members who believe there is no penalty for below-average results and there are no rewards for top performers.[14,35,36] Performance issues may result from a leader's failure to effectively communicate their expectations. As we will see later in this chapter, timely performance coaching can enable the leader to clarify expectations and resolve issues quickly and effectively.

Making hiring mistakes New leaders tend to feel very pressured to fill open positions quickly. Bowing to that pressure rather than taking the time to hire a truly qualified candidate does little to build the new leader's credibility with their team. Utilize your team's feedback on what skills or qualifications matter most in the new hire.

Failing to define goals and set expectations It is essential for new leaders to set clear goals aligned with the organization's objectives and communicate expectations with their team members. When setting expectations, be direct, clear, and specific. Ask for a recap if nonverbal behavior suggests any team member is disengaged or confused; it is not the employee or team member's job to decipher what you say.[37]

Not delegating or not asking for help Often new managers are afraid to delegate for reasons such as a fear of loss of control or a need to prove their value to their team. However, effective delegation, along with clear communication of responsibilities, timelines, and expectations, can enable a manager to be more productive and impactful. In addition, it empowers team members, aids in building trust, and gives staff opportunities to develop as individual leaders.

Not providing feedback Key tips to providing effective feedback include the following:

> Praise people or teams in public, but share negative feedback in private. This is essential in developing and maintaining the trust of your team.

> Focus on the action, not the individual. It is more helpful to say, "Your outpatient revenue is down 30% this month. What do you think has influenced that drop, and what can we do to improve it?" than to say, "Your performance has been lagging this month."

> Listen more than you talk. For example, if a previously high-performing employee starts arriving to work late, utilize the active listening skills discussed earlier in this chapter to understand what is impacting the employee's ability to get to work. Fully understanding the situation could allow you to better explore ways to address the underlying cause *with* the employee—for example, by helping the employee brainstorm transportation options or arranging a temporary shift change, rather than simply reiterating the attendance policy.

> Provide positive feedback more often than negative. The latest research on the praise ratio finds that employees perform their best when they receive at least five (and ideally six) pieces of positive feedback for every piece of negative feedback.[11,38] This approach should be utilized for everyone except any documented poor performers you anticipate terminating. Don't delay. Provide feedback as soon as possible after the incident occurs.

> Ask what you can do to help. This is especially important when addressing an issue that can be improved with training, such as correctly completing a job task or refining skills in time management or customer service.

Many of the mistakes typical of new leaders stem from ineffective communication. By being aware of these potential issues and focusing on developing their core leadership competencies, new leaders will be better prepared to succeed in their new roles. The following Stories From the Field presents a case study involving a new dietetics leader.

A registered dietitian nutritionist was recently promoted to a program manager position at their health and wellness center. One of the manager's new responsibilities was to supervise the part-time community liaison responsible for assisting with community relationships and facilitating the teen program. The new manager worked hard to develop a friendly relationship with the employee due to their role in the community. They frequently texted back and forth regarding the teen program and operations issues.

When the manager took over supervision of the employee, they were notified that the employee had a history of inconsistently completing their time sheets. After several months, the manager began to experience this issue and had to follow up with the employee multiple times to obtain and record their hours. Not wanting to sacrifice their relationship with the employee, the manager opted to remind the employee of policy and hope they would correct the situation. After a brief period of improvement, the problem resurfaced. Tired of having to constantly reach out for this information, the manager opted to begin estimating the hours worked and filling out the time sheets for the employee.

A month later, the employee worked substantially more hours than usual to assist with teen vacation camps. The busy manager overlooked this when estimating the employee's hours and the employee was substantially underpaid. The employee, upset and frustrated, used a curse word in the text they sent the manager regarding the inaccuracy of their paycheck. The manager became very upset and wanted to terminate the employee.

The manager, the employee, and the department director sat down to address the situation. When asked about the text language, the employee told the manager, "I thought we were friends. I texted you like I would my friend. I was really upset, I have bills to pay. I need my money!" The manager remained focused on the language issue and the situation became tense.

At this point, the director intervened, informing the employee that they were required to submit a time sheet every Friday by 5:00 PM or they would not be paid that week. The director also told the employee to make a copy of the time sheet so that they would always know exactly how many hours they would be paid for. The director informed the manager that managers were prohibited from entering hours for employees without a time sheet generated by the employee. The unprofessional language issue was also addressed, and the texting policy was reviewed.

Practical Ways to Develop Leadership Skills

There are many opportunities to develop leadership skills in everyday life as well as in one's career. Everyday activities with family, friends, people in your networks, or a work team all present opportunities to lead. Some ways to develop leadership skills in the workplace include these strategies.

Work with a mentor, or mentor others Mentorship is highly effective in helping develop leadership skills but is often underutilized. In a survey of 684 clinical RDNs, Patten and Sauer[39] found that working with a mentor or serving as a mentor to new RDNs or students was one of the 27 leadership behaviors practiced least frequently. The benefits of having a mentor include expanding your network of contacts, increased access to consistent feedback, opportunities to practice your core leadership skills in a safe environment, and improved self-confidence. There are several things to consider in order to find a mentor that will be beneficial to you. Most business experts recommend first deciding the specific role you'd like the mentor to provide.[40] For example, are you looking for someone within your organization to help you advance? Are you looking to transition to a new area of dietetics, such as moving from foodservice management into higher education? Other key steps include making a list of potential individuals who might mentor you and developing a concise and effective "elevator speech" to share with these potential mentors when you approach them. The Academy of Nutrition and Dietetics offers electronic mentoring resources through its professional website (www.eatrightPRO.org), and several dietetic practice groups and member interest groups offer their own mentoring and guidance resources. Mentoring is covered in greater detail in Chapters 2 and 7.

Seek out challenging projects or committee assignments Serving as a representative from your department to the Joint Commission Readiness Committee, volunteering to colead the resident advisory committee at your extended care facility, and leading a peer interview are all ways to develop leadership skills. Additional examples include agreeing to be interviewed by the media on an important and timely nutrition topic or volunteering to take the lead in revising an outdated policy and procedure and presenting it to the group for feedback; these are all ways to develop leadership capacity.

Get involved in a cause you care about Raise your hand when an opportunity to take a leadership role comes up, no matter how small. Doing well in a small role could open opportunities for larger responsibilities. Professional organizations, such as your local dietetics group and dietetic practice groups, as well as community organizations are great places to start. These groups always need volunteers, and you can start your leadership experience in ways that make you feel comfortable.

Cultivate a diverse network Get to know people at your facility in different roles, departments, or professions. This can lead to a broader perspective about your institution, expand your thinking, and teach you more about yourself. Go to lunch with the coder who worked with you on your malnutrition coding project or the pharmacist on your floor. Have coffee with the cafeteria manager.

Networks are just as beneficial outside the workplace as they are inside it. Get involved in community organizations, places of worship, or other groups where you'll encounter people of different ages, experiences, cultures, races, perspectives, and backgrounds. Box 1.6 lists examples of leadership roles and potential leadership competencies that could be developed or enhanced.

BOX 1.6 Leadership Roles and Competencies

Leadership role	Potential competencies
Secretary, Academy of Nutrition and Dietetics dietetic practice group	Communication, influence
Membership coordinator, parent–teacher association	Communication, empathy, influence
Coordinator of a holiday toy drive at your place of worship	Communication, influence, negotiation,[a] empathy, learning agility
Program reviewer—Accreditation Council for Education in Nutrition and Dietetics (ACEND)	Communication, empathy, learning agility
Joint Commission representative for your hospital department	Communication, influence, learning agility
Department safety officer	Communication, influence, learning agility, negotiation[a]

[a] See Chapter 2 for more information on negotiation.

Managing Others: Opportunities and Challenges

Whether in a formal or informal role, the thought of managing others takes many of us out of our comfort zone. In this section, we will discuss specific areas of concern.

Working Effectively With Your Supervisor

One of your most important relationships at work is the one you have with your supervisor or team leaders. Establishing an effective relationship built on trust is essential for your success in your current role, as well as for future growth and development. One reason this relationship can be challenging is that your supervisor plays two roles—supporter and evaluator.[41] Business leaders recommend to optimize your relationship with your supervisor [3,11,13,38,39]:

> Take stock of your relationship. Is it a partnership? Regardless of whether you like or admire your supervisor, it is your responsibility to ensure the relationship is a partnership that benefits both of you.

> Observe your supervisor in the workplace and ask questions to gain an understanding of their work style. For example, do they prefer written communication or verbal communication? Do they like detailed reports or brief reports condensed to bullet points? How often do they prefer to meet, and in what setting? What are their priorities for the team or the department?

> Don't be afraid to ask your supervisor for help.

> Minimize surprises. No one likes to deliver negative news, but your supervisor would rather hear it from you than be caught unaware at a meeting with their peers or supervisor.

> Don't go to your supervisor with a list of complaints; come with potential solutions to problems.

> Resist the urge to criticize your supervisor to others. It will get back to them and reflect poorly on you. This behavior also makes other people reluctant to hire or promote you, suspecting you will one day speak about them in the same way.

> Take responsibility for your own development. Speak with your supervisor to ensure there is alignment between your goals and theirs.

Coaching for Performance

Coaching for performance is a process of managing people that creates a motivational climate that helps enhance employee growth, development, and work performance through frequent feedback, recognition, and support. The goal of coaching for performance is to work with the employee to solve performance issues and improve the work of the employee, the department, and the institution or company. Coaching for performance tends to be the skill that fills new leaders with the most anxiety. There are multiple models available and the core elements of these models will be summarized here. The first step is to review your institution's policies and procedures on performance coaching to ensure you utilize the correct process. Regardless of the model you utilize, unless a serious offense has occurred that potentially requires termination, your first performance conversation with an employee should be coaching.

Ask yourself the following questions before scheduling a coaching session:

> Have you developed a relationship of trust with the employee?

> Do you know the employee well enough to evaluate whether they are in the correct position within your organization? Some potential signs of a poor fit include staff members who never get excited about their jobs, can't master job tasks despite repeated instruction, appear bored or chronically complain, and never share ideas.[7,39,40]

> Are you well prepared? Be sure you understand the coaching or progressive discipline process at your facility. Familiarize yourself with what constitutes a verbal warning, what constitutes a written warning, what forms need to be completed or signed, and so on. Until you are competent in this skill, have your supervisor, a more experienced manager, or a member of the human resources team sit in with you to observe and provide feedback afterward. They can also step in if the situation gets volatile or you make a serious error, but you should lead the conversation. After the coaching session, ask for feedback from your observer or coach. Use your self-reflection skills to note how you did and what you could have done better. This self-reflection includes asking yourself whether you listened actively, spoke clearly, checked your body language, and kept your composure, as well as whether you asked questions to confirm the employee's understanding of the situation and the repercussions of failing to improve.

Like most skills, gaining mastery in employee coaching takes practice. Don't beat yourself up if you stumble a little at first.

Method 1: Effective Coaching Blueprint

There are multiple coaching methods available in the business and human resources literature. These methods range from four to seven steps, but they all contain the following essential elements. The order of these six elements will vary slightly, depending on how the conversation flows.[40-43]

1. **Describe the performance problem to the employee.** Stick to facts, and focus on the problem or behavior. Provide accurate and specific examples to illustrate the concern. Ask questions to ensure you both are on the same page. Explain to the employee the impact their behavior has on the team and department.

2. **Ask for the employee's view of the situation.** Use your active listening skills to ensure you understand their side of the story.

3. **Determine if there are any barriers to the employee being able to perform the task effectively or fix the behavior (such as a lack of time, training, or tools, or the employee's temperament).** Do you as the leader need to assist in some way, or can the employee fix the behavior themselves?

4. **Obtain agreement from the employee that a problem exists, then discuss potential solutions.**

5. **Agree on a written action plan and discuss what the employee will do and what you will do to resolve the issue.** Complete and obtain signatures on any form your facility requires.

6. **Set a date and time for a follow-up discussion.**

Method 2: GROW Model

The second method of coaching for performance is known as the GROW model, a popular coaching method developed by Sir John Whitmore in the 1980s. It is used for all types of coaching. GROW is an acronym for the four key steps used in the model[44]:

> **Goal:** Identify a behavior that the coach and the participant agree should change, then structure a goal related to that behavior.

> **Reality:** The coaching participant describes their current reality related to this behavior.

> **Options:** Explore and decide on best options to achieve the goal.

> **Will or Way Forward:** The participant commits to specific actions that will move them forward in achieving the goal.

According to business leaders, the keys to successfully utilizing the GROW model are to ask excellent questions and to ask the right question at the right time.[44] The GROW model is further discussed in Chapter 2.

Method 3: High, Middle, and Low Conversations

The third method, developed by Quint Studer, is a process for categorizing employees into high, middle, and low performers and having targeted coaching conversations with all your direct reports, starting with those identified as high performers.[36]

High performers High performers are intrinsically motivated by performance and become frustrated when others don't work at their level. They are also most alluring to your competition. Your goal is to re-recruit them. This is especially important with Generation X and Millennial employees who may always be looking out for the next opportunity. They need to know you value them and are actively partnering with them to achieve their developmental goals.[36-38]

Middle performers Middle performers are generally reliable employees who are held back by behaviors or a lack of training. These challenges keep them from realizing their potential and becoming high performers. The goal here is to move middle performers to a higher level. Studer recommends a three-step process: First, reassure middle performers that your goal is to retain them, and then describe their good attributes. Second, provide coaching on specific developmental opportunities. Third, reassure middle performers of your commitment to their success.

Low performers The final conversations should occur with low performers. These individuals may have safety violations, customer complaints, or other job-related issues. The goal here is to move them up or out of the organization. Studer recommends taking four action steps for low performers: First, describe the problem behavior, avoiding pleasantries or small talk. Second, describe how you feel (frustrated, disappointed, etc). Third, show, demonstrate, or describe in detail how a task should be completed. Fourth, clearly state the consequences of lack of improvement, and ask questions to affirm understanding.[36]

Developing a Leadership Mindset

Concurrent with the competencies described earlier in this chapter, it is also important to develop a leadership mindset. A mindset is a mental attitude or inclination, a filter through which we see the world. Your impact as a leader stems directly from your mindset. This is because your mindset affects your behaviors, which then affect your results. A leadership mindset is a way of thinking and behaving that makes us willing to stand up and stand out, welcoming growth and seeing leadership opportunities where others may not. According to leaders in organizational change, the first step in developing a leadership mindset is having the belief that new abilities can be developed with effort.[3,45,46] Developing or advancing your core competencies of communication, self-awareness, empathy, learning agility, and influence and practicing these essential skills is important regardless of your current role or career stage. Other examples of a leadership mindset include being outward facing rather than inward facing, seeing the big picture, and thinking in terms of systems.

It's easy to have a leadership mindset when things are going well—when you're fully staffed, customer satisfaction and quality scores are high, and finances are stable, for example—but you need this mindset most during times of stress and uncertainty. While shifting your mindset and priorities can be difficult, you can substantially improve the outcomes and impact delivered by your team, and by you, both inside and outside the workplace by developing a leadership mindset.[3,45,46]

Setting the Stage for Advanced Leadership Skills

The competencies you develop with early leadership skills provide you with the tools to progress to more advanced leadership skills. Once you've mastered the basics, you will be able to learn advanced skills with additional training, experience, and practice. Early in your career, your communications skill development may be focused on writing and speaking clearly as well as using active listening skills. As you move up the career ladder or into more formal management roles, you will use the core communication skills you developed early on to achieve mastery of more advanced skills, such as building trust and conveying vision and strategic intent, which have communication at their roots.[9,11,13,16] For example, developing skills such as facilitation, change management, negotiation, and conveying vision and strategic intent may seem daunting, but they all stem from communication, empathy, and influence.

Numerous tools and methods are available to assess your leadership competencies and develop your plan for the future. The first step is to assess where you are. Tools such as the Standards of Professional Performance (SOPP) for RDNs in management of food and nutrition systems, the self-assessment available from the American College of Healthcare Executives (ACHE), and the Competency Plan Builder from the Commission on Dietetic Registration (CDR) are all excellent resources.[46-48] If you are in a leadership position currently, you may have access to a 360-degree review that provides feedback from those who supervise you, your peers, and your subordinates.

Once you have completed your self-assessment, the next step is to meet with your supervisor or mentor to share the results and determine how to proceed. The next step could be to identify projects and experiences to help you develop your leadership competencies further. For example, in a clinical setting, developing a hospital protocol for outpatient nutrition screening could help you with your influence and negotiation skills. If you work in school foodservice, you could develop a farm-to-table initiative at your school, which could enhance your communication, influence, and negotiating skills.

There are many sources for leadership training. Check with your manager, your professional association, or the place you volunteer in the community to see what resources they have. The Academy of Nutrition and Dietetics has numerous, excellent resources available including several online certificates, training programs, and learning modules. There is also a list of useful leadership books and websites available on the Academy of Nutrition and Dietetics professional website. In addition, the Academy of Nutrition and Dietetics Leadership Institute, a 12-month professional development program, offers extended leadership training and hands-on experience through a combination of self-directed study, in-person trainings, networking opportunities, small group projects, and virtual learning. More information on the Leadership Institute is available on the Academy of Nutrition and Dietetics professional website (www.eatrightPRO.org).[49]

Summary

All dietetics professionals can be leaders. Effective leadership does not require innate skills, but it is a series of competencies that can be learned through education and practice. You don't need to be in a management role or supervise others to be a leader. By focusing on developing the core competencies of communication, self-awareness, influence, empathy, and learning agility, you will be well on your way to becoming an effective leader. These core competencies will provide the fundamentals from which you can expand your skill set through increased experience and expanded roles and responsibilities.

ADDITIONAL RESOURCES

Dugan P. *Leadership Theory: Cultivating Critical Perspectives*. 1st ed. Jossey-Bass; 2017.

Lussier N, Achua C. *Leadership: Theory, Application, & Skill Development*. 6th ed. Cengage Learning; 2015.

REFERENCES

1 Boyce B. Learning to lead: developing dietetics leaders. *J Acad Nutr Diet*. 2014;114(5 suppl):S35-S39. doi:10.1016/j.jand.2014.03.003

2 Gladwell M. *Outliers: The Story of Success*. Little, Brown and Company; 2011.

3 Covey SR. *The 8th Habit: From Effectiveness to Greatness*. Free Press; 2004.

4 Leadership competencies. Accessed January 10, 2021. Society for Human Resource Management website. www.shrm.org/ResourcesAndTools/hr-topics/behavioral-competencies/leadership-and-navigation/Pages/leadershipcompetencies.aspx

5   Commission on Dietetic Registration. Introducing practice competencies. Commission on Dietetic Registration website Accessed January 21, 2021. www.cdrnet.org/competencies

6   Amanchukwu RN, Stanley GJ, Nwachukwu PO. A review of leadership theories, principles and styles and their relevance to educational management. *Management*. 2015;5(1):6-14. doi:10.5923 /j.mm.20150501.02

7   Nohria N, Khurana R. *The Handbook of Leadership Theory and Practice.* Harvard Business Publishing; 2010.

8   Leadership theories. Leadership Central website. Accessed December 28, 2020. www.leadership-central.com/leadership-theories.html

9   Kotter J. What leaders really do. *Harvard Business Review*. Accessed January 20, 2020. https://hbr.org/2001/12/what-leaders-really-do

10 Dean P. *Leadership in Everyday Life.* McGraw Hill; 2006.

11 The core leadership skills you need in every role. Center for Creative Leadership. Accessed July 30, 2019. https://ccl.org/articles/leading-effectively-articles/fundamental-4-core-leadership -skills-for-every-career-stage

12 Mitchinson A, Morris R. *Learning About Learning Agility*. Center for Creative Leadership; 2014. Accessed December 10, 2019. http://cclinnovation.org/wp-content/uploads/2020/02 /learningagility.pdf

13 Miller B. The No. 1 communication problem for new managers. Entrepreneur website. Accessed March 27, 2022. www.entrepreneur.com/article/249874

14 Benjamin B, O'Reilly C. Becoming a leader: early career challenges faced by MBA graduates. *Academy of Management Learning & Education*. 2011;10(3). Accessed February 4, 2022. doi:10.5465/amle.2011.0002

15 DiGaetani J. The Sperry Corporation and listening: an interview. *Business Horizons*. 1982;25:34-39.

16 Tracy B. Motivating employees by using effective listening skills. Leadingwithquestions website. Accessed March 27, 2022. https://leadingwithquestions.wordpress.com/2012/09/26/motivating -employees-by-using-effective-listening-skills

17 Shahin S, Thomas S. Situation, Background, Assessment, Recommendation (SBAR) communication tool for handoff in health care – a narrative review. *Saf Health*. 2018;4:7. doi:10.1186/s40886-018-0073-1

18 SBAR Tool: Situation-Background-Assessment-Recommendation. Institute for Healthcare Improvement website. Accessed December 12, 2019. http://ihi.org/resources/Pages/Tools /SBARToolkit.aspx

19 Johnson I. Communication huddles: the secret of team success. *J Contin Educ Nurs*. 2018;49(10):451-453. doi:10.3928/00220124-20180918-04

20 Huddles. Institute for Healthcare Improvement website. Accessed January 15, 2019. www.ihi.org /resources/Pages/Tools/Huddles.aspx

21 Burke K. 107 texting statistics that answer all your questions. Text Request website. Accessed December 10, 2019. www.textrequest.com/blog/texting-statistics-answer-questions

22 Whitmore J. Ask the etiquette expert: 8 rules for texting at work. Entrepreneur website. Accessed January 14, 2021. www.entrepreneur.com/article/295950

23 Frost S. About texting in the workplace. *Houston Chronicle*. Accessed December 11, 2019. https://smallbusiness.chron.com/texting-workplace-12302.html

24 Use keywords in your email subject lines. *Harvard Business Review*. Accessed January 15, 2021. https://hbr.org/tip/2017/02/use-keywords-in-your-email-subject-lines

25 Society for Human Resources Management. Twelve tips for amazingly effective subject lines. Society for Human Resources Management website. Accessed January 15, 2021. https://community.shrm.org/HigherLogic/System/DownloadDocumentFile.ashx ?DocumentFileKey=cd04ec4b-e5ef-bdd1-281e-7683d79b91f5

26 Curwen AE. Texts and emails vs. oral communication at work: which is best? Society for Human Resources Management website. Accessed December 11, 2019. https://shrm.org/resourcesandtools/hr-topics/employee-relations/pages/written-versus-oral-communication-.aspx

27 Scisco P, Biech B, Hallenbeck G. *Compass: Your Guide for Leadership Development and Coaching.* Center for Creative Leadership Press; 2017.

28 Oxford English Dictionary. Empathy. OED website. Accessed February 2, 2023. www.oed.com/oed2/00074155

29 Gentry WA, Weber TJ, Sadri G. Empathy in the workplace: a tool for effective leadership. Center for Creative Leadership website. Accessed January 23, 2019. www.ccl.org/wp-content/uploads/2015/04/EmpathyInTheWorkplace.pdf

30 Cattelan L. Impact and influence: a key competency for top performers. Linda Cattelan & Results Inc website. 2020. Accessed March 9, 2022. https://lindacattelan.com/impact-and-influence-a-key-competency-for-top-performers/#:~:text=The%20ability%20to%20impact%20and%20influence%20others%20is,competency%20in%20helping%2C%20service%2C%20managerial%20and%20leadership%20roles

31 Flaum JP, Winkler B. Improve your ability to learn. *Harvard Business Review.* Accessed January 24, 2019. https://hbr.org/2015/06/improve-your-ability-to-learn

32 Cashman K. The five dimensions of learning-agile leaders. *Forbes.* Accessed January 24, 2019. www.forbes.com/sites/kevincashman/2013/04/03/the-five-dimensions-of-learning-agile-leaders/#6325e6277457

33 Emotional intelligence. *Psychology Today* website. 2020. Accessed February 2, 2020. www.psychologytoday.com/us/basics/emotional-intelligence

34 Goleman D. *Emotional Intelligence: Why It Can Matter More Than IQ.* Bantam Books; 1995.

35 Daskal L. How to succeed as a new leader. Lolly Daskal blog. Accessed November 14, 2019. www.lollydaskal.com/leadership/succeed-new-leader

36 Studer Q. *Hardwiring Excellence.* Fire Starter Publishing; 2003.

37 Hathaway G. *Leadership Secrets from the Executive Office.* MJF Books; 2004.

38 Zenger J, Folkman J. The ideal praise-to-criticism ratio. *Harvard Business Review.* Accessed January 10, 2020. https://hbr.org/2013/03/the-ideal-praise-to-criticism

39 Patten EV, Sauer K. The framework and future opportunities for leaders in clinical dietetics. *J Acad Nutr Diet.* 2018;118(11):2017-2023. doi:10.1016/j.jand.2017.06.363

40 Ferguson M. So you want to find a mentor for your career? Here's how. Dietitian Connection website. Accessed January 20, 2021. https://dietitianconnection.com/news/so-you-want-to-find-a-mentor-for-your-career-heres-how

41 Hill LA, Lineback K. Managing your boss. In: *HBR Guide to Managing Up and Across.* Harvard Business Review Press; 2013 :3-14.

42 Hallowell EM. Set the stage to stimulate growth. In: *HBR Guide to Coaching Employees.* Harvard Business Review Press; 2014.

43 Collins J. *Good to Great: Why Some Companies Make the Leap and Others Don't.* 1st ed. HarperBusiness; 2001.

44 The GROW model. Performance Consultants International website. Accessed January 16, 2021. www.coachingperformance.com/grow-model

45 Dyess S, Sherman RO. Developing a leadership mindset in new graduates. *Nurse Leader.* 2010;8(1):29-33. doi:10.1016/j.mnl.2009.11.004

46 Berthelsen RM, Barkley WC, Oliver PM, Mclymont V, Puckett R. Academy of Nutrition and Dietetics: revised 2014 standards of professional performance for registered dietitian nutritionists in management of food and nutrition systems. *J Acad Nutr Diet.* 2014;114(7):1104-1112. doi:10.1016/j.jand.2014.03.017

47 American College of Healthcare Executives. ACHE 2020 healthcare executives competencies assessment tool. 2020. American College of Healthcare Executives website. Accessed February 14, 2020. www.ache.org/-/media/ache/career-resource-center/competencies_booklet.pdf

48 Commission on Dietetic Registration. *Competency Plan Builder Instructions*. Academy of Nutrition and Dietetics; 2021. Accessed March 28, 2022. https://admin.cdrnet.org/vault/2459/web/Competency_Plan_Builder_Instructions.pdf

49 Academy of Nutrition and Dietetics. Leadership resources. eatrightPRO website. Accessed February 14, 2020. www.eatrightPRO.org/leadership/volunteering/leadership-resources

CHAPTER 2
Advanced Leadership Skills

Julie O'Sullivan-Maillet, PhD, RDN, FADA, FAND, and
Wendy Phillips, MS, RD, CLE, NWCC, FAND

Introduction

Leadership development occurs on a continuum. There is no clear "starting line" after which advanced leadership skills emerge, so it is critical to continue to develop and master the essential skills outlined in Chapter 1. These fundamental skills of communication, self-awareness, empathy, influence, learning agility, and emotional intelligence become the building blocks for learning and honing skills needed by an advanced leader, such as building trust and conveying vision and strategic intent. While a leader may or may not possess the title of manager, a manager who practices advanced leadership skills is more likely to be effective.

Leadership skills can be learned, just like management skills. Similar to the progression for levels of practice for registered dietitian nutritionists (RDNs) as outlined by the Academy of Nutrition and Dietetics and the Commission on Dietetic Registration (CDR), individuals can progress from competent to proficient to expert across the profession.[1,2] For example, the Standards of Professional Performance (SOPP) for RDNs in clinical nutrition management present this progression.[2] Some of the differences noted between *competent* and *expert* in that reference reflect classical distinctions between managers and leaders, respectively.

Managers typically focus on planning, budgeting, supervising, communicating, and evaluating; although advanced leaders often perform these same functions, they may also mentor, write or create, present, innovate, and conduct research. For example, advanced leaders often develop and implement large projects, collaborate with or lead interprofessional teams, and develop revenue-generating services.[2] Nutrition leaders in health care need to cultivate a long-term vision of improving and expanding services and providing care to meet individual and population needs. This also includes focusing on emerging issues (eg, sustainability of the food supply and impact of food production and practices on the climate) and addressing the change drivers (eg, diversity, equity, and inclusion) for the nutrition and dietetics profession.[3] The leader creates new systems with a concentration on what is essential. The leadership skills that a manager or nutrition practitioner develops through training and experience help foster the behaviors that define an advanced leader. Core communication skills covered in Chapter 1 form the roots for the growth of other skills and traits that rely on effective communication, including building trust, conveying vision and strategic intent, and active listening. Chapter 1 also reviews leadership activities, such as facilitating change and innovation, negotiating, fostering collaboration while handling conflict, and leading in an ethical and respectful manner.

Selected Traits and Characteristics of an Advanced Leader

A clear definition of leadership remains elusive, as different people are perceived as advanced leaders for varying reasons. One approach is to define leadership based on commonly observed traits of those who are successful leaders. Although sources naturally vary in their precise definitions of advanced leadership, certain common traits come up again and again. Box 2.1 lists examples of traits that are often attributed to an advanced leader.

> **BOX 2.1** Selected Traits of an Advanced Leader
>
> **Accountable**: takes full responsibility for self and team's performance; praises and offers constructive criticism for growth but accepts ultimate responsibility
>
> **Adaptable and flexible**: able to pivot with changing environment; practices accepting and addressing challenges rather than resisting them
>
> **Critical thinker**: communicates strengths, weaknesses, and opportunities as well as threats to an organization
>
> **Communicator**: interacts with others in a genuine way; demonstrates empathy, active listening, and the ability to build relationships
>
> **Creative and innovative**: embraces new ways of thinking; willing to experiment to find solutions or paths others don't see
>
> **Empathetic**: able to sense and support emotions of team members and upper management in a constructive manner
>
> **Influential**: able to persuade others; promotes ideas and delegates
>
> **Inspirational and passionate**: conveys vision and gets others excited about it; inspires others to follow
>
> **Problem solver**: uses resourcefulness to solve small and large problems
>
> **Strategic**: possesses the ability to see where the organization or department needs to go and how to get there; sees the big picture as well as the small details needed to achieve the overall goal
>
> **Team builder and collaborator**: builds effective teams through a shared vision and passion

In 2019, Patten and Sauer presented research on a model that integrates leadership into clinicians' work (see Figure 2.1).[4] The taxonomy was developed by an expert panel of three RDN researchers and nine clinical nutrition managers and based on survey results from 684 clinical RDNs throughout the United States.[4] Leadership characteristics found to be essential included those in the five categories depicted in Figure 2.1 and described in general terms here:

> **Change:** Advocacy for change to improve work methods, with the ability to clearly communicate a strategic vision for intended results

> **Patient (Client, Customer, or Community) Focus:** Engagement in activities to improve the experience of patients, clients, customers, and communities

> **Self-Direct:** Evaluation of progress on collaborative projects while prioritizing and organizing required work functions

> **Technical:** Engagement in mastery of skills and knowledge to earn respect, build trust, and evaluate intervention outcomes with a focus on continued quality improvement

> **Relationship:** Informal and formal mentorship of others to improve efficacy of the team and oneself

FIGURE 2.1 Dietetics leadership taxonomy

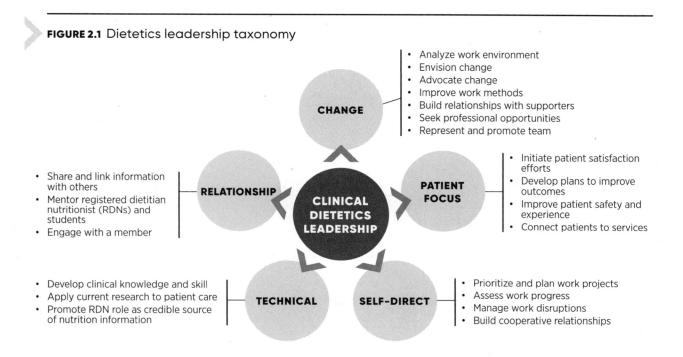

Reproduced with permission from Patten EV, Sauer K. A leadership taxonomy for clinical dietetics practice. *J Acad Nutr Diet.* 2019:119(3):369-374.

Patten and Sauer's taxonomy has relevance across the field of nutrition and dietetics. Leaders in other areas of dietetics can be described as exhibiting similar leadership traits and skills, although with slightly different projects or audiences. Leaders outside of clinical dietetics still enhance their respective fields, workplaces, and clientele through their ability to envision and advocate change, focus on the people they serve, be self-directed, stay current with technical skills and knowledge, and share that knowledge with students, colleagues, mentees, and others.

Similarly, CDR has established an Advanced Practitioner Certification in Clinical Nutrition (RDN-AP) credential; many of the competencies that characterize an RDN-AP are applicable to other practice settings and are well aligned with advanced leadership skills described in this chapter.[5] As indicated by the competencies highlighted in Box 2.2 on page 28, leadership is essential for all of these functions.[5,6]

BOX 2.2 Competencies and Associated Skills for Advanced Leaders

Competencies	Associated leadership skills
Lead an interprofessional team in designing nutrition-related services, programs, or protocols	Building trust Conveying vision and strategic intent Conducting change management Negotiating and facilitating
Direct, design, and evaluate the effectiveness of continuous quality improvement programs	Conducting change management
Evaluate existing and innovative tools, technologies, and techniques for nutrition care and stakeholder acceptance	Conducting change management
Promote a culture of proactive, patient-centered care	Conveying vision and strategic intent
Advocate for new (or modifications to) local, state, and national policies and regulations to improve nutrition care	Negotiating and facilitating
Support the growth, development, and advancement of colleagues	Building trust
Develop and implement new tools, techniques, and programs for nutrition care; create or grow programs to expand services, add value, or generate revenue	Implementing design thinking Innovating

Skills Central to Advanced Leadership

Communication Skills to Build Trust and Convey Vision and Strategic Intent

Understanding our own preferred forms of internal and external communication can lead to self-awareness and identification of priorities for professional growth. Communicating with others, including recognizing where they are in their own growth and what they already know, involves providing the right level of information to direct or influence the person or team. The fundamental skills of hearing and listening are essential components of effective communication. Leadership is about learning from others, listening, sharing ideas, designing and testing great ideas, and then planning and implementing with a continuous cycle of evaluating and improving. It is about guiding the team and facilitating collaboration. It is enabling others so that each member of the team contributes, like conducting an orchestra.[7]

As discussed in the Scope of Practice (SOP) for RDNs,[8] RDNs in management practice areas throughout the nutrition and dietetics field align people to achieve a common goal by providing a clear direction, motivating, and inspiring while allowing opportunities to give input. Strategic thinking involves aligning the individual or team plans with the mission, vision, and principles of the organization or the customer (eg, client or patient). It is important to provide proper training, mentoring, and communication and dialogue opportunities in order to set clear expectations for performance and accountability.

Founder and CEO of the online professional network Ivy Exec Elena Bajic underscores the significance of a shared vision across the team, which has allowed her company to move forward.[9] Similar to other successful leaders, she states that her company has grown fastest when communication lines are strongest, making the communication of the company's vision the single most important thing to promote success. She argues that if every employee has a clear understanding of how their work contributes to the broader company goal, including revenue enhancement, the employee is more likely to work harder to achieve those goals and feel they are vital to the company's success.[9]

Adaptability and the ability to keep pace with organizational and societal changes are required for leaders to develop and communicate strategic intent.[10] It is important to demonstrate a willingness to collaborate with key stakeholders to determine synergies in activities and vision, with a commitment to reconcile differences when possible to achieve the greater good.

Advanced leaders view strategic planning as an ever-evolving process, constantly informed by both facts and the need to shape perceptions in a collaborative manner.[10] An effective strategic plan, and therefore an effective leader, brings a united focus to a shared vision for all involved to work toward.

Building Relationships

Building effective relationships will lead to trust and learning together, which will improve performance and foster innovation. Leaders create a learning environment for improvement and for developing talent. Leaders know how to offer personalized instruction and have the ability to seize teaching and mentoring opportunities. Leadership involves setting expectations for quality work and working with the staff to evaluate competency levels and to create an educational plan to accomplish competency. A strong leader also sets an example through their behavior as a teacher by demonstrating professionalism, upholding ethics and integrity, and sharing life lessons and their vision.[11]

Successful leaders can build relationships by focusing on six factors: communication, support, safety, competence, continuous renewal, and trust.[12] Effective communication can be both complex and subtle at the same time; good communicators relay expectations with real-time feedback on whether those expectations are achieved. Support can come in many forms, such as financial, physical, emotional, and moral. Safety encompasses the basic human need to feel physically, emotionally, and psychologically safe in their environment. Leaders who recognize limitations in their own competency and who know to depend on others to fill in their knowledge gaps will have gained an invaluable skill and have built trust with their team. Continuous renewal refers to leaders who take care of themselves by making time for rest and healthy pursuits outside of work and encouraging their employees to do the same. Finally, though trust takes time to build, it is the most important thing leaders establish between themselves and their employees.[12]

Collaborative Coaching

A collaborative leader shares goals, includes the team in decision making whenever possible, asks for help, shares the problems, and uses input to build solutions.[13] Collaboration is a social skill essential to individual and group success. It involves getting to know each other, showing empathy, and fostering a culture of loyalty and trust to allow diverse or conflicting ideas to exist without personal disagreement.[14]

Boyatzis' intentional change theory (ICT)[15] promotes the idea of a leader as a coach for collaboration and change. The coach helps the individual develop competencies by guiding rather than pushing. The coach asks the right questions, listens intensively, cares about the individual, and shows compassion toward them. The leader also finds coachable moments in which to provide feedback. The leader-coach helps each staff member think through what they want to accomplish and set a personal vision, then coaches the individual to help achieve their goals. This leader-coach can be a manager or a peer. Based on a survey of managers, *Harvard Business Review* reports that coaching is somewhat rare, estimating that managers coach 9% of the time while acknowledging they should coach at least 36% of the time. However, this same study found that the time spent coaching was not strongly associated with the performance of the individual or team, but the results indicated that managers who help their team network by connecting staff with others who have expertise resulted in positive outcomes.[16]

Leading through coaching should include being supportive instead of judgmental and providing guidance rather than instructing or consulting. As noted in Chapter 1, active conversations can support these important qualities, as outlined by the GROW model to guide the conversation as follows[17]:

> **Goal:** The goal or the intent of the meeting or session; what the person wants to achieve.

> **Reality:** The facts of the situation: who, what, where, when, and how but not why, as "why" is a judgment, not a fact.

> **Options:** All the possible solutions (prompt for replies if needed); what people would ideally do if they could.

> **Will:** How committed the individual is to following through to accomplish the objective.

This conversational approach may help leaders investigate potential solutions for problems while maintaining a collaborative coaching relationship.

Collaboration Within and Among Teams

Collaboration requires working together. It requires respect and sensitivity to others, an openness to experiment, and a mission to improve.[18] In cross-silo groups, which consist of team members from different units, departments, or professions, it's essential for team members to learn about each other. The leaders of cross-silo groups should act as culture brokers to bridge connections and help build teams. Again, this is facilitated through practicing effective communication, asking open-ended questions, keeping team members focused, seeking various viewpoints, summarizing (and asking whether the summary is correct), and finally, asking the group how the process is going.[19]

Teams, especially teams of people who generally do not work together, require a shared strategic intent or reward in order to be effective.[20] Intrinsic rewards are self-generated, such as finding the work meaningful, having a sense of ownership of a project or process, being challenged by the work but doing it well, and feeling a sense of accomplishment. An effective new program, a flawless accreditation visit, or helping a client succeed are intrinsic rewards. Extrinsic rewards are external, such as a pay increase, a bonus, or public recognition.

Advanced leaders recognize and address the challenges inherent in cross-silo teamwork. Management pressure, individual feelings of anxiety, inadequate breadth or depth of skill sets, and limited resources may influence a team's ability to work together to design and implement change. A request to work on one of these collaborative teams may trigger a fear of loss, power, autonomy, or job, so team members may retreat and become protective of their ideas and knowledge. This may be interpreted as criticism of other team members, blocking or ignoring otherwise good ideas. When cross-silo teams are used, the meetings should occur early on to understand each individual's role and foster trust within the group. Ideally, a threat analysis should be conducted before the group forms, including thinking about or listening to why the collaboration might seem threatening, why the partnership is essential, and what potential losses might be perceived. This discussion may provide ideas for strategies to encourage nondefensive behavior once the team begins its work.[21] Good leaders can then reinforce each person's fundamental role to minimize the perception of threats.

Commitment and shared values and vision help teams stay focused on the required steps to achieve goals, which builds trust that their work will help achieve the desired outcome.[22] Leaders who are successful help teams make the space and time for new ideas to emerge and maintain an overall sense of direction and purpose.[23]

Change Management and Innovation

A leader has a substantial role in keeping abreast of changes influencing their work. Change is constant, and it is occurring at an accelerated pace. One current example of change in our field is the decline of 50% to 20% in emergency room visits and hospitalizations, even before the COVID-19 pandemic began.[24] The decrease was due to advances in technology that enabled care and monitoring at home through wearable devices, smart videos, home-based laboratory tests, and virtual office visits for routine health care. This phenomenon was predicted as a change driver in the Academy of Nutrition and Dietetics Visioning Report 2017.[3] The concepts in that 2017 report remain valid today and in the future; they can serve as a roadmap for advanced leaders skilled at harnessing change.

Furthermore, nutrition and dietetics leaders can embrace VUCA—the managerial acronym referring to volatility, uncertainty, complexity, and ambiguity in an environment—to thrive in practice and lead meaningful, relevant change.[25] The Academy of Nutrition and Dietetics provides guidance for RDNs to build trust and manage unpredictable changes in the Leadership section of its member website (www.eatrightPRO.org/leadership); the leadership concepts discussed in this chapter expand on those ideas.

Change models can provide guidance on creating innovation or managing change. Change management is a process or a series of tasks that is influenced by every part of the business system to which it belongs. For a change management process to be successful, collaboration is essential between each individual, each group, and (hopefully) any outside forces that are most likely to be affected and involved in the change. Box 2.3 on page 32 includes questions that need to be anticipated and ultimately answered throughout the process.[26]

Advanced leaders have learned to determine if they are creating or reacting to change and should strive to proactively create change that is beneficial for self-development or team development and organizational effectiveness rather than wait to be reactive. For success, leaders must initialize the change process, obtain buy-in from stakeholders, implement the change in a collaborative manner, and monitor the process and outcomes. Change management works when the leader focuses on results, identifies solutions to overcome barriers, communicates often, and monitors the situation closely.

Change Theories or Models

Change is inevitable, and advanced leaders use this fact as an opportunity to create changes that will improve and evolve an organization and themselves on an ongoing basis. Many organizational psychologists and other researchers have created change theories or change models to provide guidance on how to effectively lead change for positive results on an individual, team, communal, and societal level.

ADKAR Model

The ADKAR model focuses on an individual employee's change, which is important to ensure that the employee buys into an organizational change.[27] The five elements of this model include the following:

> **Awareness:** ensuring that the individual and everyone else involved understands the reason why the change is needed

> **Desire:** creating momentum and inspiration so that everyone wants to become involved

> **Knowledge:** providing each individual with the information they need to complete their part of the change process

> **Ability:** teaching skills and providing mentoring and training for the employee to be successful

> **Reinforcement:** after the change is attained, working with employees to ensure the changes are sustained

Nudge Theory

Another change model is the nudge theory,[27,28] which relies more on communicating and fostering a mindset than on particular change management steps. Employees are persuaded to want the change on their own after being presented with information as a recommendation (as opposed to in a commanding manner) that illustrates how the expected change will both benefit and affect them. Nudge theory involves getting people to think in new and different ways to promote innovation. Advanced leaders who communicate well and can convey vision and strategic intent will be most successful using nudge theory to develop engaged employees who will support change.

Kübler-Ross Change Model

Similar to the stages of grief, the Kübler-Ross change model explains how employees may react to a departmental or company change that they do not support.[27] The stages include the following:

> **Denial:** refusal to believe change is coming
> **Anger:** frustration at having change forced upon them
> **Bargaining:** pushing for compromise that avoids having to accept the entire change
> **Depression:** a sense of helplessness to influence the coming change
> **Acceptance:** realization that one must adapt to the change in order to keep their job

Leaders should design the change to expect and address these feelings directly in order to gain buy-in for the change.

Lewin Phases of Change

The Lewin phases of change model summarizes change occurring in three steps[29]:

1. Unfreezing the process.
2. Creating the change.
3. Refreezing the process where the monitoring, revising, and follow-up occur.

Leaders may find that the most difficult yet most important step is the unfreezing step, as it involves overcoming inertia and the defense mechanism to avoid change for fear of the results. Once the need for change becomes urgent or inevitable, the actual change occurs in the second stage. Clear, timely, and accurate communication is most important during this second phase; advanced leaders who have practiced and refined this skill via experience will be the most successful in leading change through this step. If the change is successful, the third step is when the change becomes the standard. An advanced leader will help people understand that success often depends on this continuous cycle of change, with an effort to avoid the return to complacency. Although the model is organized into phases or steps, it is important to note that Lewin was clear that change should be thought of as a *process*, not as individual discrete stages.[29] Thinking of change as a process contributes to an individual or team's ability to adapt more quickly to future change.[17] An example of applying Lewin's phases of change model to a real-life scenario is described in the Stories From the Field box on page 34.

Kotter Model: Eight-Step Process for Leading Change

John Kotter, DBA, studied successful change management leaders, extracted the success factors, and combined them into an eight-step methodology described next to lead change.[30] Each step builds on the one before it, with each one being unique and vital to success in a stepwise manner.

1. **Create a sense of urgency.**

   Help others see the urgency by creating a bold opportunity statement that clearly communicates the need to act quickly. This step is essential and advanced leaders can build on existing communication skills to convey the vision. It is important to spend substantial time and energy building urgency before moving on to the next steps.

2. **Build a guiding coalition.**

   Even advanced leaders should recruit fellow powerful change leaders to persuade others that change is needed. This collaboration can support step 3, as more effective strategic change coalitions can be built.

3. **Form a strategic vision and initiatives.**

   Clearly conveying vision and strategic intent will ensure that people with shared passion and inspiration join the coalition.

4. **Communicate the vision.**

   Large numbers of people with a common goal, inspired by advanced leaders who have adequately communicated the vision, will be more effective. Leaders can best communicate the vision through their actions.[31]

5. **Empower broad-based action.**

   This step involves identifying obstacles that inhibit change and making a plan to overcome those obstacles to achieve a unifying vision. Inefficient processes, silos, and hierarchies can be barriers to change, as can ineffective leaders. The guiding coalition established early on in the process can remove philosophical and financial barriers if the coalition was assembled correctly.

6. **Generate short-term goals and wins.**

   Advanced leaders routinely communicate immediate wins, early and often, to keep track of progress and encourage team members to persist in the change effort. Short-term wins validate the effort, maintain an appropriate level of urgency, and provide an intrinsic reward to the coalition.

7. **Sustain acceleration by consolidating gains and producing more change.**

   Building on early successes increases the credibility of leaders and the guiding coalition. After every win, analyze what went right and what needs improving. Set goals to continue building on the momentum of success.

8. **Anchor new approaches in the culture.**

   Share connections between new behaviors and organizational success and reinforce new behaviors consistently until they become habits. Develop a leadership succession plan.

   Box 2.4 on pages 36 and 37 includes an example of how to apply Kotter's steps to leverage community and stakeholder involvement to address food insecurity at a population health level.[30,32,33]

BOX 2.4 Using Kotter's Eight-Step Process for Leading Change to Describe a Change Effort to Address Food Insecurity[30,32,33]

In 2018, 7.3% of older adults were food insecure and 2.7% were very low food secure.[32] The National Poll on Healthy Aging in December 2019 showed that adults aged 50 to 80 years had an overall prevalence of food insecurity·at 14%.[33] The social isolation and economic devastation of the COVID-19 pandemic worsened the problem.[32] The issues of financial hardship and food insecurity took center stage of the national conversation in 2020, leading to important congressional actions impacting existing federal food assistance programs. Public-private partnerships are needed to better meet the needs of the US population.

The Kotter Eight-Step Process for Leading Change can be used to demonstrate how nutrition and dietetics leaders can develop innovative ways to help meet these needs.[30]

1. **Create a sense of urgency**

   Statistics, such as those shared here, can create a compelling case for action to implement strategies to reduce food insecurity if they are accompanied by real-life examples of affected individuals who would be served with innovative programs.

2. **Build a guiding coalition**

   Many health care and community/public health professionals are passionate about meeting the needs of people in their communities, and these people are essential to include in the coalition as they share the passion and inspiration needed. It is important to ensure that people with enough power and resources to create the change are included. Advanced leadership skills are needed to help the coalition work together effectively to achieve the common goal (in this example, the goal is to reduce the incidence of food insecurity).

3. **Form a strategic vision and initiatives**

   The people who have joined the coalition likely have shared passions and inspirations, and these need to be directed toward a concise and clearly communicated vision, with strategies for achieving that vision. For example, the overall shared passion may be "Reduce the number of people who are hungry." The strategic vision should be more concise, such as "Older adults living in the northeast Ohio communities who screen positively on the Hunger Vital Sign screening tool will receive food assistance with an educational component to sustain the change." Strategies would then be developed to provide both food and education.

4. **Communicate the vision**

   Communication is the most important step in a change process, and it is also the most challenging one. Multiple communication channels need to be used for both internal and external communication, and all members of the coalition should be involved in implementing the communication plan.

5. **Empower broad-based action**

   Obstacles to change will always exist. Effective leaders will recognize the obstacles and work with the coalition to change the systems or structures that undermine the vision. Obstacles commonly encountered in addressing food insecurity interventions include funding, conflicting priorities for programs, the ability to measure baseline and postintervention data to show a return on investment, and participant-level concerns such as program acceptance and adherence. Leaders will work together to develop nontraditional ideas and are willing to take the risks to implement them and monitor for change.

6. **Generate short-term goals and wins**

   Coalition members will stay more engaged and work toward expanding programs if there are short-term, visible, and measurable "wins." Advanced leaders will plan ahead for this by creating goals that can be achieved with relatively little time and effort, which serve as benchmark goals along the way to the strategic vision. For example, when developing food insecurity interventions, the first goal may be related to program adherence over the planned time for intervention, with a longer-term goal being related to a change in hospitalization rates.

continued on next page

continued from previous page

7. **Sustain acceleration by consolidating gains and producing more change**

Short-term wins usually encourage existing coalition members to remain engaged and attract new members. This can reinvigorate the process with new projects and change agents. For example, a food insecurity intervention that meets program goals for participant adherence and completion may encourage key stakeholders to extend that intervention to more people or extend the length of time for the intervention to the existing participants.

8. **Anchor new approaches in the culture**

This is another step in which clear communication is essential. Advanced leaders can articulate the connection between the interventions and results with the strategic vision in order to create an ongoing culture of change and expansion. An effective leader will always have a focus on mentoring and developing the next team of leaders so as to ensure that the intervention and vision is scalable and transcends one individual.

Design Thinking

The use of design thinking is worthwhile for any substantial change.[23] The goal of design thinking is to see problems in a human-centered way—from a customer, patient, or client perspective—and challenge assumptions while redefining problems to identify alternative strategies. It is a solution-based approach; it allows failure and ambiguity and tests various options. The focus of design thinking is always on the customer needs, not the employee needs.

Design thinking goes beyond managing change to discovering and designing the difference that is needed. It involves five phases that are not necessarily sequential. (1) Empathy is required to see the problem and develop a solution with the needs of the end user in mind. (2) The problem must be defined and may be continuously redefined to drive new potential solutions. (3) A third phase encourages leaders to ideate, which allows for assumptions to be challenged and innovation to be made, (4) leading to the prototype phase where solutions are created. (5) Importantly, the test phase is critical at multiple steps of the process, as solutions should continuously be tested for sustainability and results.

Design management and design leadership can be differentiated. Design managers optimize resources to implement programs in the most effective and profitable way, while design leaders also integrate innovation, design, and strategy to achieve an organization's goals.[34] Design leadership promotes business success since it helps to envision the future, provides strategy, directs funding while maximizing the return on investment, creates a sustainable innovative business environment, and organizes training for design within a business.

Innovation

Change management and innovation are interrelated. Identifying the need for change is often the impetus for innovation. One way to challenge conventional thinking is to create "disturbances"[35] to stimulate new ideas and break down assumptions. This is done by addressing weaknesses and then strengths as an assumption or problem and investigating how other disciplines handled similar issues. Advanced leaders create environments that dare employees to try and reward their trials with incentives for trying new approaches rather than for their successes or failures. The goal is to encourage a learning environment.[36]

Zenger and Folkman interviewed 33 innovative individuals, identified by their coworkers and bosses, to determine the actions or behaviors that caused them to be perceived as innovative.[37] Distinctive behaviors emerged, including displaying strategic vision, seeking to get inside the customer's mind to discern needs and wants, cultivating an upward communication organizational culture, and emphasizing speed while reaching for stretch goals.

Negotiation and Facilitation

When a dispute occurs in the workplace, the conflict can escalate to the level of costly litigation, hostile work environments, high turnover, and reduced workplace productivity. Negotiation is often necessary to reach agreements without the help of an outside facilitator. Successful negotiation requires appropriate communication and a commitment to reach a common goal.[38] Three negotiation strategies can help involved persons mend their partnership and get back to the business of creating value:

> Avoid being provoked into an emotional response by taking a physical and mental break from the situation, identifying the abuse of the situation, then diverting attention back to the issues at hand.

> Hold fast to value-creating strategies and avoid public awareness of the conflict.

> Use time to one's advantage, as disputes can be constantly in flux. In addition, time often provides perspective and a recommitment to the common goal.

Ideally, all involved will be flexible and willing to compromise; this is more likely if rapport and trust have been built prior to the conflict that necessitated the negotiation. Advanced leaders can create an environment of curiosity, flexibility, and openness to listening and understanding each point of view.[38]

Facilitation differs from negotiation in that it requires the participation of someone who is not directly involved in the negotiation.[38] The facilitator would stay neutral, leading the negotiation. Effective managers and leaders will recognize the need for facilitation early, and work to resolve disputes before they become insurmountable. The following characteristics of advanced leaders are important for effective facilitation:

> commitment to remain neutral so that participants can work out mutually agreeable solutions

> creation of an inclusive environment that respects group dynamics

> clear communication of guidelines and the ability to uphold them throughout the process

> maintenance of participation and momentum toward the common goal

Skills for negotiation and facilitation are developed over time, and leaders who are willing to embrace the risks associated with these roles will be most likely to hone communication skills, build trust with their teams, and be able to convey strategic vision and intent to build effective teams and coalitions.

Ethics and Leadership

Leaders are looked to as role models, so their actions, failures, and triumphs generally carry greater importance in the work environment.[39] An ethical leader will recognize when certain priorities, such as employee safety or environmentally sound business practices, are more important than profits. They will use their power for the good of the employees and the company as a whole rather than only in their best self-interest.

Advanced leaders are aware that people are watching and, therefore, consistently behave in an ethical manner. Beyond the question as to whether something is right vs whether it is legal, incorporating ethics into personal and organizational values will set the stage for ethical behavior and promote doing good for others, being just, and showing integrity.[40] A good resource for acting ethically within the field of nutrition and dietetics is the Code of Ethics for the Nutrition and Dietetics Profession, jointly published by the Academy of Nutrition and Dietetics and the Commission on Dietetic Registration.[41] The code is updated periodically to reflect the changing needs of the country and the nutrition and dietetics profession; the most recent update was in 2018.

The code outlines four categories of principles and standards that provide guidance for RDNs and nutrition and dietetics technicians, registered (NDTRs), to adhere to core values of customer focus, integrity, innovation, social responsibility, and diversity—all of which are characteristics of advanced leaders.[41]

Competence and Professional Development in Practice (Nonmaleficence)

Consistent with this ethical principle, advanced leaders continuously develop their expertise by assessing the validity of scientific evidence and how to apply it to create a knowledgeable and collaborative team. By acting in an empathetic and respectful manner, seeking counsel from others as needed, and incorporating perspectives from diverse individuals, advanced leaders can generate innovation, research, and discovery to enhance practice.

Integrity in Personal and Organizational Behaviors and Practices (Autonomy)

Advanced leaders do not require direct oversight or constant monitoring to comply with applicable laws and regulations, respect intellectual property rights, or provide accurate and truthful communications. Acting ethically enables leaders to build the trust that is essential to gain respect and develop a platform from which advanced leadership can be built.

Professionalism (Beneficence)

People are more likely to join collaborative teams when the leader consistently demonstrates respect for the values, rights, knowledge, and skills of other professionals while contributing to the advancement and competence of others through mentorship.

Social Responsibility for Local, Regional, National, and Global Nutrition and Well-Being (Justice)

Justice focuses on being fair and equitable. It suggests that as leaders, we have responsibilities to help in reducing health disparities and protecting human rights, promoting diversity and inclusion, and contributing time and expertise to food security and sustainability of the food supply and climate needs. Collaborations with a shared purpose and vision are more likely to attract like-minded individuals to achieve the common goal. Advanced nutrition and dietetics leaders naturally seek leadership opportunities in professional, community, and service organizations to enhance health and nutritional status while protecting the public.

Cultural Humility, Diversity, and Inclusion

Cultural humility involves an active and ongoing commitment to a lifelong process that includes striving for cultural competence.[42] Nutrition and dietetics professionals should continually engage in self-reflection and self-critique, and advanced leaders model this for others in their words and actions. It is impossible for RDNs to know everything about every culture, but they can develop an underlying understanding of how stereotypes that a practitioner holds for certain populations can affect decision making and influence interactions, with a commitment to be inquisitive and continuously learn more about other cultures and individuals.

Similarly, advanced leaders are skilled at creating personal and professional environments that celebrate diversity and practice inclusion by not assuming that they have all of the answers.[43] It is important to seek input from employees, patients/clients, and colleagues on which processes and behaviors need to be corrected or developed to support an inclusive workplace that does not impede performance but rather fosters collaboration among the team. Leaders act with humility and courage to create the change that is needed with a commitment to action.

See Chapter 3 for more details on this important topic.

Advocacy and Leadership

RDNs and advanced leaders should engage in nutrition- and health-related advocacy efforts. Advocacy is any action that argues for a cause or supports, defends, or pleads on behalf of others. The SOPP for RDNs[1] states that RDNs "advocate for provision of quality food and nutrition services as part of public policy" through multiple avenues. The SOP[8] encourages RDNs to advocate to decrease health disparities and promote health policies that improve the patient/client experience of care, improve population health, and reduce costs associated with care. It also states that RDNs will advocate for sound food and nutrition legislation, policies, and programs. Some examples of avenues that can be used to advocate for nutrition services include legislative action at the local, state, or federal level; participation in committees, workgroups, and task forces that develop nutrition policies; and involvement in coalitions that address populations with special needs and chronic conditions.

An example of a grassroots advocacy effort that involved a large coalition of RDNs and health care professionals in multiple states gained full momentum in 2011, resulting in success in 2014.[44] Academy of Nutrition and Dietetics staff and member leaders recognized that hospital regulations published by the Centers for Medicare & Medicaid Services (CMS) created an impediment to expanding the scope of practice of RDNs and posed unnecessary burden on physicians and other health care practitioners, while delaying access to nutrition interventions for patients. In 2011, the Academy of Nutrition and Dietetics submitted public comments to CMS requesting revision to the hospital regulations backed by research showing that nutrition care is safer, provided in a timelier manner, and often costs less when provided by RDNs. These comments were followed by 2 years of advocacy by member leaders of dietetic practice groups, state affiliates of the Academy of Nutrition and Dietetics, and individual RDNs providing care to patients. These advocacy efforts included building coalitions by meeting with local and state elected officials; by leaders for other health-related organizations, such as the state affiliates for the American Hospital Association and the American Academy of Pediatrics; and by hundreds of people writing letters and submitting comments to CMS to garner support. In May 2014, CMS published their final ruling on the applicable hospital regulations, removing restrictions and allowing RDNs to write nutrition-related orders when permitted by state law and local hospital policy.[42]

This is one of many grassroot efforts that has led to major advancements in patient/client access to care and expanded the scope of practice for RDNs. The success of these types of broad-scale efforts relies on the concepts discussed throughout this chapter, such as using communication skills to build trust and convey vision and strategic intent, building relationships and collaborations, negotiating and innovating, and developing leadership capabilities through practice.

Summary

Being a leader is multidimensional. This chapter shares ways to approach change, focuses on the profession's key issues, and encourages the reader to think of the big picture (mission, vision, and values) and continuously innovate. It talks about the need to communicate, dialogue, and respect the values and views of others. Being a leader involves varying one's approach based on the situation and acting ethically in all circumstances while using the skills to advocate for beneficial changes in the nutrition and dietetics field.

REFERENCES

1   Academy Quality Management Committee, Academy of Nutrition and Dietetics. Revised 2017 Standards of Practice in Nutrition Care and Standards of Professional Performance for Registered Dietitian Nutritionists. *J Acad Nutr Diet.* 2018;118(1):132-140.e15. doi:10.1016/j.jand.2017.10.003

2   Doley J, Clark K, Roper S. Academy of Nutrition and Dietetics: Revised 2019 Standards of Professional Performance for registered dietitian nutritionists (competent, proficient, and expert) in clinical nutrition management. *J Acad Nutr Diet.* 2019;119(9):1545-1560.e32.

3   Kicklighter JR, Dorner B, Hunter AM, et al. Visioning Report 2017: a preferred path forward for the nutrition and dietetics profession. *J Acad Nutr Diet.* 2017;117(1):110-127. doi:10.1016/j.jand.2016.09.027

4   Patten EV, Sauer K. A leadership taxonomy for clinical dietetics practice. *J Acad Nutr Diet.* 2019;119(3):369-374. doi:10.1016/j.jand.2018.01.011

5   Brody RA, Skipper A, Chaffee CL, Wooldridge NH, Kicklighter JR, Touger-Decker R. Developing an advanced practice credential for registered dietitian nutritionists in clinical nutrition practice. *J Acad Nutr Diet.* 2015;115(4):619-623.

6   Commission on Dietetic Registration. *Advanced Practitioner Certification in Clinical Nutrition.* Commission on Dietetics Registration website. Accessed April 28, 2020. https://admin.cdrnet .org/vault/2459/web/CDR%20AP%20Test%20Specification%20for%20Publication.pdf

7   Gleason PM, Harris JE. The Bayesian approach to decision making and analysis in nutrition research and practice. *J Acad Nutr Diet.* 2019:119(12):1993-2003.

8   Quality Management Committee. Academy of Nutrition and Dietetics: revised 2017 scope of practice for the registered dietitian nutritionist. *J Acad Nutr Diet.* 2018;118(1):141-165.

9   Bajic E. Why communicating vision is the single most important thing you can do. Forbes website. Updated December 27, 2017. Accessed February 6, 2022. www.forbes.com/sites /elenabajic/2017/12/27/why-communicating-vision-is-the-single-most-important-thing-you -can-do/?sh=188f0c171e64

10 Stein K. The Academy's governance and practice: restructuring for the challenges of the turn of the 21st century. *J Acad Nutr Diet.* 2017;117(10S3):S166-S191.e14.

11 Rogers M. My approach to 1-on-1s. Marco Rogers blog. Updated January 1, 2020. Accessed February 6, 2022. https://marcorogers.com/blog/my-approach-to-1-on-1s

12 Hensley PA, Burmeister L. Leadership connectors: a theoretical construct for building relationships *Educational Leadership and Administration: Teaching and Program Development.* 2008;20:125-134. Updated 2010. Accessed February 6, 2022. https://Eric.ed.gov/fulltext/ej965151.pdf

13 Plummer M. A short guide to building your team's critical thinking skills. Harvard Business Review website. October 11, 2019. Accessed February 6, 2022. https://hbr.org/2019/10/a-short-guide-to -building-your-teams-critical-thinking-skills

14 Brooks A, John L. The surprising power of questions. *Harvard Business Review.* 2018;96(3):60-67.

15 Boyatzis R, Smith M, VanOosten E. Coaching for change: how to help employees reach their potential. *Harvard Business Review.* 2019;97(5):151-155.

16 Managers can't be great coaches all by themselves. *Harvard Business Review.* 2018;96(3):22-24.

17 Ibarra H, Scoular A. The leader as coach. *Harvard Business Review.* 2019;97(6):110-119.

18 Gino F. Cracking the code of sustained collaboration. *Harvard Business Review.* 2019;97(6):72-81.

19 Casciaro T, Edmondson A, Jang S. Cross-silo leadership. *Harvard Business Review.* 2019; 97(3):130-139.

20 Haas M, Mortensen M. The secrets of great teamwork. *Harvard Business Review.* 2016;94(6):70-76.

21 Kwan L. The collaboration blind spot. *Harvard Business Review.* 2019;97(2):66-73.

22 Ogbonnaya C. When teamwork is good for employees – and when it isn't. *Harvard Business Review.* August 29, 2019. Accessed April 27, 2020. https://hbr.org/2019/08/when-teamwork-is -good-for-employees-and-when-it-isnt

23 Bason C, Austin RD. The right way to lead design thinking: how to help project teams overcome the inevitable inefficiencies, uncertainties, and emotional flare-ups. *Harvard Business Review.* 2019;97(2):82-91.

24 Pearl R, Madvig P. Managing the most expensive patients. *Harvard Business Review.* 2020;98(1):68-75.

25 Academy of Nutrition and Dietetics. Navigating future practice: VUCA. eatrightPRO website. Updated May 2020. Accessed February 6, 2022. www.eatrightPRO.org/leadership/governance /governance-resources/visioning-process

26 Javidi M. Collaborative change management: a systematic approach. *Intercultural Communication Studies.*2003;12(2):83-92. Accessed February 6, 2022. web.uri.edu/iaics/files/08 -Mitch-Javidi.pdf

27 Hicks K. Organizational change management: 8 proven models to help navigate change. Zendesk website. Updated January 19, 2022. Accessed February 6, 2022. www.zendesk.com /blog/change-management-models/

28 John P, Cotterill S, Moseley A, et al. *Nudge, Nudge, Think, Think*. 2nd ed. Manchester University Press; 2020. Accessed February 20, 2022. doi:10.7765/9781526153487

29 Tang KN. Change management. In: Tang KN. *Leadership and Change Management*. Springer, Singapore; 2019:47-55. doi:10.1007/978-981-13-8902-3_5

30 Kotter JP. Why transformation efforts fail. *Harvard Business Review*. 1995;73(2);59-67.

31 Rose KH. *Leading Change: a Model* by John Kotter. SIRIUS Meetings website. Accessed February 6, 2022. www.siriusmeetings.com/files/Leading_Change_by_Rose1.pdf

32 Ziliak JP, Gundersen C. *The State of Senior Hunger in America in 2018: An Annual Report*. Feeding America; 2020. Accessed April 19, 2021. www.feedingamerica.org/sites/default/files/2020-05 /2020-The%20State%20of%20Senior%20Hunger%20in%202018.pdf

33 Leung CW, Kullgren JT, Malani PN, et al. Food insecurity is associated with multiple chronic conditions and physical health status among older US adults. *Prev Med Rep*. 2020;20:101211. doi:10.1016/j.pmedr.2020.101211

34 Gloppen J. Perspectives on design leadership and design thinking and how they relate to European service industries. *DMI*. 2009;4(1):33-47. doi:10.1111/j.1942-5074.2009.00005.x

35 Brandenburger A. Are your company's strengths really weaknesses? Harvard Business Review website. August 22, 2019. Accessed February 6, 2022. https://hbr.org/2019/08/are-your -companys-strengths-really-weaknesses

36 Anthony S, Cobban P, Nair R, Painchaud N. Breaking down the barriers to innovation. *Harvard Business Review*. 2019:97(6):92-101.

37 Zenger J, Folkman J. Research: 10 traits of innovative leaders. Harvard Business Review website. Updated December 15, 2014. Accessed February 6, 2022. https://hbr.org/2014/12/research-10 -traits-of-innovative-leaders

38 Gallagher L. ADR: negotiation and facilitation. MRSC website. Updated September 14, 2020. Accessed February 6, 2022. https://mrsc.org/Home/Stay-Informed/MRSC-Insight/September -2020/ADR-Negotiation-and-Facilitation.aspx

39 Ciulla JB. *The Ethics of Leadership*. Wadsworth/Thomson; 2003. Accessed February 6, 2022.

40 Epley N, Kumar A. How to design an ethical organization. *Harvard Business Review*. 2019;97(30):144-150.

41 Commission on Dietetic Registration, Academy of Nutrition and Dietetics. *Code of Ethics for the Nutrition and Dietetics Profession*. Academy of Nutrition and Dietetics; 2018. Accessed April 28, 2020. www.eatrightPRO.org/-/media/files/eatrightPRO/practice/code-of-ethics /codeofethicshandout.pdf

42 Hook JN, Davis DE, Owen J, Worthington EL Jr, Utsey SO. Cultural humility: measuring openness to culturally diverse clients. *J Couns Psychol*. 2013;60(3):353-366. doi:10.1037/a0032595

43 Ramirez R. 5 inclusive leadership traits that will improve organizational diversity. University of San Diego website. Updated April 6, 2020. Accessed February 9, 2022. www.sandiego.edu/news /detail.php?_focus=76018

44 Phillips W. Timeline of events leading to allowance of RDN order writing privileges by CMS. *Future Dimensions*. 2016;35:10-12.

CHAPTER 3

Embracing Diversity & Embodying Inclusive Leadership in Nutrition & Dietetics

Camille Range, MPH, RDN, and Deanna Belleny Lewis, MPH, RDN

Introduction

The year 2020 illuminated the existing inequities in our current systems and ways of thinking while forcing us to persevere through unprecedented times. Injustices for people of color and marginalized groups continued to plague our world as the COVID-19 global pandemic tested our systems and ability to navigate through public health crises. Americans witnessed hospitalization, case, and death rates from the pandemic disproportionally impacting Black, Brown, and Indigenous communities[1]; unarmed Black people losing their lives at the hands of police; an increase in racist hate crimes and discrimination against Asian Americans[2]; and a record amount of violence against transgender and gender-nonconforming individuals.[3] Practitioners need sustainable solutions that advance health and racial equity for every community and our shared future, but we must commit to action. To be successful in any arena—including in the field of nutrition and dietetics—there is a need to embrace your role as a leader, a leader that puts in the work to understand their foundation, to embrace diversity, to advocate for equity, and to embody inclusive leadership. Increased efforts in leadership are vital for an equitable, sustainable future for ourselves, our profession, and the next generation.

Inclusion, Diversity, Equity, and Access

Health and nutrition professionals have an ethical responsibility to advocate for inclusion, diversity, equity, and access (IDEA) within the field and for the health and well-being of the people they serve. Without this commitment, prejudice, discrimination, racism, and bias from health care providers will continue to be contributing factors to inequities in health care.[4]

Two prevailing strategies are necessary to advance this goal. First, we must increase the diversity of the workforce and remove the systemic norms that have supported a lack of diversity in the field.[5] Second, there is a paramount need for all dietitians to be equipped to provide equitable and culturally humble care to diverse patients, clients, and communities. To accomplish these goals, we must embrace diversity in our field but also commit to lifelong learning to become inclusive and equity-centered leaders.

This chapter will provide strategies to support the development of leadership at any level, with a focus on advancing IDEA in the nutrition and dietetics field. The chapter leads explicitly, though not exclusively, with race. We recognize that marginalization occurs based on many factors including gender, sexual orientation, size, income, and age, just to name a few. It is important to address all areas of marginalization; by deepening our ability to eliminate racial inequity, we will be better equipped to transform systems and institutions that impact other marginalized groups.

To maximize the lessons shared in this chapter, the reader must view diversity, in all its forms, as an asset. The definition of *diversity* used by the Academy of Nutrition and Dietetics recognizes the presence of differences among individuals within a given setting, including differences in ability, age, creed, culture, ethnicity, gender, gender identity, political affiliation, race, religion, sexual orientation, size, socioeconomic characteristics, and other factors.[6] Diversity can also include thought and experiences. Second, the reader must also understand that although diversity is often viewed as a quantitative measure (for example, how many people are aged 65 years or older or identify as belonging to a given religion), these attributes only represent the tip of the diversity iceberg. These numbers fail to capture the quality of an individual's experiences. To catalyze real, impactful, systemic change, there must be a focus on equity, justice, and access while promoting diversity and inclusion. Lastly, one must understand that strengthening inclusive leadership skills to support diverse, accessible, and equitable spaces is a lifelong process. Open-mindedness and a desire to learn are essential traits. According to social justice scholar D-L Stewart, PhD, the concepts of diversity and inclusion and issues based in equity and justice ask fundamentally different questions[7]:

Diversity asks, "Who's in the room?"

Equity responds, "Who is trying to get in the room but can't? Whose presence in the room is under constant threat of removal?"

Inclusion asks, "Have everyone's ideas been heard?"

Justice responds, "Whose ideas won't be taken as seriously because they aren't in the majority?"

The future of nutrition and dietetics requires leaders who think about these questions and help work toward solutions. Our field needs leaders who can support the recruitment and retention of diverse practitioners; who help students and professionals of all backgrounds gain proficiency in working with diverse populations; and who build and promote diverse, inclusive, and equity-centered teams. All of these efforts are critical for today and for the future of the profession and the public. Box 3.1 provides working definitions of common terms used in this chapter.[6,8-13]

BOX 3.1 Common Terms Related to Diversity and Inclusion[6,8-13]

Access	*Access* refers to giving equitable access to everyone regardless of human ability and experience.[6]
Bias » Bias » Conscious bias » Implicit bias/ unconscious bias	*Bias* is defined as a disproportionate weight in favor of or against an idea or thing, usually in a way that is closed minded, prejudicial, or unfair. Biases can be innate or learned. People may develop biases for or against an individual, a group, or a belief. Bias may be conscious or unconscious.[6] *Conscious bias* in its extreme is characterized by overt negative behavior that can be expressed through physical and verbal harassment or through more subtle means, such as exclusion.[8] *Implicit bias* or *unconscious bias* operates outside of a person's awareness and can be in direct contradiction to a person's espoused beliefs and values. Implicit bias is dangerous because it automatically seeps into a person's affect or behavior and is outside of the full awareness of that person.[8]
Diversity	*Diversity* is defined as the presence of differences within a given setting. These differences may be with respect to race/ethnicity, religion, color, gender, national origin, disability, sexual orientation, age, size, education, geographic origin, skill characteristics, or other qualities or attributes. Diversity refers to the composition of a group of people from any number of demographic backgrounds, identities (innate and selected), and the collective strength of their experiences, beliefs, values, skills, and perspectives.[6]
Equity	*Equity* exists when cultural identity and social classification no longer predict outcomes, and the reality that historical oppressions have caused systemic differences in access to resources and opportunities is recognized.
Justice (social)	*Social justice* constitutes a form of activism based on principles of equity and inclusion; it encompasses a vision of society in which the distribution of resources is equitable and all members are physically and psychologically safe and secure.[10]
Inclusion	*Inclusion* is defined as a process of intentional, ongoing effort to ensure that diverse people with different identities can fully participate in all aspects of the work of an organization, including leadership positions and decision-making processes. It is about engaging each individual and making everyone feel valued. Inclusion is the act of establishing philosophies, policies, practices, and procedures so that organizations and individuals contributing to organizations' success have a more level playing field on which to compete and equal access to opportunities and information.[6]
Dominant culture	A *dominant culture* is any culture that historically had, and currently has, greater access to resources and influence.[11] For example, *white supremacy* refers to the dominant, unquestioned standards of behavior and ways of functioning, which may be seen as mainstream, dominant cultural practices.[9]
Nondominant culture	A *nondominant culture* is defined as any culture that historically had, and currently has, reduced access to resources and influence.[11]
Culture	*Culture* is defined as a social system of meaning and customs developed by a group of people to ensure its adaptation and survival. Cultural groups are distinguished by a set of spoken or unspoken rules that shape values, beliefs, habits, patterns of thinking, behaviors, and styles of communication.[9]
Cultural humility	*Cultural humility* refers to the ability to maintain an interpersonal stance that is other-oriented (or open to the other) in relation to aspects of cultural identity that are most important to the client. It requires practitioners to engage in self-reflection and self-critique as lifelong learners.[6] Cultural humility requires a lifelong commitment to performing self-evaluation and critique, redressing power imbalances in the practitioner-patient dynamic, and developing mutually beneficial and nonpaternalistic partnerships with communities on behalf of individuals and defined populations.[12]
Positionality	*Positionality* places an individual in the sociocultural context of their environment, identifying the power they are either afforded or denied based on their cultural identities.[13]

Aligning the Foundation

On the first day of their coordinated graduate program in dietetics, eager students file into their seats excited to continue their journey to becoming registered dietitian nutritionists (RDNs). Professor Aida Miles, EdD, MMSc, RDN, CSP, LDN, FAND, starts with a story. It's her personal story of what brought her to dietetics and why. She shares the highs, the lows, the challenges, and the successes of her journey, often bringing a flood of emotions and vulnerability to the classroom. She then invites students to participate in a reflective activity that is timed to precede their clinical training. She asks them to share their response to a fundamental, two-part question: "How did you get here, and where do you want to go?" When this activity is introduced, students spend at least 2 hours engaged in learning about themselves and their classmates. Subsequently, students are led through individual reflective exercises throughout their training, with opportunities to share during cohort meetings, based on their comfort level. Students share diverse stories about food insecurity, family meal dynamics, body image issues, class, race, ethnicity, and the future of dietetics. According to Miles (personal communication, March 11, 2021), trust is built, awareness is developed, and perspectives are broadened.

Self-Awareness and Education

Developing awareness is the foundation of effective, inclusive, equity-centered leadership. Self-awareness is a pillar for managerial effectiveness and leadership success.[14] An awareness or recognition of your own strengths, weaknesses, behaviors, biases, and preferences starts with education and introspection. Similar to the experiences in Miles' classroom, exploring questions around who you are, why you are here, and where you want to go helps clarify your unique frame of reference. Self-awareness is connected to an ability to build stronger relationships, strengthen emotional intelligence, communicate effectively, and lead teams with higher staff satisfaction.[15,16] Tools such as the CliftonStrengths Assessment,[17] the Myers-Briggs Type Indicator,[18] the Implicit Association Test from Harvard University,[19] and the Emotional and Social Competence Inventory[20] can facilitate self-awareness by providing information about how you make decisions, where your strengths lie, how you perceive the world, and how you may interact with others. The Academy of Nutrition and Dietetics also has a hub of resources to support current and aspiring leaders with the goal of improving equity and access for everyone.[21]

As an effective, equity-centered, inclusive leader, it is important to reflect regularly on your identity in various contexts. As mentioned previously, a few examples of social identity groups include gender, race, ethnicity, age, (dis)ability, class, and religion, although this is not a comprehensive list. These groups range in their degree of obviousness or ambiguity as well as in the sense that some social identity groups are self-proclaimed and others are ascribed by people other than the individual.[22] It is also important to consider whether an identity is part of the dominant culture or of a nondominant culture. A dominant culture is any culture that historically had, and currently has, greater access to resources and influence and defines the cultural norms for an environment or profession.[11] Dominant social identities also come with inherent privileges and power. Nondominant cultures historically had, and currently have, reduced access to resources and influence. People with nondominant cultural identities are typically expected to conform to dominant cultural norms.[11] People often have a combination of dominant and nondominant identities. For example, Janet is a bilingual Latina RDN working in a leadership role at a large foodservice company in San Antonio, TX. In the context of the dietetics field, she holds a dominant identity as a woman, but she holds a nondominant identity as a Latina. In the context of her neighborhood, her race, ethnicity, and language are part of the dominant culture. When she attends leadership meetings, she is one of the only women and one of the only people of color at the table. Leaders who are aware of their positionality, or how their differences in social position and power shape identity and access in society, are best equipped to recognize and redress power imbalances.[12] This awareness and skill is important for building cultural humility and crucial for creating more inclusive and equity-focused environments. Box 3.2 contains examples of reflective questions and exercises to increase individual identity awareness.[19,22-25]

BOX 3.2 Identity Awareness Exercises[19,22-25]

"I am" exercise: a personal identity exercise[22,23]
Complete the sentence "I am …" using as many different descriptors as possible in 1 minute.

Next, reflect on your list using the following questions:

» Which of the listed characteristics do you identify with most?

» Which of the listed characteristics do you identify with least?

» In reviewing your responses, are there any other characteristics that come to mind but you did not list?

» How have your responses changed (or stayed the same) over the course of your life?

Voices of discovery social identity wheel exercise[24]
This individual and group exercise can support a greater understanding of intergroup and diversity issues and intergroup dialogues and is available online: https://sites.lsa.umich.edu/inclusive-teaching/wp-content/uploads/sites/355/2018/12/Social-Identity-Wheel-3-2.pdf

Implicit association test from Harvard University[19]
This series of free online assessments can be used to help educate about hidden biases and is available online from Harvard University's Project Implicit website: https://implicit.harvard.edu/implicit/

Values assessment[25]
There are free tools for assessing personal values. Each requires you to select from a list of common values and further focus on ones most important to you. The following is widely used, is broadly accepted in the field, and is available online: http://webmedia.jcu.edu/advising/files/2016/02/Core-Values-Exercise.pdf

---

After developing awareness of yourself, the second form of awareness is gaining insight into how others view you. How would your coworkers, supervisors, clients, patients, or employees describe your strengths, weaknesses, biases, and leadership style? Do their descriptions align with your own? Alignment between how you, as a leader, see yourself and how others see you creates better relationships, better communication, and a perception of leaders as being more effective.[15] As a leader takes on higher formal leadership roles, it is common for them to become less self-aware, overestimate their skills, and be less likely to receive honest feedback.[15,26,27] Gathering honest feedback on these topics is essential but can be difficult. As leaders continue to grow, they must frequently seek feedback from peers, employees, supervisors, and friends. One way to do this is to build a personal advisory board—a small group of trustworthy colleagues who can provide constructive feedback and support your journey to being an inclusive and effective leader. Another way to encourage feedback is to advocate, participate in, or institute 360° feedback in a formal review process within your organization. Engage a diverse group of coworkers, supervisors, and those you manage to get a well-rounded perspective.

Cultural Knowledge and Cultural Humility

Leaders should learn about themselves from others but, more importantly, they should seek to learn more about others. This can help build relationships and broaden perspectives. Relationship building is vital to effective leadership and building trust. Leaders with strong, trusting, authentic relationships influence job satisfaction, well-being, and engagement.[28] Learning more about others will inevitably expose gaps in your knowledge, but leaders should feel comfortable admitting what they don't know and seek answers from others. This vulnerability can promote psychological safety between the team and impact the entire workplace culture. Admitting when you don't know something and seeking understanding from others not only elevates different perspectives but can also encourage others to voice their opinions and similarly admit gaps in knowledge without fear of judgment or penalty. The ability to listen to and learn from others is especially important in the field of dietetics and in the provision of quality care for all; providing quality care that addresses health inequities is contingent on providers minimizing bias, maximizing cultural humility, and understanding power differentials and racial inequity.[5]

Coupling cultural competence with practicing cultural humility is key. Cultural competency (defined as understanding, appreciating, and working with individuals from cultures other than one's own[29]) has previously been promoted as the strategy to address health inequities. While this is important, it can also imply that there is an end point to the learning, but you can never be fully competent in any culture. Cultural competency alone is not enough. *Cultural humility* is a term originally introduced by Melanie Tervalon, MD, MPH, and Jann Murray-García, MD, MPH. Its primary principles include ongoing and critical self-reflection, focusing on individual experience rather than a body of knowledge or set of skills, redressing power imbalances, and developing mutually beneficial and nonpaternalistic partnerships with communities.[12] Tervalon and Murray-García describe cultural humility "not as a discrete end point but as a commitment and active engagement in a lifelong process that individuals enter into on an ongoing basis with patients, communities, colleagues, and with themselves."[12]

Although cultural humility emphasizes learning through interactions and critical self-reflection, it does not overlook the importance of increasing knowledge and cultural intelligence through formal training and education. Learning more about the history of various forms of oppression in this country (including racism, sexism, classism, xenophobia, homophobia, heterosexism, ageism, ableism, sizeism, and others) provides valuable information that increases awareness and cultural knowledge. Other specific topics and skills to research include the history of health care in your surrounding communities, the history of organizations with which you work or volunteer, the definition and impact of social determinants of health on care, trauma-informed care, and the food preferences and practices of various groups.

All of these topics impact health and are important to advancing IDEA. Other topics and opportunities for research will arise from interactions with patients, clients, and colleagues; use those opportunities to question thoughtfully and do independent research.

Leaders should recognize and value individualism and avoid using new knowledge to stereotype individuals. What is common for one person from a certain group may or may not be for another. Stereotyping disregards the heterogeneity of groups and wrongly assumes that cultural beliefs and behaviors always go along with a given ethnic identity.[30] Refer to Box 3.3 for a list of strategies for increasing and valuing diverse perspectives. For example, learning about the historical and cultural foods of the Pakistani community does not translate to knowing about the customs and food preferences for an individual Pakistani patient. Avoid this pitfall, and "be flexible and humble enough to assess the cultural dimensions of the experiences of each person."[12]

BOX 3.3 Strategies for Increasing and Valuing Diverse Perspectives

Personal strategies for learning and experiencing different perspectives

» Engage in curious and respectful questioning (open-ended questions that seek to understand the other person's views, values, and motivations).

» Ask opinions from those who think differently from you.

» Hear at least one other perspective before you make a decision.

» Identify whose voice is *not* involved in the decision-making processes, and work to ensure that voice is included going forward.

» Use patient-focused interviewing to highlight the voice of patients and clients; they are the experts on themselves.

» Admit when you do not have the answer or are wrong.

Strategies for consciously learning a new and different perspective

» Seek out opportunities to experience culturally diverse environments.

» Use mobile applications such as Native Land to increase territory awareness, learn about the Indigenous communities from that land, and then read about the history of those lands.[31]

» Identify and attend training and workshops taught by diverse speakers on topics relevant to your work.

» Invite and pay speakers from diverse groups to provide various training or webinars to your team.

» Research and catalog foods your clients eat that are unfamiliar to you.

» Visit grocery stores that specialize in foods from specific cultures.

» Use social media to expand your perspectives and connect with other people with perspectives and experiences different from your own.

» Leverage other forms of media (books, podcasts, blogs, and television) to learn from individuals who don't have the same identities as you.

Strategies for understanding personal limitations, combatting biases, and valuing different ideas and experiences

» Listen attentively to learn rather than to respond.

» Defy the tendency to judge other cultures as inferior to your own.

» Demonstrate the ability to see things from others' viewpoints, and solicit feedback on how well you're doing in this effort.

» Assess equity in pay, promotions, and hiring, and take action to correct any identified inequities.

Awareness of Systems

Lastly, equity consciousness and systems awareness are necessary for growing and inspiring effective, inclusive, equity-centered leaders. Equity consciousness includes being aware of individual-level biases and recognizing systems of oppression and institutional bias.[32] One way to increase equity consciousness is through intentional questioning. For example, asking, "What conditions have we created that maintain certain groups as the perpetual majority?"[11] may help expose inequities in the system and begin conversations about addressing challenges and enacting solutions. Engaging with internal and external stakeholders and asking about their perspectives on existing inequities provides another opportunity to increase equity consciousness. This can happen formally, through surveys, focus groups, or organizational equity assessments. A list of additional strategies and tools for data collection are outlined in the section Leveraging Data and Resources, which appears later in this chapter.

Increasing awareness of inequitable systems also involves understanding the culture of an organization and its impact on creating diverse, inclusive, and equitable environments. Leaders are often responsible for helping to create that culture, whether for the organization as a whole or within their work teams. This can be challenging work, as culture is not always named, often consisting of "unspoken rules that shape values, beliefs, habits, patterns of thinking, behaviors, and styles of communication."[9] The dominant culture that shapes most institutions in American society is that of the White middle and upper class.[33] This has evolved from the United States' history of white supremacy (for example, chattel slavery and the Ku Klux Klan) and continues to be reinforced by systems including the media and public education. According to the definition offered by scholars Tema Okun, PhD, and Kenneth Jones, white supremacy culture describes a series of characteristics that institutionalize whiteness and Westernness as normal, right, and superior to other ethnic, racial, and regional identities and customs.[9] This can unfold in many ways, including the characterization of women as less emotionally stable and less effective as leaders,[22] discrimination in the hiring process because of an applicant's name, or the association of hairstyles that are part of Black culture with unprofessionalism. White supremacy culture is often described as the water we all swim in: the longer we swim in it, the less we notice it. This is why awareness is of foremost importance in cultivating inclusive and equitable spaces.

A multifaceted example of the impacts of white supremacy culture in dietetics appears when we examine food items and patterns that are historically and currently most highlighted. This is not the fault of any one person but of a system developed based on the dominant culture's perspective and then continuously reinforced over time. The dominant-culture bias is reinforced in how various cultures and foods are researched, by lessons and perspectives taught in the curriculum, by images and foods highlighted in educational resources, and in the discussion of these foods and cultures in the media. In 2020, the Food4Health Alliance conducted a study examining the systematic reviews overseen by the 2020-2025 Dietary Guidelines Advisory Committee.[34] The group examined the evidence base for the *Dietary Guidelines for Americans, 2020-2025* (DGA), which is meant to shape the eating patterns for all Americans. The researchers looked specifically at the reviews' consideration of minority and low income populations and found that of the 56 reviews, 91% to 95% neglected to take into account race, ethnicity, or socioeconomic status, or used a sample that could not be generalized to the larger US population.[34] Knowing this, here are some questions to ask yourself: How do you think these limitations might impact the recommendations of the DGA? Does this create an equitable and inclusive perspective of foods for all Americans? What recommendation would you give to the Dietary Guidelines Advisory Committee to create a more inclusive process? What role can you personally play, now that you are aware of these limitations? Box 3.4 provides another example of institutional bias that has positive intent but exclusionary impact.

BOX 3.4 An Example of Institutional Bias and Its Impact

History	The National Health and Nutrition Examination Survey (NHANES) is used to understand the eating habits of the US population.[35] These data inform the Dietary Guidelines for Americans.[35]
Policy	Interviews for the NHANES study are conducted in English and Spanish.
Immediate impact	The foods and preferences of individuals who don't speak English or Spanish are not accounted for in this important data set.
Secondary impact	Not all people, practitioners, or aspiring nutrition professionals see their foods represented in what is depicted as healthy eating.
Opportunities for improvement	seek and center the diverse perspectives from communities and individuals most impacted by systemic inequities. Mentor, hire, support, equitably pay, and promote diverse voices in your work. As reported in *Kaiser Health News*, "Nutrition science would benefit from scientists in the field conducting primary research in more diverse populations with varying age groups and different racial, ethnic, and socioeconomic backgrounds."[36]

Awareness of personal, interpersonal, and organizational attitudes and practices that promote homogeneity makes it possible to challenge those practices and create change. Although it might feel intimidating to challenge the status quo, inclusive leaders are courageous. They "act on convictions and principles even when it requires personal risk-taking."[37] As you work to increase awareness, you may experience feelings of discomfort and defensiveness. When these feelings come up, reflect on where the feelings are coming from and why. Seek out other perspectives. It's important to remember that we are all part of a problematic system, and we must stay engaged to create more equitable systems. This has an impact on ourselves, on the field as a whole, and on the individuals and communities we serve. We all have the power to catalyze change in our local and national systems.

Activating Inclusivity

Leveraging the Power of Diversity Through Inclusive Leadership

Diversity in all its forms is an asset to the country and the field of dietetics, but inequities as well as bias, prejudice, and stereotyping in health care can contribute to negative health outcomes for various groups.[38] A more diverse workforce can have a positive impact on health disparities and advance health equity.[39] Given the increased diversity of younger generations in the US workforce as well as in the demographic profile of students and interns enrolled in dietetics programs,[40] leaders who are effective, equity centered, and inclusive have the ability to support and accelerate a substantial shift in the field.

Organizations increasingly rely on multidisciplinary and diverse teams, but research proves that diverse teams do not automatically foster high-performing, productive, and effective teams.[41-44] A study conducted by researchers at Leiden University of 45 teams in the public sector found that greater team diversity does not automatically yield an inclusive climate. Inclusive leadership is needed to support an inclusive climate in which different team members are valued for what they bring to work practices. This study found that inclusive leadership serves as a facilitating bridge between team diversity and an inclusive climate. When a team's ethnic-cultural diversity is high, inclusive leadership also needs to be high in order to minimize the creation of a noninclusive climate. Although this study focuses on ethnic and cultural diversity, the results and concepts can be applied to a broad spectrum of diverse attributes and emphasizes the importance of creating an inclusive climate.[41]

Inclusive leaders must ensure everyone on the team agrees they are being treated fairly and respectfully, are valued, have a sense of belonging, and feel psychologically safe.[44] Inclusive leaders are intrinsically motivated to grow and facilitate an inclusive environment because they know these environments are where everyone (including themselves) can perform most effectively. To optimize the benefits of inclusive leadership, individuals, organizations, and systems need to embody "leadership with a little *L*."[45] Sylvia Escott-Stump, MA, RDN, LDN, FAND, past president of the Academy of Nutrition and Dietetics, notes the importance of the adoption of small-*L* leadership and expands on leadership traits we all can develop and practice. Specifically, Escott-Stump notes that being committed, being open, and encouraging others' perspectives are key traits of inclusive leadership and require emotional intelligence to practice.[45] Given the prevalence of RDNs in diverse sectors, specializations, industries, and countries, it is critical to the evolution and sustainability of the profession that RDNs be diligent in embodying inclusive leadership skills now and in the future.

Inclusive Leadership: Definition and Application

How is inclusive leadership different from other types of leadership, such as transformative or authentic leadership? A review of the literature of leadership styles finds that inclusive leadership is distinct in the demonstration of behaviors that support team members' full integration and create a norm for all to foster inclusiveness.[42] It might be helpful to imagine inclusive leadership as the mortar between the bricks that build strong, sturdy foundations of monuments of success. An inclusive leader seeks to engage diverse perspectives and strengths to interact, be effective, and be productive. Inclusive leadership is a way of being for all members on a team to embody. Everyone has a role in creating and facilitating a positive, inclusive environment.

Inclusion itself is composed of two distinct concepts: belongingness and uniqueness. Balancing these two concepts leads to overall cohesiveness and effectiveness. Belongingness involves individuals seeking similarities with and validation of others, and uniqueness honors individuality in comparison to others.[41] Inclusive leadership considers team members' differences and supports their belongingness to facilitate individual engagement and contributions rather than encouraging the need to assimilate toward collective needs or goals.[42] Research by both the *Harvard Business Review*[44,46] and Deloitte[47] agreed on six common traits of inclusive leaders and how to become one. Box 3.5 lists these characteristics of inclusive leadership and examines how to apply them regardless of your position of power, your position in a given hierarchical structure, or your role on a team.[44,46,47]

BOX 3.5 Inclusive Leadership Characteristics and How to Apply Them[44,46,47]

Commitment
» Believe in your individual ability to create a welcoming culture.
» Value and prioritize diversity and inclusion of thoughts.
» Possess a strong responsibility for positive change.

Courage and humility
» Challenge the status quo.
» Acknowledge personal limitations and seek to overcome them.
» Create space for others to contribute and provide their feedback.

Cognizance or self-awareness
» Work to identify personal blind spots and prevent biases from influencing your decision-making processes.
» Seek to implement policies and processes to prevent organizational biases.
» Advocate for meritocracy—a power structure determined by an individual's skills, talent, and achievements rather than their wealth or social status.

Curiosity
» Be hungry to learn from other perspectives to minimize personal biases and improve your ability to make inclusive decisions.
» Keep an open mind, and engage in respectful questioning and active listening.
» Listen without judgment and demonstrate empathy.

Cultural intelligence or mindfulness
» Remain curious about all cultures and norms.
» Strengthen your ability to adapt your communication style in response to different cultural norms.
» Demonstrate self-awareness of your own culture and how it shapes your worldview.
» Identify power imbalances between you and the people with whom you interact.

Collaboration
» Be willing to share your own perspective.
» Create an environment where others are empowered to express their opinions with the group.
» Pay close attention to team composition, processes, and cohesion.

In reading the traits of inclusive leadership, you will be reminded of the lifelong learning process required for personal growth. Processing and practicing individual traits is a journey that takes time—your personal time, time at work, or time spent with a group. You can start your journey toward inclusive leadership today. Share your learning journey about recognizing and overcoming biases. Explore opportunities for personal reflection and begin building your confidence and willingness to share. Immerse yourself in new or uncomfortable environments. Choose growth over comfort by learning about stakeholders, perspectives, and experiences that differ from your own.

Cultivating an Inclusive Climate

Importance of Inclusive Leadership in the Workplace

The benefits and importance of inclusive leadership practices in the workplace can be found in business administration and personnel management studies. Employees working in settings perceived as inclusive report higher levels of "fit" with their coworkers, their skills, and the demands of the job and higher levels of engagement; they receive higher performance ratings and are more likely to perceive support from their managers.[41,44,46,47] Employees in inclusive workplace environments also report less harassment and discrimination and experience less turnover in the workplace.[44,48] Surprisingly, despite the observed benefits of inclusive leadership, research revealed leaders were unaware of the specific behaviors influencing whether they were rated more or less inclusive.[44] This is an alarming result given that the highlighted research studies analyze the impact of inclusive leadership through the ability of the executive or supervisor.[41,44] The current research in inclusive leadership only assesses the skills and attributes of leaders in a formal supervisory role. Future studies should use this opportunity to educate those in positions of organizational leadership on the definition and application of inclusive leadership as well as to educate and study the application of associated traits by all team members.

Not only can inclusive leadership enhance performance and employee satisfaction but it can also save lives. Researchers studied the impact of diversity, inclusive leadership, and health outcomes in 10 hospitals and found a substantial decrease in mortality rates through the work of guiding coalitions.[43] These diverse teams or guiding coalitions were able to accelerate creative problem solving and innovation. The guiding coalitions shared three attributes: they included staff from different disciplines and levels of organizational hierarchy, encouraged authentic participation from all members, and used distinct methods of conflict management.[43] RDNs in clinical health care settings and on multidisciplinary teams are in a unique position to embody inclusive leadership with their knowledge of social and environmental factors impacting a patient's nutrition and health status.

Let's look at an example of how an RDN can use inclusive leadership to improve patient care. Gerald, an RDN in a private hospital, observed his new care team operating under the assumption that patients would not need additional financial support based on the hospital's status and reputation for treating patients who could afford high-quality care. Gerald encouraged members of his care team to work to identify local food access resources and other support services for patients who may be experiencing food insecurity. These resources included print and electronic forms translated into multiple languages. The team also collaborated with patient navigators to share the new resources with patients and other care teams in the hospital. During and after this experience, Gerald and his care team members participated in reflective conversations about the self-awareness gained and lessons learned about their team dynamics. The team members were thankful for Gerald's suggestion to better serve their patients and become more effective health care providers. It is vital for future RDNs and health care practitioners to learn and embody inclusive leadership practices to remain competent and effective in serving clients and communities.

Dimensions of an Inclusive Climate

Inclusive leadership traits represent necessary steps in the creation of an inclusive climate. An inclusive climate, in turn, is a prerequisite for inclusion and promotes the application of diverse perspectives and ideas to enrich the decision-making process, thereby boosting the performance of diverse teams.[41] An inclusive climate consists of employees' shared perceptions of expected and rewarded behaviors, thus influencing their experience and behaviors in the workplace. Everyone should embrace these conditions of inclusive climates, and those in supervisory positions must be doubly aware and committed to strengthening their role as climate engineers.[48]

Previous research outlines two distinct dimensions that help the cultivation of an inclusive climate: the cultural integration of differences, and the inclusion of differences in decision making. Both of these have a direct impact on individual team members' experiences of uniqueness and belongingness in a given environment. The cultural integration of differences emphasizes a norm of openness, value, and respect of differences, which contributes to individuals' feelings of uniqueness.[49] When effectively implemented, teams and organizations can avoid simplistic assumptions and stereotypes in problem solving and developing solutions. The cultural integration of differences relies heavily on effective communication regarding an individual's values, strengths, perspectives, and ideas.

The second dimension of an inclusive climate is the inclusion of differences in decision making. This concept demonstrates the importance of an individual's contributions to enhance work practices and can support an individual's feeling of belongingness.[48] The combination of group biases and exclusion of those with different perspectives can disrupt the full integration of team members and hinder the utilization of their diverse strengths.[46] In contrast, the facilitation and integration of different perspectives allows team members to focus their energy on deeper levels of problem solving and critical and systems thinking, fostering more effective solutions. As Nishii notes, "Facilitating inclusions requires more than preventing bias; leaders need to proactively create workgroup norms that counteract intergroup tensions commonly arising in diverse groups to enable and motivate group members to leverage cognitive diversity effectively."[49] Motivating all team members to integrate different perspectives requires those in supervisory roles to embody and model doing so in a conscious and intentional process.

Box 3.6 outlines action steps in communication and decision making that will help leaders and team members alike cultivate an inclusive environment featuring effective communication, integration of diversity in processes including decision making, and inclusive leadership.

BOX 3.6 Actions Steps in Communication and Decision Making to Cultivate an Inclusive Environment

COMMUNICATION

Individuals

» Deepen your experiences and interactions by engaging in open and honest dialogue; diversify who you share with and seek perspective from.

» Communicate with your team and organization when you notice your department is benefitting from diversity. It's important to speak up!

» Build awareness around the words you use. Are you using words (such as pronouns) that include or exclude? Do your words signal organizational improvement or constructive feedback?

» Disturb the peace when you do not agree. Don't be afraid to speak up; chances are someone else agrees with you.

Teams

» Engage in active listening to better understand and engage with your diverse team.

» Share your team's experiences in creating an inclusive climate with other departments and key stakeholders.

» Embrace inevitable differences of opinion and engage in respectful communication to seek better mutual understanding.

» Support team members in their journey along the diversity continuum. Allow people to change without questioning their motives.

DECISION MAKING

Individuals

» Seek out constructive criticism and feedback from new and different sources before making a decision.

» Join an employee resource group to learn more about how you can partner and advocate for a more inclusive climate.

» See and acknowledge how your own biases influence your decision making.

» Intentionally change the way you do a repetitive action or carry out a responsibility.

Teams

» Bring innovation to existing or routine meetings by inviting new people to attend and participate, letting others lead the meeting, ensuring everyone is heard, and sharing meeting notes with a more diverse distribution list.

» Assess whose voices are heard, trusted, or listened to most often. Whose voices are often left out or not even at the table?

» Challenge each team or department to increase the diversity of traditional suppliers and business partners.

» Consider different perspectives and needs when selecting the date, time, and menu for a group function, and make a point of offering group functions at different times of day or on different days of the week.

» Ensure your team activities link your diversity strategy to the core business strategy.

Leveraging Data and Resources

The commitment to creating an inclusive climate and the curiosity to learn how to do so can be enhanced by leveraging data and subsequent collection of feedback. In order to understand the current climate and learn the perceived steps needed to create a more inclusive climate, team members must be offered ways to provide this feedback. The processes and spaces conducive to providing such feedback must be updated continuously to integrate diverse perspectives, thoughts, and modes of communication.[50] When this feedback is applied, systems can change for the better and learning will propel the skills and development of all associated team members. Tools that leaders and teams can use to assess organizational readiness and measure inclusive, diverse, equitable, and accessible spaces include the following:

> Academy of Nutrition and Dietetics IDEA Resources[22]

> American Public Health Association "Equity, Diversity, Inclusion: Action Toolkit for Organizations"[51]

> Annie E. Casey Foundation "Advancing the Mission: Tools for Equity, Diversity and Inclusion"[52]

> Bay Area Regional Health Inequities Initiative "Organizational Self-Assessment for Addressing Health Inequities Toolkit" for local health departments [53]

> Western States Center Assessing Organizational Racism tool[54]

These resources have a variety of helpful questions at the individual and organizational levels and define best practices to assess the current state of IDEA and track progress over time. After collecting any data, it is important for leaders to make the results available and create a plan of action from the findings. Transparent data can be an effective way to create a sense of urgency and build collective power to advance goals.

This chapter demonstrates what can be learned and done to advance IDEA goals, even in low- or no-cost ways. However, it is important to note that historically, the responsibility of IDEA initiatives often falls on a small group of individuals, volunteer diversity committees, or a single position, such as the chief diversity officer. In many cases, these individuals lack the power or resources (or both) needed to promote and sustain the goal of advancing IDEA initiatives, which then fail to gain traction, slow what momentum they had, or come to a complete halt.[55] Executive leaders should support IDEA work in words and in action. They must advocate for the allocation of the resources vital to sustaining and integrating IDEA principles throughout the entire organization. They must also be involved in supporting the identified actions.

Box 3.7 highlights the work of FoodCorps, an organization that has integrated IDEA work into its daily mission to promote health and nutrition in communities and schools across the United States.[56]

BOX 3.7 FoodCorps: An Example of Communication and Implementation of Equity, Diversity, and Inclusion Goals[56]

With the vision of connecting all children to healthy food and overcoming health inequities, FoodCorps views equity, diversity, and inclusion work as a moral imperative. As the group's website explains, "We are convinced that for FoodCorps to be effective, we must not replicate the inequality we see in society at large; we must become a model for the change we seek."[56]

In 2020, FoodCorps revised its commitments to diversity and inclusion, equity, social justice, and antiracism. In many circumstances, these statements live only on websites, but FoodCorps wanted to communicate these commitments in a way that drove their day-to-day work. The FoodCorps SHIFTING framework was developed to support the integration and operationalization of equity into all aspects of the organization's work. This framework is applied in establishing organizational strategies, planning and evaluating projects and programs, setting individual and departmental goals, and guiding both major and minor decisions. It also informs how employees communicate with stakeholders and share their values with those with whom they work. Providing this framework for how to live the commitments by "shifting" gave employees at all levels a shared language to work toward diversity, equity, inclusion, and justice.

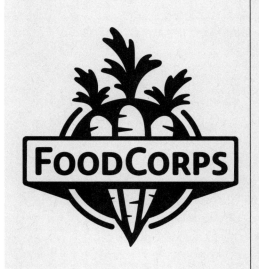

S = Shift power, resources, and access to those most impacted by systemic oppression and closest to the work that needs to be done.

H = Honor and trust the wisdom and expertise of grassroots leadership in the communities where we work.

I = Interrupt internalized, interpersonal, and systemic oppression.

F = Foster an environment that reflects the diversity of our partner communities and in which everyone can show up and feel brave, supported, and valued for their contributions.

T = Try to create the world we want to see even when we know we might fail.

I = Invest in equity when it comes to budgeting, contracts and vendors, compensation, leadership development, recruitment, and promotions.

N = Name and frame racism, transphobia, ableism, and other forms of oppression and marginalization when we see it.

G = Grant ourselves the time necessary to make decisions and do work that advances justice and minimizes harm.

Adapted with permission from FoodCorps.

Inclusive Leadership in Action

The 2016 experience of the nutrition department at Metropolitan State University of Denver (MSUD) is an example of how inclusive leadership traits and strategies can enhance the experience of the next generation of RDNs, public health professionals, and systems responsible for cultivating their success (Jessica Torro, personal communication, March 16, 2021).[57] In 2016, MSUD was designated as a Hispanic-Serving Institution (HSI). Although the university qualified quantitatively for this distinction, the nutrition department looked within its programs and realized that, year after year, a large majority of its students were White women. Was their program an inclusive space for the growing number of Latino students on campus? Was it welcoming for all students? Why was the demographic profile of the nutrition program not matching that of the university? These questions catalyzed a movement to ensure the nutrition department's program increased its diversity and provided a space where all students felt they belonged.

Aligning the Foundation

For MSUD, the HSI designation was the impetus to learn more about the student experience. In 2018, the nutrition faculty and staff sent out a survey to assess students' perceptions and attitudes of the nutrition program. The survey results found that many Latino students did not feel welcome. Many of those surveyed mentioned qualitative factors, such as "not looking the part," specifically expressed as not being White or not being skinny. Others mentioned that their cultural foods did not fit into what the textbooks recommended as part of a healthy diet. Overall, the surveyed students felt discouraged.

The nutrition faculty and staff began a journey of discovery and education reflecting on their own identities and the dynamics of the team. They completed the Intercultural Development Inventory,[58] which provided information about individual mindsets and skill sets around cultural differences and commonalities. They participated in workshops that focused on recruiting, retaining, and supporting diverse students in their program. They hosted webinars for faculty, staff, preceptors, and students on topics including race and nutrition, the impact of implicit bias on disproportionate disease burden, and microaggression. Lastly, they critically examined accessibility policies and practices within their dietetic internship program.

Activating Inclusivity

After gathering data and building awareness, the MSUD nutrition department was ready to move into action. Bruce Rengers, PhD, RDN, a professor of nutrition at MSUD, sought out resources that would move the department's diversity, equity, and inclusion efforts forward. He identified a pivotal grant opportunity from the Department of Education. If the department were awarded the grant, the funding could provide substantial resources to support new programming and hopefully create a more inclusive nutrition program. Before moving forward, Bruce collaborated with students, faculty, and staff. He created space for others to express their opinions and share whether they were ready to use this funding to build a more inclusive department. The answer was a resounding "yes." The team was committed, ready to challenge the status quo, curious to learn, and on the path to building more self-awareness and mindfulness.

Cultivating an Inclusive Climate

In September 2019, MSUD was awarded the Department of Education grant. The financial support enabled the nutrition department to create the Post-Baccalaureate Opportunity for Hispanic Americans (POHA)-Denver Diversify Nutrition Grant. Led by their new POHA grant manager, Jessica Torro, MS, RDN, the grant provided financial support for students from diverse backgrounds as well as those seeking to serve diverse populations. The grant also provided numerous other resources that the department hoped would cultivate an inclusive climate. Torro's voice brought a new and diverse perspective to the team. She shared her vision of where MSUD could welcome diversity by thinking outside the box. The textbooks might still need updating for more inclusive representation, but the missing content could be brought into the classroom in other ways. Research might have provided one perspective, but there should also be opportunities to share lived experiences. When put into action, the grant provided students with skill-building workshops on nutrition and nonnutrition-related topics, an RDN speaker series showcasing diverse RDNs in traditional and nontraditional careers, and a mentorship program. The department began to see positive changes in its organizational culture. All staff received cultural competency education every quarter. Uncomfortable conversations and open discussions about IDEA became increasingly common. Students expressed their need for a space in which they felt like they belonged and for easier access to faculty. As a result, students were supported in forming a Diversity in Dietetics club, and faculty members adjusted their schedules to facilitate more student connections. While the staff at MSUD realize they still have a way to go, they are a shining example of what effective, equity-centered, inclusive leadership can look like in the field of dietetics.

Pathways to Leadership

Becoming a leader focused on advancing IDEA can be an exciting and challenging process to navigate. Whether you are interested in stepping into a leadership role for the first time or are an experienced leader looking to grow into a senior-level position, you will find there are multiple pathways to leadership. Sometimes opportunities will present themselves; for example, a new project or role might become available in the organization where you work or volunteer. Other times, you can propose and create opportunities. In either situation, you need to be ready to excel—but how do you prepare? Conversations with a group of leaders in dietetics yielded five major themes for identifying and excelling in leadership opportunities: (1) discover what you want and how to get there, (2) let your voice be heard, (3) step up and improve your skills, (4) build your network and find mentors, and (5) be yourself and build confidence. See Box 3.8 for more information.

BOX 3.8 Major Themes for Excelling in Leadership Opportunities

Discover what you want and how to get there.
"When seeking leadership opportunities, ask, 'Have you figured out what field you want to be in within the profession? Have you then looked at the job descriptions and figured out what those skills are that you need to do that job well? Have you assessed what skills you have and what skills you don't have? What proof do you have that you possess those skills? What type of organization do you want to work for? What are the values that are really important [for you to] see in an organization?' Once you do that, you then can start creating a path for yourself." (Shanon Morris, MS, RD, CDN, personal communication, August 27, 2021)

"Put yourself in situations to learn everything you can about your job, the job of others, and the job you want. Unfortunately, people with nondominant identities have to learn more in order to be seen as the same." (Zachari Breeding, MS, RDN, CSO, LDN, FAND, email communication, August 30, 2021)

continued on next page

continued from previous page

Let your voice be heard.

"I speak the truth as I see it, and I've learned as a leader to speak the truth as necessary." (Evelyn Crayton, EdD, RDN, LDN, FAND, personal communication, September 6, 2021)

"Ask to be included in the conversation. Most of the time, upper-level leaders do not think about including others because they are focused on the mission or task at hand. Being included gives you the opportunity to share your perspectives and show off your skills or knowledge to leadership." (Zachari Breeding, MS, RDN, CSO, LDN, FAND, email communication, August 30, 2021)

Step up and improve your skills.

"If you're looking to be a leader, then you need to step up and start proving yourself without the title. That could be both at your job and externally, as well. If you're looking for leadership opportunities, it doesn't hurt for you to [help the organization with] social media, write articles, perform research, join a committee, or volunteer to be part of a special project. Whatever it is, that's going to help build your credibility." (Shanon Morris, MS, RD, CDN, verbal communication, August 27, 2021)

"Embrace new opportunities and learn from them, even if they are not traditional dietetics skills." (Evelyn Crayton, EdD, RDN, LDN, FAND, verbal communication, September 6, 2021)

Build your network and find mentors.

"While some may underestimate you, seek to tokenize you, or marginalize you, learn to recognize allies. Build your network and make sure it includes peers, mentors, sponsors, and professionals at all places in their careers—just starting out, mid-career, and seasoned veterans. Be curious and open to things that will help you along your path but may be a little out of your comfort zone." (Winona Bynum, RDN, PMP, email communication, September 2, 2021)

"There has to be someone encouraging you and mentoring you. Get with someone who has the leadership skills that you are looking for and doing some of the things you are looking [to do]." (Evelyn Crayton, EdD, RDN, LDN, FAND, verbal communication, September 6, 2021)

Be yourself and build confidence.

"Stay true to yourself no matter what anybody else says about you. No matter what they do to discourage you, ignore it. You can't allow others' [negative] ideas and thoughts [to] shake who you are or what you're supposed to do. You have to follow the plan you have in your heart and in your spirit. Stay persistent, stay focused and don't let others define you." (Evelyn Crayton, EdD, RDN, LDN, FAND, verbal communication, September 6, 2021)

"Be aware of the challenges related to holding a nondominant identity in a society built to benefit the dominant culture, but don't let the challenges define you. Don't let the challenges put you on the defensive or lure you into putting the majority of your energy into disputing negative stereotypes. Be yourself unapologetically. Know your worth [and] your strengths, be clear about what you uniquely offer, and look for opportunities to build your skills." (Winona Bynum, RDN, PMP, email communication, September 2, 2021)

"Many cultures teach us to be modest. Sharing your expertise with your colleagues will lift all around you. Consider your unique perspective as an advantage to the profession. You have varied and valuable experiences to share." (Manju Karkare, MS, RDN, LDN, CLT, FAND, email communication, September 2, 2021)

"Continue to exude confidence and strength. Allow others to have their own expectations of you—it is not your job to change anyone's mind. Just be yourself and let your own charisma, talent, knowledge, and skills shine through. Eventually, people will start figuring out the real you and adjust their own perceptions and feelings without any of your own effort." (Zachari Breeding, MS, RDN, CSO, LDN, FAND, email communication, August 30, 2021)

Finally, know that you don't need a title to lead. "Great leaders don't set out to be a leader, they set out to make a difference. It's about the goal, not the role. Titles and positions don't always identify leadership; you have the ability to lead through your actions." (Manju Karkare, MS, RDN, LDN, CLT, FAND, email communication, September 2, 2021)

As mentioned earlier in this section, those who hold nondominant identities in the field of dietetics may face unique barriers as they pursue leadership roles and grow into leadership positions. The following Stories From the Field box highlights two personal stories of leadership pursuit and navigating challenges.

STORIES FROM THE FIELD: Facing Challenges and Growing as a Leader

Manju Karkare, MS, RDN, LDN, CLT, FAND

Attending graduate school as an international student posed some challenges that continued into my career. First and foremost, the awkward feeling of "otherness" felt with turning heads upon hearing my accent, and then specific pronunciation training as a teaching assistant, highlighted my nondominant identity. I thought it might have been typical of small, university towns, although moving to larger and more populated states did not ease that feeling.

It took intentional efforts to "fit in" with learning the local lingo and workplace culture in my clinical jobs. At my very first clinical job, I met two other RDNs [registered dietitian nutritionists] of my heritage. I learned about belonging and networking through the affiliates and expanded my personal knowledge of the world of dietetics in the United States. It was clear to me that international RDNs must go above and beyond the ordinary to be noticed. I took the initiative to expand my clinical skills through acquiring CNSD [certified nutrition support dietitian] credentials. Good relationships with the nursing and pharmacy [teams] helped me establish comprehensive nutrition support protocols. While advancing the clinical knowledge and leadership within the workplace seemed possible, I also believe I happened to be at the right place at the right time [to take advantage of the growth opportunities].

Recognizing opportunities in the professional organization was much harder, as I did not see any leaders who looked like me. I pursued my social justice passion and got involved at the leadership level within my local community. It was years later [that] it occurred to me that the leadership skills and experience I had gained at community nonprofits could be applicable to enhance our professional diversity. I gained significant organizational knowledge as a diversity leader. Yet, leaders who looked like me were few and far between. Intentional networking, getting comfortable with the discomfort of "otherness," and choosing to educate my colleagues all took extra effort. Applying leadership skills in any situation or organization is not different. However, I found that positions held within the professional organizational system (DPGs [dietetic practice groups], affiliates, or national committees) were valued more than leadership experience from other organizations. Getting selected for such positions seemed like a popularity contest. It was all about who you know rather than what you know. I felt that I had to prove myself through my words and actions. Learning the acceptable and influential words was another challenge, as English is my second language.

When I was elected to the Board of Directors of the Academy of Nutrition and Dietetics, I did not know other board members (except one). I assumed that was normal, since it was my first time serving at the national level. I was surprised to learn that almost all other members were familiar with each other, and some had served in the past, as well. I made it my mission to identify other potential leaders from the nondominant identities. Encouraging them to seek leadership opportunities and offering support through the process has been very fulfilling to me.

continued on next page

continued from previous page

Zachari Breeding, MS, RDN, CSO, LDN, FAND

Getting others to acknowledge or believe in my skill set has been challenging, based on the fact that I carry myself differently or speak differently in the workplace (not in an unprofessional way, just in my own unique way). Dealing with this perception others have of me has been a challenge that I have had to face head on while trying to elevate into leadership positions. I think this stems from the preconceived notion that leaders look and act in certain ways, and those who do not fit into that standard have their skill set questioned. Having your skills and knowledge questioned can be really demotivating, so it became really important to me that I not only knew what I had to know but that I was confident in my answers.

Being more effeminate than the average heterosexual male created a challenge of being seen as weak, demure, and/or able to be taken advantage of. Walking into the department I was soon going to manage showed me that people I work with may sometimes see that inner quality (a male being more effeminate) as an opportunity to break policy and procedures in my presence. I did not change who I was because of this perception—instead, I used it to my advantage to soften the blow of the critical conversations I had to have to enforce the rules of the operation and hold people accountable without seeming like a dictator. I do not aim for leadership positions to create friendships, but the more I can show my department the various facets of my personality, the more I feel I can garner trust more easily by just being myself. I feel people are more easily able to follow directions from someone that they admire and respect than from someone they do not feel connected to. I aim to establish inter-personal working connections by staying true to myself and my identity.

Action Steps

The Code of Ethics of the Academy of Nutrition and Dietetics cites social responsibility and diversity as two core values that should guide dietetics education and practice.[59] For these reasons, adopting a leadership philosophy that centers onIDEA is pivotal to creating a more inclusive and diverse field. While impactful and rewarding, the work of advancing IDEA is hard. It is not a smooth or linear process and may be met with resistance. The following key points will help you manage the challenges of leading change through IDEA efforts:

1. Start small and SMART (specific, measurable, achievable, realistic, and time bound) when planning out your first goals.

2. Identify a support system: build a small team of similarly interested individuals or join a group of other IDEA advocates.

3. Increase the visibility and recognition of the IDEA work by taking the following steps:

   a. Create an IDEA report outlining goals, successes, and progress.

   b. Share your story of successes, failures, and lessons learned.

Still wondering where to start? The Academy of Nutrition and Dietetics has established diversity and inclusion impact goals with corresponding strategies.[21] Consider what strategies you can put into action, using what you've learned from this chapter. Use Figure 3.1 to identify what you want to keep doing, stop doing, and start doing now that you've read this chapter.

FIGURE 3.1 Final reflection and next steps

Goals	What you can start doing	What you want to stop doing	What you want to keep doing
Establish infrastructure and resources to achieve optimal and sustainable inclusion, diversity, equity, and access (IDEA) outcomes.			
Increase recruitment, retention, and completion of nutrition and dietetics education and leadership for individuals from underrepresented groups.			
Cultivate organizational and professional values of equity, respect, civility, and antidiscrimination.			
Advance food and nutrition research, policy, and practice through a holistic IDEA lens.			

Summary

While we know the importance and effectiveness of diverse teams and inclusive environments, building and supporting them requires buy-in at every level. Leaders play a role in cultivating buy-in, communicating a vision, and sustaining support. They are able to manage change by understanding the people and stakeholders involved and adequately communicating in a transparent way.[60] This is of paramount importance to those in the field of dietetics, as food and nutrition intersect with culture, health, and justice.

REFERENCES

1   Centers for Disease Control and Prevention. Risk for COVID-19 infection, hospitalization, and death by race/ethnicity. CDC website Accessed September 10, 2021. www.cdc.gov/coronavirus /2019-ncov/covid-data/investigations-discovery/hospitalization-death-by-race-ethnicity.html

2   Ruiz NG, Edward K, Hugo Lopez M. One-third of Asian Americans fear threats, physical attacks and most say violence against them is rising. Pew Research Center website. April 2021. Accessed September 10, 2021. www.pewresearch.org/fact-tank/2021/04/21/one-third-of-asian-americans -fear-threats-physical-attacks-and-most-say-violence-against-them-is-rising

3   Human Rights Campaign Foundation. Violence against the transgender and gender non-conforming community in 2020. Human Rights Campaign wesbite. Accessed September 10, 2021. www.hrc.org/resources/violence-against-the-trans-and-gender-non-conforming -community-in-2020

4   Bailey ZD, Krieger N, Agénor M, Graves J, Linos N, Bassett MT. Structural racism and health inequities in the USA: evidence and interventions. *Lancet.* 2017;389(10077):1453-1463.

5   Lund A, Yoder Latortue K, Rodriguez J. Dietetic training: understanding racial inequity in power and privilege. *J Acad Nutr Diet.* 2021;121(8):1437-1440.

6   Academy of Nutrition and Dietetics. List of IDEA term definitions. eatrightPRO website. Accessed July 13, 2021. www.eatrightPRO.org/practice/practice-resources/diversity-and-inclusion/list -of-d-and-i-definitions

7   Stewart D-L. Language of appeasement. *Inside Higher Ed.* March 30, 2017. Accessed February 17, 2021. www.insidehighered.com/views/2017/03/30/colleges-need-language-shift-not-one -you-think-essay

8   Conscious and unconscious biases in healthcare: two types of bias .National Center for Cultural Competence website. Accessed September 13, 2021. https://nccc.georgetown.edu/bias /module-3/1.php

9   Racial equity tools glossary. Racial Equity Tools website. Accessed February 17, 2021. www.racialequitytools.org/glossary

10 University of Washington College of the Environment. Diversity, equity and inclusion glossary. Accessed April 11, 2021. University of Washington College website. https://environment.uw.edu /about/diversity-equity-inclusion/tools-and-additional-resources/glossary-dei-concepts

11 Foundations of culture and identity. In: *Communication in the Real World.* eLearning Support Initiative: University of Minnesota Libraries; 2016.

12 Tervalon M, Murray-García J. Cultural humility versus cultural competence: a critical distinction in defining physician training outcomes in multicultural education. *J Health Care Poor Underserved.* 1998;9(2):117-123.

13 Misawa M. Queer race pedagogy for educators in higher education. *Int J Crit Pedagogy.* 2010;3(1):26-35.

14 Showry M, Manasa KVL. Self-awareness — key to effective leadership. *IUP J Soft Skills.* 2014;8(1):15-26.

15 Eurich T. What self-awareness really is (and how to cultivate it). *Harvard Business Review.* January 2018. Accessed February 21, 2021. https://hbr.org/2018/01/what-self-awareness-really -is-and-how-to-cultivate-it

16 Van Velsor E, Taylor S, Leslie JB. An examination of the relationships among self-perception accuracy, self-awareness, gender, and leader effectiveness. *Hum Resour Manage.* 1993;32(2-3):249-263. doi:10.1002/hrm.3930320205

17 Learn how the CliftonStrengths assessment works. Gallup website. Accessed February 21, 2021. www.gallup.com/cliftonstrengths/en/253676/how-cliftonstrengths-works.aspx

18 MBTI basics. Myers & Briggs Foundation website. Accessed January 21, 2021. www.myersbriggs .org/my-mbti-personality-type/mbti-basics

19 Project Implicit website. Accessed February 27, 2021. https://implicit.harvard.edu/implicit /takeatest.html

20 Emotional and social competence inventory (ESCI). Consortium for Research on Emotional Intelligence in Organizations website. Accessed March 27, 2021. www.eiconsortium.org /measures/eci_360.html

21 Academy of Nutrition and Dietetics. Inclusion, Diversity, Equity and Access. eatrightPRO website. Accessed February 24, 2023. www.eatrightPRO.org/idea/inclusion-diversity-equity-and-access

22 Tatum BD. The complexity of identity: "who am I?" In: Adams M, Blumenfeld WJ, Castañeda C, Hackman HW, Peters, ML, Zúñiga X, eds. *Readings for Diversity and Social Justice: An Anthology on Racism, Sexism, Anti-Semitism, Heterosexism, Ableism, and Classism.* Routledge; 2020:9-14.

23 Diversify Dietetics. Self-study program. (Paid e-learning course). Diversity Dietetics website. Accessed February 24, 2023. https://diverisfydietetics.lpages.co/supporting-equitable -dietetics-education-self-study

24 Social Identity Wheel Resource. LSA Inclusive Teaching Initiative website. Accessed February 24, 2023. https://sites.lsa.umich.edu/inclusive-teaching/social-identity-wheel

25 *Core Values Exercise.* John Carroll University. Accessed on March 28, 2021. http://webmedia.jcu .edu/advising/files/2016/02/Core-Values-Exercise.pdf

26 Gunsalus CK, Lickman E, Burbules N, Easter R. The self-aware leader. *Inside Higher Ed.* August 7, 2019. Accessed February 28, 2021. www.insidehighered.com/advice/2019/08/07/importance -understanding-yourself-academic-leader-opinion

27 Kaplan RS. Top executives need feedback—here's how they can get it. *McKinsey Q.* September 2011. Accessed February 27, 2021. www.mckinsey.com/featured-insights/leadership/top -executives-need-feedback-and--heres-how-they-can-get-it

28 Allas T, Schaninger B. The boss factor: making the world a better place through workplace relationships. *McKinsey Q.* September 2020. www.mckinsey.com/business-functions /organization/our-insights/the-boss-factor-making-the-world-a-better-place-through -workplace-relationships

29 DeAngelis T. In search of cultural competence. *Monit Psychol.* 2015;46(3):64.

30 Yeager KA, Bauer-Wu S. Cultural humility: essential foundation for clinical researchers. *Appl Nurs Res.* 2013;26(4):251–256. doi:10.1016/j.apnr.2013.06.008

31 Native Land app. Native Land Digital. Accessed March 1, 2021. https://native-land.ca

32 National Equity Project. Leading for equity framework. National Equity Project website. www.nationalequityproject.org/framework/leading-for-equity-framework

33 Okun T. White supremacy culture. Dismantling Racism website. February 2021. Accessed February 28, 2021. www.dismantlingracism.org/white-supremacy-culture.html

34 Food4Health Alliance. *Limitations of the Evidence on Race, Ethnicity, and Socio-Economic Status in the Report by the 2020 Dietary Guidelines Advisory Committee.* 2020. Food4Health Alliance website. https://food4health.org/wp-content/uploads/2020/08/F4H-report-113p.pdf

35 US Department of Agriculture, Department of Health and Human Services. Data analysis for the 2020 Dietary Guidelines Advisory Committee. Dietary Guidelines for Americans. Accessed February 28, 2021. www.dietaryguidelines.gov/advisory-committee-approaches-to-examine -the-evidence/data-analysis

36 Giles C. Food guidelines change but fail to take cultures into account. *Kaiser Health News.* February 1, 2021. Accessed March 27, 2021. https://khn.org/news/article/food-guidelines -change-but-fail-to-take-cultures-into-account

37 Bourke J. The six signature traits of inclusive leadership: thriving in a diverse new world. *Deloitte Insights.* April 14, 2016. Accessed February 28, 2021. www2.deloitte.com/us/en/insights/topics /talent/six-signature-traits-of-inclusive-leadership.html

38 Nelson A. Unequal treatment: confronting racial and ethnic disparities in health care. *J Natl Med Assoc.* 2002;94(8):666-668.

39 Wilbur K, Snyder CR, Essary A, Reddy S, Will KK, Saxon, M. Developing workforce diversity in the health professions: a social justice perspective. *Health Professions Education.* 2020;6(2):222–229. doi:10.1016/j.hpe.2020.01.002

40 Accreditation Council for Education in Nutrition and Dietetics. *Accreditation Council for Education in Nutrition and Dietetics Education Program Statistics 1998-2021.* eatrightPRO website. Accessed March 3, 2022. www.eatrightPRO.org/-/media/files/eatrightPRO/acend /about-acend/acend-data/1998-2021-diversity-enrollment-trends.pdf6

41 Ashikali T, Groeneveld S, Kuipers B. The role of inclusive leadership in supporting an inclusive climate in diverse public sector teams. *Rev Public Pers Adm.* 2020:1-23. doi:10.1177 /0734371X19899722

42 Randel AE, Galvin BM, Shore L, Ehrhart K, Chung BG, Dean MA, Kedharnath U. Inclusive leadership: realizing positive outcomes through belongingness and being valued for uniqueness. *Hum Resour Manag Rev.* 2018;28:190-203. doi:10.1016/j.hrmr.2017.07.002

43 Bradley EH. Diversity, inclusive leadership, and health outcomes. *Int J Health Policy Manag.* 2020;9(7):266-268. doi:10.15171/ijhpm.2020.12

44 Bourke J, Titus A. Why inclusive leaders are good for organizations, and how to become one. *Harvard Business Review.* March 29, 2019. Accessed January 2, 2021. https://hbr.org/2019/03 /why-inclusive-leaders-are-good-for-organizations-and-how-to-become-one

45 Escott-Stump SA. Leadership with a little "L." *J Acad Nutr Diet.* 2014;114(5):S6. doi:10.1016/j.jand .2014.02.020

46 Bourke J, Titus A. The key to inclusive leadership. *Harvard Business Review.* March 6, 2020. https://hbr.org/2020/03/the-key-to-inclusive-leadership

47 Dillon B, Bourke J. Six characteristics of inclusive leadership. *Wall Street Journal.* May 4, 2016. Accessed January 2, 2021. https://deloitte.wsj.com/cio/2016/05/04/6-characteristics-of -inclusive-leaders

48 Nishii LH, Leroy HL. Inclusive leadership: leaders as architects of inclusive workgroup climates. In: Ferdman BM, Prime J, Riggio RE, eds. *Inclusive Leadership: Transforming Diverse Lives, Workplaces, and Societies.* Routledge; 2020:162-178.

49 Nishii LH. The benefits of climate for inclusion for gender-diverse groups. *Acad Manage J .* 2013;56(6):1754-1774. doi:10.5465/amj.2009.0823

50 Porter J. How leaders can get honest, productive feedback. *Harvard Business Review.* January 8, 2019. Accessed February 28, 2021. https://hbr.org/2019/01/how-leaders-can-get-honest -productive-feedback

51 Oyetunde T, Boulin A, Holt J. *Equity Diversity Inclusion Action Toolkit for Organizations.* American Public Health Association; 2020. www.apha.org/-/media/Files/PDF/affiliates/equity_toolkit .ashx

52 Annie E. Casey Foundation. *Advancing the Mission: Tools for Equity, Diversity, and Inclusion.* Annie E. Casey Foundation; 2009. https://drive.google.com/file/d/1yPt4jGqkwVihrYqUPB95 6heWNXTx6JDz/view

53 Bay Area Regional Health Inequities. *Local Health Department Organizational Self-Assessment for Addressing Health Inequities: Toolkit and Guide to Implementation.* Bay Area Regional Health Inequities; 2010. Accessed March 3, 2022. https://bd74492d-1deb-4c41-8765-52b2e1753891 .filesusr.com/ugd/43f9bc_d4d3dcc60ab1412a913b296353719b3f.pdf

54 Western States Center. Assessing organizational racism. *Western States Center Views.* 2001:14-15. Accessed February 3, 2023. https://drive.google.com/file/d/1iki01-yjMkTdG2b7augs RksU6ovtkHn3/view

55 Creary S. How to elevate diversity, equity, and inclusion work in your organization. Knowledge at Wharton website. July 20, 2020. Accessed February 16, 2022. https://knowledge.wharton.upenn .edu/article/elevate-diversity-equity-inclusion-work-organization

56 FoodCorps. Equity, diversity, inclusion. FoodCorps website. Accessed March 28, 2021. https://foodcorps.org/about/equity

57 Metropolitan State University of Denver. *The Voice of Hispanic Higher Education.* Winter 2020. Accessed March 27, 2021. https://issuu.com/hacunews/docs/thevoice29.4_winter2020issuu

58 Intercultural Development Inventory. The roadmap to intercultural competence using the IDI. IDI website. Accessed April 12, 2021. https://idiinventory.com

59 Academy of Nutrition and Dietetics. Code of Ethics for the Nutrition and Dietetics Profession. 2018. Accessed April 12, 2021. eatrightPRO website. www.eatrightPRO.org/-/media/files /eatrightPRO/practice/code-of-ethics/codeofethicshandout.pdf

60 National Association for County and City Health Officials. Change management. National Association for County and City Health Officials website. Accessed April 12, 2021. www.naccho.org/programs/public-health-infrastructure/performance-improvement/change -management

CHAPTER 4
Clinical Nutrition Management

Susan Renee Roberts, DCN, RDN, LDN, CNSC, FAND;
Ashley Mullins, MS, RDN, LD, CNSC; and Kristin Ringo, RDN, LD, CNSC

Introduction

Clinical nutrition managers (CNMs) are essential leaders in the health care setting. They have a challenging role due to the many responsibilities—and sometimes competing priorities—related to management and leadership. CNMs often are responsible for both inpatient and outpatient nutrition teams, which adds another layer of complexity to the position. In some organizations, the leader who manages the clinical nutrition team may also manage patient services and may have a different title, such as Director of Patient Services (see Chapter 5, Foodservice Management and Leadership). Effective CNMs have a good understanding of the "why" behind crucial activities required to meet organizational goals and regulatory requirements. In order to be successful, CNMs must establish themselves within the organization as the nutrition experts and build professional relationships within and outside of their department that foster ongoing collaboration and efforts to ensure evidence-based nutrition practices are followed. This chapter aims to provide CNMs with practical tips on activities unique to the role.

Staffing Models and Competency Assessment

One of the most important responsibilities of the CNM is ensuring that patients receive timely, high-quality care. Competent and adequate clinical nutrition staffing is key to meeting this essential goal. Therefore, CNMs must establish standards and methods of assessing competency and determining the staffing model. The number of clinical staff members necessary is influenced by the scope of care, as are the types of care provided by clinical staff members as well as their responsibilities. Thus, the necessary competency assessment process and tools will vary depending on the types of clinical staff and their responsibilities.

Determining the Appropriate Staffing Model

Standardized clinical staffing models have been difficult to establish, partly because of an evolving and varied dietetics profession and limited validated research to support an accepted standardized model. In the clinical nutrition setting, policies, procedures, practice norms, and expectations are inconsistent across organizations. Some organizations' registered dietitian nutritionists (RDNs) may provide elevated services, such as nutrition support, order writing (OW), and bedside feeding tube placement, along with more traditional activities. Elevated practice should and will impact both staffing needs and the competency process. Clear and reliable clinical benchmarks linked to patient outcomes would assist in determining ideal staffing models. Substantial efforts from the profession have made headway in closing this gap.[1] However, CNMs are still challenged with the task of determining the optimal number of RDN full-time equivalents (FTEs), as well as nutrition and dietetics technician, registered (NDTR) FTEs, if they are part of the staffing model.

To create a viable staffing pattern, CNMs must understand and analyze multiple variables, including the policies and procedures related to nutrition screening and assessment, patient population mix (population served and complexity), interdisciplinary interactions, participation in patient care rounds, RDN OW privileges, RDN feeding tube placement, and accreditation standards. A comprehensive review of accreditation and regulatory standards is provided in Chapter 10, Statutory and Regulatory Issues. The CNM must also consider staff competency and skills, additional staff responsibilities beyond direct care including teaching other health care providers, precepting dietetic interns, participation in interdisciplinary committees, quality improvement activities and research, and maintaining a relationship between food services and the clinical nutrition services team when determining staffing levels.

Nutrition Policies and Regulatory Standards

Ensuring compliance with all accreditation standards related to clinical nutrition services is a key CNM role. These standards are in place to promote timely, evidence-based care (eg, nutrition screening, assessment, interventions, monitoring, education, and care coordination with other disciplines). The CNM, in collaboration with other disciplines, must establish policies and procedures to address and maintain compliance.

The screening tools and processes in place at an organization influence the volume of patients referred to and assessed by clinical nutrition staff. The CNM is responsible for monitoring compliance with the organization's policy for nutrition screening, assessment, and reassessment. In addition, if noncompliance with a policy is identified, the CNM must address it with a corrective action plan and demonstrate that compliance has been reestablished. Nutrition screening within the first 24 hours of admission helps capture patients at nutrition risk, and it was historically a mandatory procedure required by regulatory agencies such as The Joint Commission (TJC). However, in 2016, TJC eliminated the standard requiring nutrition screening within 24 hours of admission, because nutrition screening had become an accepted and consistent practice within health care organizations. Nutrition risk screening continues to be a part of screening in hospitals and is an accepted best practice.[2,3] Organizations are now expected to establish policies and procedures defining criteria and timeframes for nutrition screening based on patients' conditions and needs.[2,3] Frequently, a nutrition screening tool is utilized by nursing staff, with additional screening or patient prioritization conducted by clinical nutrition staff.

While validated nutrition screening tools exist and should be implemented for first-line nutrition screening,[4,5] organizations may decide to add additional screening processes to capture other high-risk patients who may not be captured by a short screening tool. It is important to note that this is not mandatory and, if implemented, should be used in conjunction with a validated screening tool. The criteria and conditions included in the clinical nutrition screening process may vary across organizations but often include patients with high nutrition risk diagnoses. Because the screening criteria and process impact the type and number of patients seen by the clinical nutrition staff, the CNM should evaluate whether all patients should be assessed by RDNs or if some can be evaluated by NDTRs. If NDTRs are a part of the staffing structure, the CNM should determine which criteria are commonly associated with lower nutrition acuity and assign those to the NDTR. The NDTR can conduct an initial evaluation, determine the patient's risk level, and determine if a full assessment by the RDN is warranted. Box 4.1 provides an example of the division of screening criteria for RDNs and NDTRs. For sites without NDTRs, all patients meeting screening criteria would receive care from the RDN. If this additional screening tool is implemented, it is important for the CNM to monitor its effectiveness.

BOX 4.1 Suggested Distribution of Patients to Nutrition Staff

Conditions and criteria for registered dietitian nutritionist assessment	Conditions and criteria for nutrition and dietetics technician, registered evaluation
Parenteral nutrition	Acute renal failure
Enteral nutrition	Congestive heart failure
Burns on more than 25% of body surface area	Colon or rectal cancer (active)
Large nonhealing wound or pressure injury	Chronic obstructive pulmonary disease (unstable)
Cancer of head or neck	Fractured jaw
Cancer of upper gastrointestinal tract	Difficulty chewing or swallowing
Diabetes (new diagnosis or uncontrolled)	Unintentional weight loss (amount or percentage over specified timeframe)[a]
Eating disorder	Poor appetite over a specified timeframe
Malabsorptive gastrointestinal disease	Multiple food allergies
Malnutrition	Extended length of stay (based on facility's average length of stay)
Pancreatitis	

[a] If substantial weight loss is noted suggesting risk of malnutrition, the patient is passed to a registered dietitian nutritionist for immediate assessment.

Policies that address the timeliness of nutrition assessments and reassessments must also be monitored by the CNM and can also impact staffing needs. Depending on the type of consult, nutrition assessments may take place within 24 to 48 hours of notification of receiving the consult. The timeframes of reassessments are usually determined by the organization and can occur between 1 to 7 days after the initial assessment depending on the care level of the patient. There are no established standards at this time; however, an example of an accepted practice for reassessment timeframes is as follows: 1 to 4 days for patients requiring high-level care, 3 to 5 days for patients requiring moderate-level care, and 5 to 7 days for patients requiring low-level care.

Patient Population Mix

The makeup of an organization's patient population can also influence staffing needs. For example, hospitals with many high-acuity patients and more patients requiring nutrition support will likely need a different staffing model compared to a hospital with lower acuity, and very few patients requiring nutrition support. In addition, hospital lengths of stay (LOS) have decreased over time due to measures intended to reduce costs and improve efficiencies. The high inpatient acuity level combined with shorter LOS can increase resources required to provide nutrition care. Clinical nutrition staff must assess high-risk patients as soon as possible in order to intervene in a timely and meaningful way before discharge.

Clinical RDNs often spend time beyond direct patient care; they participate in interdisciplinary rounds, management of nutrition orders, interventions such as enteral nutrition (EN) and parenteral nutrition (PN) support orders, and quality improvement and research in order to measure and improve patient outcomes. To identify the characteristics of the patient population served, the following parameters can be evaluated:

> patient acuity level

> average length of stay

> types of diagnoses and procedures

> specialty patient populations (such as organ transplant, burns, or short bowel rehabilitation)

> prevalence of malnourished patients

> most common diet prescriptions

> number of patients receiving nutrition support

This information can be used to develop a nutrition acuity profile of an organization's patient population and can assist in capturing the number of patients needing medical nutrition therapy (MNT). The nutrition acuity can be monitored utilizing an assigned nutrition risk level, which can be determined from a variety of parameters in the nutrition assessment. Patients are frequently categorized as having a low, moderate, or high nutrition risk based on the complexity of their conditions and the care they require. An example of a nutrition acuity prioritization model and the indications and interventions for each level of care is found in Box 4.2.[6]

Patients at high risk and those with malnutrition require more frequent RDN reassessment than patients at low or moderate risk. In addition, complex high-risk patients typically require more RDN time and expertise.[6] By tracking the number of patients from each risk category who require nutrition care, the average percentages of patient encounters for each risk level can be used to determine the anticipated workload for the year. If an entire year of data is not feasible, the CNM can use data from several months and extrapolate for an annual requirement. If this method is used, the CNM should select months that—when averaged—are representative of the year, as opposed to months with a very low or high census. This exercise can be combined with the average amount of time spent by acuity level obtained from a productivity time study (discussed later in this chapter). This method of projecting the number of patient encounters does not account for the number of patients the RDN should have seen but was not able to due to potential time restrictions. Nor does

BOX 4.2 Indications and Common Interventions Influencing Nutrition Acuity

	High complexity (3)	Moderate complexity (2)	Low complexity/ noncompromised (1)
Indications	Providing nutrition interventions that warrant frequent comprehensive reassessments	Providing nutrition interventions that warrant early evaluation	No nutrition intervention is needed
	Document impact of the intervention, which includes evidence-based nutrition outcomes	Less frequent comprehensive reassessment	Palliative/comfort care only
Common nutrition interventions	Comprehensive nutrition assessment of patients presenting with a chronic/complex disease(s) that impacts nutritional status	Nutrition assessment of patients deemed at nutritional risk	
	Enteral/parenteral nutrition—new, modified	Enteral/parenteral nutrition—stable	
	Comprehensive nutrition education—new, complex	Brief nutrition education	Brief nutrition education

Adapted with permission from Hand RK, Jordan B, DeHoog S, Pavlinac J, Abram JK, Parrott JS. Inpatient staffing needs for registered dietitian nutritionists in 21st century acute care facilities. *J Acad Nutr Diet.* 2015;115(6):985-1000.

the total FTE count incorporate additional minutes required for essential clinical care beyond time spent in the direct encounter. Additional monitoring to evaluate the number of consults and screened patients as well as the time spent in clinical care and other value-added tasks will provide important insight. Table 4.1 provides an example of how data related to nutrition acuity for a large hospital and a small hospital can assist with determining staffing needs.

TABLE 4.1 Sample Clinical Nutrition Staffing Projection Based on Nutrition Risk Levels

	Tertiary care hospital (1,000 Beds)			Community hospital (160 Beds)		
Annual number of patient encounters	63,000			8,200		
Annual encounter metrics	*Low*	*Moderate*	*High*	*Low*	*Moderate*	*High*
Percentage of annual encounters by risk level	15%	65%	20%	35%	50%	15%
Total annual patient encounters by risk level	9,450	40,950	12,600	2,870	4,100	1,230
Average time per patient encounter (minutes)	30	40	50	30	40	50
Total time spent on patient encounters (minutes)	286,500	1,638,000	630,000	86,100	164,000	61,500
Total time spent annually for all patient encounters for all risk levels (minutes)	2,554,500			311,600		
Time per week (annual minutes spent divided by 52 weeks)	49,125			5,992		
Total full-time equivalents (FTEs) (2,400 minutes per 1 FTE)	20.5 FTEs			2.5 FTEs		

Staffing Mix

CNMs can use their organization's nutrition acuity profile and other services provided by the clinical nutrition team to assist with determining the appropriate staffing mix. The budget for clinical staff salaries and FTE count allowance should also be considered. The staffing mix refers to the type of clinical nutrition staff in place (eg, full-time, part-time, as-needed RDNs and NDTRs). After analyzing these elements, the CNM can determine if the staffing should only include RDNs; whether RDNs are full-time, part-time, or working on an as-needed basis; and if NDTRs can fulfill some patient care duties.

Nutrition and Dietetics Technicians, Registered

Depending on the organization's size and needs, the addition of NDTRs to the clinical staff can allow RDNs to focus more on higher-acuity patients and tasks such as participating in interdisciplinary collaboration, placing feeding tubes, and managing EN and PN. NDTRs work under the supervision of the RDN when providing direct patient care.[7] NDTRs can assist RDNs with gathering information for evaluating low-risk patients, implement and monitor nutrition interventions, provide nutrition education per institution guidelines, and complete nutritional analyses of menus. They may also participate in responsibilities related to monitoring the quality and accuracy of food service to patients.[8]

Pro Re Nata Registered Dietitian Nutritionists

Utilization of pro re nata (PRN) RDNs (which usually means *working only when needed*) can be a creative way to provide patient care coverage and improve job satisfaction of the full-time staff. The PRN RDN schedule can vary greatly depending on the organization's needs. Some PRN RDNs may work a set schedule each week, whereas others may work on an as-needed basis only. PRN RDNs can provide patient care when full-time staff take time off during the usual workweek or on the weekends. While full-time staff often cover weekends in many organizations, the obligatory days off during the week may lessen the continuity of care supported by having the same RDN FTEs Monday through Friday. It is important to note that not all organizations have the ability to provide full weekend coverage with PRN or full-time RDNs and may need to provide coverage on just one weekend day or follow an on-call protocol in order to comply with policy. Another benefit of utilizing PRN RDNs is that they are often ideal candidates when full-time openings arise. There are also advantages for the PRN RDN. Those who are new to the profession can enhance their confidence and skills as well as obtain more exposure to different patient populations. The PRN role is also a good opportunity for experienced RDNs who desire part-time hours and the ability to maintain their clinical skills.

Determining the best staffing mix for an organization may involve some trial and error. Ongoing evaluation of the staffing model may be necessary, as what works best for one time period may not work best in the future, especially if the variables that impact clinical nutrition staffing needs change. For example, if the current staffing mix is based on physicians writing nutrition support orders and the RDNs are going to take on this responsibility, the CNM will need to evaluate whether additional RDNs are needed, if RDNs with different skills or credentials should be added, or if the staffing pattern for the week needs to be altered. The availability of RDNs and NDTRs in a geographical region is another factor that may influence which type of clinical nutrition staff is providing care. Both internal and external variables will play a role in the staffing mix. Overall, while the right staffing mix is important, the competency of the staff in place is likely more important.

Competency Assessment of Clinical Staff

Competency assessment of clinical staff is a regulatory requirement and, therefore, a high priority for CNMs. In its Definition of Terms document, the Academy of Nutrition and Dietetics defines *competence* as "a principle of professional practice, identifying the ability of the provider to administer safe and reliable services on a consistent basis."[9] The Definition of Terms also states the following about competency within the nutrition and dietetics profession[9-11]:

> *In keeping with the Academy [of Nutrition and Dietetics]/CDR [Commission on Dietetic Registration] Code of Ethics, RDNs and NDTRs practice in areas in which they are qualified and have demonstrated and documented competence. RDNs and NDTRs understand and practice within their individual scope of practice; use up-to-date knowledge, skills, judgment, and best practices; make sound decisions based on appropriate data; communicate effectively with patients, clients, customers, and others; critically assess their own practice; identify the limits of their competence; and improve performance based on self-evaluation, applied practice, and feedback from others.*

The US Office of Personnel Management states that "competencies are used for assessing and selecting candidates for a job; assessing and managing employee performance; workforce planning; and employee training and development."[12] While an individual RDN or NDTR may have achieved their respective credentials through completion of required education, training, and successful examination, they may or may not be competent to perform a specific clinical position or activity, especially if the position or activity requires expertise in a specialized patient population (eg, neonates, critically ill patients, transplant recipients) or an activity, such as nutrition support OW. This concept speaks to the individual scope of practice vs general RDN or NDTR scope of practice and is essential for the CNM to keep in mind when establishing competencies for clinical staff. Chapter 10 provides additional information about RDN standards of practice (SOP) from a regulatory standpoint.

In addition to education and credentialing requirements, RDNs and NDTRs are required to maintain registration by acquiring 75 and 50 hours, respectively, of continuing education every 5 years, documented in the Commission on Dietetic Registration (CDR) Professional Development Portfolio. The Essential Practice Competencies released by CDR in 2015 provide overarching validated standards for RDNs and NDTRs. These practice competencies define the knowledge, skill, judgment, and attitude requirements throughout a practitioner's career and provide a structured guide to help identify, develop, and evaluate the behaviors required for maintaining competence.[10,11] CNMs can work with their clinical staff to establish performance metrics and professional development activities that align with competency assessment results, the individual's professional development goals, and the organization's anticipated needs. For example, if an organization is anticipating the need for an inpatient RDN with the Certified Diabetes Care and Education Specialist (CDCES) credential, the CNM can identify an RDN with this interest and partner with them to determine the pathway to meet the need. This type of activity benefits the organization, the patients, and the individual RDN.

CNMs must assess and maintain documentation of credentials and competency requirements for RDNs and NDTRs according to the organization's policies, procedures, and job descriptions. Independent verification of credentials, including specialty credentials (eg, Board-Certified Specialist in Pediatric Nutrition [CSP]), should be conducted prior to the individual's first day in the organization and expiration of the credential. To independently verify credentials, the CNM must access proof of the credential directly from the accrediting body or source. Accepting a copy of the RDN's registration card as proof is not sufficient. It is important to note that regulatory organizations will not accept anything but an independent verification. The RDN and NDTR credentials are verified through CDR. For state licensure, contact the state agency that oversees RDN licensing for verification of licensure. Usually, the source, whether CDR or another accrediting organization, has an online mechanism that allows the CNM to print, sign, and date the verification document for the employee's file. The verification date must be prior to the credential expiration. Frequency of verification will vary depending on the credential, but the RDN and NDTR credentials must be verified annually. Most specialty credentials must be reverified every 5 years, and state licensure credential expiration is set by the respective states.

The initial competency assessment should be completed within 30 days of the hire date and repeated annually. The CNM should encourage and facilitate continuing education opportunities related to the clinical nutrition staff's roles and responsibilities, and should require documentation of continuing education from clinical staff. CNMs may determine in advance specific clinical areas, skills, and knowledge in which the RDN or NDTR must obtain continuing education, based on the responsibilities of the clinical staff at their organization. For instance, if RDNs practice in a specialized area such as oncology or trauma, they should have continuing education documented in this area to demonstrate that they are staying up to date on current practice in order to maintain competency. CNMs should also routinely conduct quality monitoring activities, such as chart audits, as a means of evaluating competency and determining skill development needs.

Figures 4.1 and 4.2, respectively, are examples of RDN and NDTR competency assessment tools. Each competency may be validated by one or more methods, including observation, demonstration, or verbal explanation of how to complete a task or meet the expectations of the job. Observation and demonstration are preferred over verbalization, as these allow the CNM to verify competency of clinical staff during actual patient care. Clinical staff should only be allowed to practice in areas in which they are qualified and have demonstrated and documented competence to achieve ethical, safe, and quality outcomes in the delivery of food and nutrition services.

FIGURE 4.1 Registered dietitian nutritionist competency assessment

Clinician Name: _____

Patient Population (circle one): Neonate / Pediatric / Adolescent / Adult / Geriatric

Competency	Validation Method: Observed, Demonstrated, Verbalized (O/D/V)	Competent: Yes, No, Not Applicable (Y/N/NA)	Evaluator Initials	Date of Review
Cultural and religious variables, disabilities, lifestyle components, and learning needs are addressed.				
Evidence that a nutrition focused physical exam is performed or attempted is documented. Exam findings are documented and micronutrient deficiencies are addressed appropriately.				
Laboratory values are assessed and documented.				
Medications are assessed and documented.				
Nutritional needs (calorie, protein, and fluid) are calculated appropriately.				
A plan for nutrition therapy is developed using an interdisciplinary approach.				
Oral diets are assessed and modified appropriately (if applicable).				
Patient-centered, measurable, time-based goals for the patient are identified.				
An appropriate diagnosis is identified and documented using the PES format.				
The chosen intervention(s) are geared to resolve the patient's nutrition diagnosis.				
Monitoring and evaluation relate to the nutrition diagnosis, goals, and interventions, and change over time if appropriate.				
Progress toward achievement of goals is addressed, including comparison of intake to established nutrient needs.				
Malnutrition diagnosis (if applicable) is determined based on established criteria and documented appropriately.				
Documentation and communication address the nutrition plan of care for patient discharge or transition of care.				

Clinician Signature: _____ Date: _____

Evaluator Signature: _____ Date: _____

PES = problem, etiology, signs and symptoms

FIGURE 4.2 Nutrition and dietetics technician, registered competency assessment

Clinician Name: _____

Competency	Validation Method: Observed, Demonstrated, Verbalized (O/D/V)	Competent: Yes, No, Not Applicable (Y/N/NA)	Evaluator Initials	Date of Review
Accurately completes screening of patient lists				
Correctly documents nutrition care in the electronic health record using the approved format				
Consistently and appropriately communicates patient observations to the registered dietitian nutritionist				
Addresses cultural and religious variables, disabilities, and lifestyle factors				
Correctly interprets diet orders and the appropriate menu items				
Correctly completes nutritional analysis of food recalls				
Appropriately communicates with patient or client, family, or caregiver				
Provides appropriate nutrition information and education per facility guidelines				

Clinician Signature: _____ Date: _____

Evaluator Signature: _____ Date: _____

Training should incorporate competency-based education focused on the learning style of the clinician. The competency-based education approach involves assessing skill sets by evaluating real-life situations vs the traditional use of a standardized test. In addition, the observer evaluating the clinician in training should be deemed competent in the skill set they are evaluating. For example, a CNM or another RDN determining whether an EN support order was prescribed safely and accurately must have demonstrated their own competency in this task before assessing the competency of another individual. The CNM may need to reach out to another CNM within the same health care system and coordinate a competency assessment.

The Academy of Nutrition and Dietetics Quality Management Committee (QMC) has developed SOP for RDNs and standards of professional performance (SOPP) for RDNs and NDTRs.[10,11] These documents provide standards and indicators for practice and professional performance at the minimum level of competence. In addition, the QMC works closely with experts in various practice areas, including clinical nutrition management, oncology, diabetes, and nutrition support, to develop SOPs and

SOPPs addressing the needs in those areas.[13] The focus area standards are meant to be used for "self-assessment, professional development and advancement of practice."[13] The focus area standards indicate three levels of competence: competent, proficient, and expert. A *competent* practitioner is an RDN who is a new practitioner or an experienced RDN who is changing to a new focus area. A *proficient* practitioner is an RDN whose operational skills are more developed and who has a deeper understanding of complex situations. An *expert*-level RDN is recognized as having mastered the highest degree of skill in and knowledge of nutrition and dietetics.[14] When completing competency assessments, the SOP or SOPP, as well as the job tasks assigned to the clinician, should be considered.

CNMs should also develop competencies constructed around their organization's goals and patient population. For example, if an organization has an initiative to reduce the number of hospital-acquired pressure ulcers (HAPUs), the CNM should ensure the clinical staff is receiving adequate training on nutritional care related to HAPUs. In addition, both the initial and annual competency plans should be based on the activities carried out by the clinical staff. Supplementary competency assessment processes may be necessary for RDNs with specific specialty or advanced roles and for those who carry out activities such as OW or feeding tube placement. For example, if a CNM manages RDNs who write PN orders, the CNM should review and consider adopting the OW competency model for PN developed by the American Society for Parenteral and Enteral Nutrition (ASPEN).[15] The model can be adopted as is or adapted to meet the needs of the particular organization.[15,16] RDN OW privileges will be discussed in more detail later in this chapter. The SOP and SOPP documents for the various focus areas are also valuable in determining key competencies for RDNs.[13]

In the case that an RDN fails to meet any of the criteria in the competency assessment, further training and reassessment of the criteria should be completed within 30 days of the first competency assessment. Routine chart evaluations that include a specific focus on the area of deficiency should also be completed monthly to ensure the deficiency has been corrected.

Competency assessment of clinical nutrition staff is an essential CNM responsibility that contributes to regulatory compliance, quality of care, and staff development (see Chapter 7, Professional Staff Development). Like other CNM duties, competency evaluations may require revision as practice at an organization evolves. In addition, the CNM should be mindful of changes in practice or high-impact issues that arise internally or externally. Once these issues are identified, the CNM can provide continuing education opportunities for staff and make appropriate additions or adjustments to the competency assessment process.

Staffing Model and Productivity Evaluation

After gaining an understanding of the variables that influence staffing, the CNM should monitor and evaluate productivity. Effective productivity and a high level of clinical staff knowledge and skills competency are important achievements. Ideally, these are tied to improved patient outcomes and meeting the overall goals of the department and organization. Opportunities for quality improvement and quality assurance initiatives are explored in greater detail in Chapter 13.

Identification of relevant clinical performance measures is key to conducting effective benchmarking. *Performance measurement* refers to the process of collecting and reporting data on practices, clinical processes, and outcomes; *benchmarking* refers to the process of comparing performance to an external standard.[17] Benchmarking requires standardized monitoring tools and can be accomplished through a variety of methods including third-party companies, internal automated or customized tools, and productivity time studies. Identifying relevant clinical performance measures is crucial to demonstrate the value of the RDN in connection with improved patient outcomes. Box 4.3 provides some common clinical performance and productivity metrics influencing clinical staffing and outcomes.

> **BOX 4.3** Suggested Clinical Performance and Productivity Metrics
>
> **Inpatient nutrition care metrics**
> - » Ratio of direct to indirect patient care time per day, week, or month
> - » Average minutes spent per patient encounter
> - » Average minutes spent per patient encounter by risk level
> - » Number of patient encounters per clinician per day or hour
> - » Acuity levels of patients per registered dietitian nutritionist
> - » Time spent on patient care rounds or team conferences
> - » Percentage of patients receiving nutrition care, by census or care units
> - » Volume of patients receiving nutrition support (enteral or parenteral), and percentage of calorie and protein needs met
>
> **Outpatient nutrition care metrics**
> - » Appointments per day, week, or month (completed vs scheduled)
> - » Cancellation and no-show rates
> - » Percentage of time spent in billable tasks (eg, medical nutrition therapy visit)
> - » Percentage of time spent in nonbillable tasks (eg, scheduling, phone calls, correspondence with providers)
> - » Ratio of direct to indirect patient care time per day, week, or month
>
> **Hospital and organizational metrics**
> - » Readmission rate
> - » Occupancy rate of facility
> - » Average length of stay
> - » Prevalence of malnutrition
> - » Population mix

Clinical Productivity

Productivity studies facilitate informed decisions regarding comprehensive nutrition care. To contain costs, clinical staff must document that procedures and services are both efficient and effective. Goals of productivity studies are to discover all tasks being performed, estimate or validate the time each task takes, and obtain objective data to establish appropriate staffing ratios. As patient LOS declines and criteria for insurance reimbursement practices change, the focus on doing things in a timely and accurate way intensifies. An evaluation of current practices is an integral part of an effective clinical nutrition program. Evaluation of current practices may indicate specific areas in which role changes could improve the quality of nutrition care provided. Findings from a productivity study may lead to staff reassignment, altered processes, or the elimination of specific clinical activities.

Clinical productivity can be defined qualitatively or quantitatively. Qualitative measurement requires comparing services to accepted standards of care and impact on patient outcomes. Quantitative measurement requires selection of a method to collect data, usually in the form of a time management study. Time estimates can be obtained through time-sampling procedures to determine the average time required to perform a specific task or Nutrition Care Process (NCP) step. Clinical productivity studies should have an identifiable beginning and end, characterize activities (not skills or knowledge), be performed by individual staff members, differentiate between activities that involve different kinds of knowledge and skills, be neither too broad nor too specific, and be expressed in clear and unambiguous statements that have the same meaning to all staff.

Direct vs Indirect Care

Time spent in direct vs indirect patient activities at each nutrition risk level can be tracked and analyzed to determine the average amount of services required for each level. For example, a high-risk patient may require a comprehensive nutrition assessment and several reassessments during an admission, whereas a low-risk patient may only require one visit by a clinical nutrition staff member. Specialty patient populations, such as patients in the intensive care unit or solid-organ transplant unit, may also influence the amount of time the nutrition staff member will spend on patient care. These patients typically require more visits by the clinician and additional activities such as medical rounds are often a part of the patient's care. According to the Academy of Nutrition and Dietetics productivity study conducted in 2017, RDNs see an average of 59% of patients admitted to the hospital for at least an initial nutrition assessment and care plan development.[1,8] According to both the 2014 and 2017 Morrison Healthcare productivity benchmarking studies, 16% to 23% of the RDN's time is spent completing indirect care activities.[1,8] It is critical that this segment of time during the RDNs', workday be preserved, as it is often used to complete skill-enhancement training and quality improvement activities and to provide trainings to other members of the health care team. These activities are among many others necessary to ensure the RDN is providing high-quality care that leads to improved patient outcomes.[1] Box 4.4 provides further examples of direct vs indirect activities.[6,8] In addition, RDNs are becoming more involved in quality improvement initiatives than ever before due to the increased focus on patient safety and the provision of quality care by accrediting agencies such as TJC.[8]

> **BOX 4.4** Direct vs Indirect Care Activities[6,8]

Direct care

- » Screening
- » Patient rounds (individually or with the multidisciplinary team)
- » Patient education
- » Patient assessment or reassessment

Indirect care

- » Foodservice tasks, such as meal rounds
- » Presentations
- » Meetings and committee responsibilities
- » Required trainings
- » Administrative tasks
- » Precepting
- » Research or quality improvement

Clinical Productivity Benchmarks

Three publications highlight efforts made to gain a better understanding of clinical benchmarks for RDNs.[1,6,8] In 2014, the Academy of Nutrition and Dietetics established a work group composed of the Clinical Nutrition Management Dietetic Practice Group and the Nutrition Research Network. The primary goal was to analyze RDN productivity within adult and pediatric acute care facilities to establish comparison benchmarks, which could be used to evaluate RDN time in relation to patient outcomes. Key productivity benchmarks studied were time required per inpatient encounter and ratio of direct to indirect care time.[6] Morrison Healthcare also contributed to the body of knowledge by publishing outcomes collected from a standardized productivity monitoring tool across 420 facilities in 2014.[8] This study was further expanded in 2017 with additional benchmarks including the percentage of patients seen on each patient care floor.[1] Table 4.2 summarizes outcomes of interest observed in these three studies.[1]

Researched outcomes such as these can provide helpful comparisons for benchmarking; however, internal benchmarking and monitoring of productivity remains essential due to organizational variation. The dietetics profession continues to gain valuable insight on important productivity metrics that should be monitored to improve standardization and for greater opportunity to conduct external benchmarking.

Third-party companies provide strategic planning and performance measurement to achieve internal and external benchmarking.[18] These platforms may collect both qualitative and quantitative data to guide organizational decision making. Hospitals participate in benchmarking programs to help them compare their performance with the performance of other similar organizations (eg, level I trauma centers or freestanding children's hospitals), typically in the key areas of cost and

> **TABLE 4.2** Clinical Productivity Benchmarks

Measurement	Morrison Healthcare Benchmarks 2014 (n = 420 hospitals)	Academy of Nutrition and Dietetics Benchmarks 2015 (n = 78 adult, 42 pediatric hospitals)	Morrison Healthcare Benchmarks 2017 (n = 19 hospitals)
Average minutes spent per *comprehensive* assessment			40
High-complexity encounters	Not collected	31.7	
Moderate-complexity encounters	Not collected	25.6	
Average minutes spent per *limited* assessment (low-complexity encounters)	Not collected	17.4	22
Average number of inpatients seen per 8-hour day			10.2
All	12-15	9.5	
Pediatric		8	
Adults		9.7	
Total assessments that were comprehensive (%)	Not collected	Not reported	74
Minutes spent in rounds	Not collected	50	19
Minutes spent screening	Not reported	35	34
Minutes spent in indirect care activities	77	Assumption made[a]	84
Patients seen on each patient care unit	Not collected	Not collected	59

[a] Direct and indirect care was not defined the same in the Academy of Nutrition and Dietetics study as the two Morrison Healthcare studies.

Adapted with permission from Phillips W, Janowski M, Brennan H, Leger G. Analyzing registered dietitian nutritionist productivity benchmarks for acute care hospitals. *J Acad Nutr Diet*. 2019;119(12):1985-1991.[1]

quality. Such benchmarking programs provide varying levels of specificity in terms of types of performance compared. Performance is evaluated for the organizations as well as at the department and subdepartment levels. An organization may elect to collaborate with one or more high-performing facilities in its benchmarking group.

As previously outlined, benchmarking requires obtaining key productivity metrics from one's own organization and department. These metrics can be collected and evaluated by conducting productivity time studies. CNMs, whether benchmarking with another organization or working to establish appropriate staffing for their own organization, will need to conduct productivity time studies.

Conducting a Clinical Productivity Study

Results of a productivity study can help identify specific tasks or activities needed to fulfill patient care responsibilities and to whom those activities should be assigned. Tasks or activities that require flexibility and judgment should be assigned to staff with greater knowledge and comprehension of the patient population, appropriate interventions, and overall goals of the department and organization. Results may have the following outcomes:

> reduction or increase in FTEs
> altered use of support personnel (eg, NDTRs or diet clerks)
> redesign of job descriptions
> evaluation of priorities with current staffing level
> cost-control measures
> evaluation of peak admission days and appropriate adjustments to staffing

Results may reveal the need for more flexible scheduling to ensure nutrition staff is in the assigned work area at the most beneficial time for patient care and interaction with the interdisciplinary team. In situations where clinical staff members are paid an hourly wage rather than a salary, flextime can decrease overtime. For example, if a staff member works 9 hours on one day due to high patient volume, they can be assigned fewer hours on another day within the same pay period in order to keep the total hours worked during the pay period at the level allocated in the budget.

Scheduling a Productivity Time Study

The timing of productivity studies is important. Studies need to be planned around a time when the organization has a normal census and circumstances; do not choose the week of the winter holidays or a time during the launch of a new electronic health record (EHR) system. Initially, studies should run for a period that can capture normal census variations—generally about 3 to 4 weeks. This duration provides adequate data to evaluate the number of times a task or activity is typically repeated and includes weekend as well as weekday activities. Follow-up time studies can be completed monthly or quarterly for continued evaluation of changes.

Data Collection

The collection of accurate and reliable data is essential in conducting a time study, which can be challenging considering the data are typically self-reported by the clinician. Clinicians providing clinical care will need to track time spent on various tasks, including direct and indirect patient care as well as additional activities. Differentiating direct and indirect care tasks and accurately tracking time spent on each type of task can become challenging since many RDNs prioritize their day by grouping tasks together—for example, gathering data for multiple patients, visiting and assessing patients, and only then completing documentation for multiple patients. The time study should also record nutrition risk levels, so an assessment can be made of time spent in correlation to patient acuity. A total count of patient encounters is also essential. The elements of importance for the CNM to collect will be influenced by the clinical nutrition policies unique to the facility. Refer to Box 4.3 for suggested clinical performance and productivity metrics. Figure 4.3 provides a sample daily time log clinicians can use to track their productivity.

FIGURE 4.3 Daily clinical nutrition time log

Name:	Clinician Type:
Facility:	Encounters Due But Not Seen:
Date:	Total Minutes Logged
Total Hours Worked:	(Sum of Direct, Indirect, & Other)

Direct Care Activities

Time Spent on Interventions by Risk Level (minutes)

Patient Room	Patient Care Unit	Initial Assessment			Reassessment			Education		
		Low	Moderate	High	Low	Moderate	High	Low	Moderate	High

Totals by Risk Level	Low	Moderate	High
Total Time by Risk Level (minutes)			
Total Encounter Count by Risk Level			

Total Direct Care Time (minutes)	
Total # Encounters	

Totals by Intervention	Initial Assessment	Reassessment	Education
Total Time by Intervention (minutes)			
Total Encounter Count by Intervention			

Daily Indirect Patient Care Activities

Activity	Description	Time Spent (minutes)
	Total Time (minutes)	

Other Daily Activities

Activity	Description	Time Spent (minutes)
	Total Time (minutes)	

Evaluation of Time Study

The data for the entire evaluation period should be sorted by clinical position and by individual. The data can be entered into a computer program, such as a spreadsheet, by each staff member. The program can be designed to provide the percentage of time spent in patient care and other activities by each person and the total time spent by each type of position. The program should be designed around the FTEs allocated. The analysis will show the individual's percentage of time in patient care and the average FTEs allocated to daily care. The total FTEs can demonstrate what staffing is actually needed by incorporating the work not accomplished and any hours beyond expectations (eg, an 8-hour paid workday vs an actual 10-hour workday without monetary compensation for the additional 2 hours). The efficiency of each staff member must be considered.

The evaluation should assess weekdays separately from weekends. When analyzing weekend time, the level of care and ability to achieve standards for providing care (as defined in policies) should be assessed. If activities are moderate or basic care, the staff assigned to weekend shifts should reflect that level of care. Consideration should be given to regulatory standards that require the same level of care on all days of the week in a facility. Standards of care of the nutrition department will mandate the staffing on the weekend. For example, once a patient is identified to be at nutritional risk, most regulatory agencies require a nutrition assessment be completed and documented in the patient's medical record within a certain timeframe. The timeframe is usually determined by the organization but must be supported with a rationale for why this timeframe was chosen. This should be considered when determining whether on-site RDN staffing is required both Saturday and Sunday or if having one or more on-call RDNs available is an option for one or more weekend days.

Time Study Outcomes

The outcome of the time study can justify maintaining the current staffing level or adding staffing to meet the mission statement of the department, the facility, and established standards of care. When analyzing the data, CNMs should look for inefficiencies in indirect and nonpatient care activities. Inefficiencies may include time spent in rounds that may not be necessary, attending patient care conferences that do not have a nutrition implication, or socializing in unproductive ways. After analyzing the data, decisions can be made to eliminate or reassign activities. The following Stories From the Field box demonstrates how a clinical productivity time study can be used to adjust the staffing model.

> **STORIES FROM THE FIELD:** Use of Clinical Productivity Data to Change the Staffing Model
>
> A 1,000-licensed-bed teaching hospital has an average daily census of 800 employed registered dietitian nutritionists (RDNs) and nutrition and dietetics technicians, registered (NDTRs) to provide clinical nutrition care. The organization budgeted for 15 RDN full-time equivalents (FTEs) and three NDTR FTEs for clinical care. The NDTR scope within this organization was to conduct a nutrition evaluation of patients and provide ongoing care for all patients assessed to be at low complexity or
>
> *continued on next page*

continued from previous page

risk. Patients assessed as moderate or high complexity or risk required ongoing monitoring by an RDN. The policy required the RDN to conduct an initial nutrition assessment within 24 hours of receiving notification from the NDTR of the patient's need. Nutrition screening and assessment policies were developed to minimize duplicated efforts and achieve efficient prioritization of patients to the appropriate clinician type. Using a daily log, the clinicians of the department conducted a clinical productivity study for 7 days each month, the results of which were reported to the clinical nutrition manager (CNM).

The CNM summarized the daily productivity logs and identified that the NDTRs spent 50% of their time conducting initial evaluations for moderate- and high-risk patients. (See data below.) The CNM reviewed additional time studies from other months, which confirmed this pattern. The CNM reviewed the nutrition screening policy that defined conditions assigned to RDNs vs NDTRs. The CNM wanted to determine whether a certain condition or diagnosis was contributing to patients at moderate or high risk being referred to the NTDR instead of the RDN for an initial evaluation. The CNM also conducted monthly chart audits to monitor quality and accuracy of care, which confirmed the clinicians were correctly classifying patient risk levels. The CNM concluded the overall patient acuity was high; in order to reduce the rate of patient handoff and duplicate assessments and to ensure timely care of high quality, an adjustment in the number of FTEs of NTDRs and RDNs was needed.

The CNM used the data to support adding one RDN FTE to account for the approximate 1.3 FTE of NTDR time spent on initial evaluations of patients at moderate or high levels of complexity or risk. The CNM also recommended reducing the number of NDTR FTEs from three to two. The proposal was accepted, and the staffing model was changed. The RDNs, although initially hesitant about the change, quickly saw the benefits in terms of more timely interventions for patients at moderate or high levels of complexity or risk.

Clinician Full-Time Equivalent (FTE) by Risk Level

Registered Dietitian Nutritionist (RDN)	Percentage of Direct Care	Encounter Count	Total FTEs	Direct Care Activities or Interventions		
				Initial Assessments	Reassessments	Nutrition Education
Total Low 1	3%	32	0.29	0.15	0.09	0.05
Total Moderate 2	69%	548	6.47	2.60	3.84	0.03
Total High 3	28%	217	2.67	0.41	2.23	0.03
Total Direct Care		797	9.43	3.16	6.16	0.11
Total Indirect Care			3.78			
Total Other			2.72			
TOTAL (Direct/Indirect/Other)			15.92			

Nutrition and Dietetics Technician, Registered (NDTR)	Percentage of Direct Care	Encounter Count	Total FTEs	Initial Assessments	Reassessments	Nutrition Education
Total Low 1	50%	103	1.10	0.50	0.40	0.20
Total Moderate 2	32%	75	0.70	0.80	0.00	0.00
Total High 3	18%	20	0.40	0.50	0.00	0.00
Total Direct Care		198	2.20	1.07	0.33	0.25
Total Indirect Care			0.30			
Total Other			0.50			
TOTAL (Direct/Indirect/Other)			3.00			

Productivity studies facilitate intelligent and informed decisions about comprehensive nutrition care. To contain costs, clinical staff must document that procedures and services are both efficient and effective. Goals of productivity studies are to discover all tasks being performed, estimate or validate the time each task takes, and obtain objective data to develop appropriate staffing ratios. Selection of essential staff is vital to achieving the goals and objectives of the organization. Therefore, CNMs must evaluate staffing levels and requirements using productivity reports and time management studies in both inpatient and ambulatory settings.

Implementing Clinical Nutrition Practices to Elevate Registered Dietitian Nutritionists and Improve Patient Outcomes

Demonstrating the value of the RDN and optimal nutrition delivery in health care overall is not a "one-and-done" activity. As patients and health care evolve, so must the role of the RDN to meet the needs of the patients and organizations. As CNMs assess the landscape at their organization, they should evaluate whether opportunities exist to either raise the level of clinical nutrition practice or improve on documentation and communication of how the RDNs' interventions contribute to improved patient, quality, or financial outcomes.

Improving Nutrition Delivery and Practices

CNMs should lead activities that improve delivery of nutrition through EN, PN, or oral nutrition. CNMs can also work to change practices, protocols, and policies to improve nutritional intake and outcomes for patients and elevate the role of the RDN within the health care team. Implementing change takes time and requires extensive collaboration and the ability to negotiate the best outcome for all (see Chapters 1 and 2 on leadership and management skills). Practices shown to improve nutrition delivery and demonstrate the value of RDNs are discussed next.

Registered Dietitian Nutritionist Order-Writing Privileges

RDNs, due their expertise in nutrition, are the optimal health care professional to write and manage nutrition-related orders, including EN and PN orders. RDN OW has led to improved outcomes for both patients and organizations. Positive outcomes associated with RDN OW include more timely implementation of nutrition interventions, improved delivery, appropriate use of EN and PN, fewer complications and errors, and increased cost savings.[16,19-24] With the aim of capitalizing on these improvements and efficiencies in patient care, in 2014 and 2016 the Centers for Medicare & Medicaid Services (CMS) made changes to allow more RDNs to obtain OW privileges within their organizations (see Chapter 10, Statutory and Regulatory Issues, for details on these rule changes).[25-27] The CNM can advocate for RDN OW privileges. State regulations may still preclude RDN OW despite the CMS ruling at the federal level. However, most states' regulations allow for health care facilities to grant RDN OW privileges.[28] Even so, CNMs must thoroughly investigate and understand their state's regulations prior to implementing RDN OW. In addition, each individual organization must establish, via policy or privileging, what type of orders RDNs can write and what competencies must be met to do so.

Although most states allow RDN OW, many RDNs have not been able to take advantage of this practice. Dietitians in Nutrition Support (an Academy of Nutrition and Dietetics dietetic practice group) and ASPEN conducted a survey of more than 500 RDNs to better understand RDN OW practices and barriers preventing RDNs from writing orders.[29] The study included RDNs who provided nutrition care for adult patients; the majority of the RDNs in the sample were practicing in a community or academic medical center. A nutrition specialty credential, most commonly the Certified Nutrition Support Clinician (CNSC) credential, was more prevalent in those with OW privileges. Although about 50% of all RDNs in the study had some level of PN ordering privileges, 47% did not. Among the RDNs with full or partial PN OW privileges, 68% had a nutrition specialty credential. RDNs reported they were denied or had not applied for OW privileges due to opposition from other disciplines, lack of education or experience, liability concerns, or limitations due to state regulations (to name just a few of the reasons). More encouraging was the finding that approximately 80% of RDNs had some degree of EN OW privileges. Of RDNs with complete or partial EN OW privileges, 65% had a nutrition specialty credential. This study demonstrates that RDNs have made progress in OW privileges, but several challenges still exist. CNMs can collaborate with their clinical nutrition team, their organizational leaders, and externally with CNMs in neighboring facilities to address barriers to obtaining OW privileges. Figure 4.4 on page 90 addresses common barriers and considerations related to each one.[15,16,25-29]

Research supports RDN OW as a practice that improves patient and organizational outcomes. In addition, RDNs with OW privileges report increased job satisfaction and recognition from physicians and others on the health care team. Therefore, unless they are in a state with regulations preventing RDN OW, CNMs should consider pursuing approval for RDN OW privileges. However, some organizations may need time to establish policies and workflows as well as develop current staff or hire the right staff to ensure competency. A stepwise approach may build confidence among RDNs and other providers and offer a foundation for expansion of OW in the future.

Registered Dietitian Nutritionists and Feeding Tube Placement

Enteral feeding tube placement has been within the RDN scope of practice for decades, and some RDNs adopted this into their practice in the early 2000s.[30-34] However, while the exact number of RDNs in the United States placing feeding tubes is not known, it is not a common practice at most organizations. The reasons for this vary from organization to organization but may be related to lack of comfort with or interest in tube placement by RDN staff, insufficient RDN staffing to perform existing tasks, low awareness by other disciplines that RDNs can place feeding tubes, or the presence of an effective process whereby feeding tubes are placed by another discipline or department.

Like RDN OW, RDN involvement in bedside feeding tube placement requires assessment of internal and external factors. The CNM should determine if the current tube placement process could be improved and if RDN staff have an interest in tube placement. If the organization already has a process that promotes timely, efficient, effective, and safe feeding tube placement, there may not be a case for changing practice. However, if one or more of these elements is of concern, it represents an

FIGURE 4.4 Barriers to and considerations for achieving registered dietitian nutritionist order-writing privileges[15,16,25-29]

Organizational	Professional	Regulatory

Determine how to obtain order-writing privileges either through credentialing or a policy.
» What is the approval process?
» What committees are involved?
 	
Establish need for registered dietitian nutritionist (RDN) order writing with data from the organization.
» Timely interventions?
» Enteral nutrition and parenteral nutrition delivery adequate and used in the appropriate patients?
» Are patients, especially those who are malnourished, receiving the most liberalized diet possible?
» Is glycemic control managed well?
 	
Establish trust with other health care professionals.
» Multidisciplinary rounds— demonstrate knowledge
» Participate in relevant committees
» Identify physician, nurse, or pharmacist champions
 	
Educate other health care professionals about:
» RDN scope of practice
» Organizational data supporting RDN order writing
» Research demonstrating improved outcomes related to RDN order writing
 	
Consider a pilot study to demonstrate value of RDN order writing
	Experience and competency
	» Develop a training program and policy outlining steps and competency evaluation required prior to an RDN being allowed to write orders.
	» Consider requiring a specialty certification, such as the Certified Nutrition Support Clinician (CNSC), for nutrition support order writing.
	
	Build on success
	» Start with less complex orders, such as oral nutrition supplements and diets. Collect data to demonstrate a positive outcome of interest.
	» Providers may be more open to RDN nutrition support order writing if a co-signature is required.
	» Partner with pharmacists or providers on electrolyte and medication additives, such as insulin, to gain experience and confidence.
	
	RDNs need to be willing to take responsibility along with order-writing privileges—invest time in great communication with other health care team members and willingness to write orders, especially nutrition support, 365 days a year.
	» Additional liability insurance may be needed.
		Scope of practice
		» State licensure regulations both for RDNs and other health care professionals
		  » State licensure laws for other health care providers, such as pharmacists, may prohibit RDNs from writing orders for medications, such as parenteral nutrition or vitamins and minerals.
		» Academy of Nutrition and Dietetics Scope Of Practice And Standards Of Professional Performance
		» Individual Scope Of Practice
		  » Utilize the Academy of Nutrition and Dietetics Scope of Practice Decision Algorithm
		
		Does the state adopt Centers for Medicare & Medicaid Services regulations for hospitals or have its own?
		» Request assistance from the appropriate department (legal or regulatory) in the organization with the regulations impacting clinical nutrition activities
		
		Which regulatory or deemed status organization accredits the hospital? Determine whether their standards impact order-writing privileges or requirements for competency.
		
		State regulations may be under revision. State affiliates and their advocacy or public policy group are a resource for this information.

opportunity for change and improvement.[33] Even if there is a case for change, adoption of feeding tube placement by RDNs requires RDNs who are willing to become competent in this skill. Also, a specific competency process and documentation of competency for feeding tube placement is necessary.

Dietitians in Nutrition Support developed a toolkit to assist with implementation of RDN feeding tube placement. The toolkit, titled Small Bowel Feeding Tube Insertion by Registered Dietitian Nutritionists: A Toolkit for Success, provides resources for making the case for a change, RDN SOP, training guidance, a competency checklist, and information on how to obtain approval within an organization.[35] Simulation and working under the guidance of another clinician with tube placement experience are also useful for RDNs seeking to become competent in tube placement.[35-37]

Benefits associated with RDN feeding tube placements will vary by organization based on which elements require improvement. Several RDNs who place feeding tubes have demonstrated positive outcomes including improved timeliness of tube placement and initiation of EN, a higher success rate with tube placement into the small bowel, and a reduction in the number of x-rays for confirmation of tube location.[33,38-40] While RDN tube placement may not be an option for some organizations, the opportunity warrants exploration, especially if the current practice is causing delayed EN, inadequate EN delivery due to intolerance of gastric feedings, or inappropriate PN use because of lack of ability to place a small bowel feeding tube.

RDNs can be the "one-stop shop" for nutrition support when both OW privileges and tube placement are under their scope of practice within an organization. Imagine a severely malnourished patient who is not tolerating gastric feedings. In some organizations, without an RDN tube placement team, the patient (who has already gone some period without adequate nutrition) may have to wait a day or more for tube placement in the radiology department. Or the patient may receive PN because small bowel feeding tube placement is not an option. In an organization with an RDN involved in tube placement, the RDN is already aware of the severity of malnutrition and lack of EN adequacy. The RDN can communicate this information to the health care team, get approval and an order for a tube placement, place the tube, obtain an x-ray if necessary, and then order EN feeding within the same day. RDNs who can practice at a higher level in collaboration with the health care team to ensure patients receive the nutrition they need are highly valued by the rest of the health care team.

Related Nutrition Support Practice Changes

Along with OW privileges, CNMs and RDNs can implement other practices aimed at optimizing EN delivery. Volume-based EN (as opposed to rate-based EN) has been shown to safely and effectively improve EN delivery in multiple studies involving both medical and surgical patients.[41-46] Volume-based EN involves an EN order for a 24-hour period rather than specifying an hourly rate. For example, a traditional rate-based order directs the nurse to infuse 60 mL/h without any means to compensate for EN cessation. Conversely, an example of a volume-based order directs the nurse to deliver 1,440 mL during a 24-hour period. If EN is held due to procedures, tests, or surgery, the nurse is provided with guidance on increasing the rate of infusion to make up for EN cessation.[41,42] While this may seem to be a logical and practical approach, it is not familiar or intuitive for many nurses.

Gastric residual volume (GRV) monitoring has long been a practice to assess EN tolerance and prevent aspiration. However, routine GRV monitoring is no longer recommended.[47,48] Studies have shown that eliminating routine GRV checks improves EN delivery without increasing complications such as aspiration, pneumonia, and mortality.[49-51]

To successfully implement practice changes such as these, CNMs will need to be familiar with and able to articulate the published literature on these topics. In addition, extensive collaboration with and education of other health care professionals will be necessary. Once changes are implemented, CNMs should conduct monitoring to assess nursing compliance, share data, and determine whether additional strategies are necessary to reinforce practice changes as the "new normal" (see Chapter 13, Quality Management and Improvement). The CNM can also positively influence adoption of evidence-based practices by working with informatics specialists to incorporate desired practices into EHR order sets (see Chapter 14, Nutrition Informatics).

Outpatient Nutrition Services

The information presented thus far has focused on the CNM's role in inpatient settings. However, in many organizations, CNMs also manage outpatient RDNs and clinics. Therefore, the remainder of this chapter addresses topics relevant to the CNM's responsibilities in outpatient settings and is adapted from previous work by Julie Grim, MPH, RDN, LD, in *The Clinical Nutrition Manager's Handbook: Solutions for the Busy Professional.*[52]

Implementing Revenue-Generating Services

Outpatient clinical nutrition staff often report to the CNM. Therefore, CNMs should become knowledgeable about the role of MNT in preventive care and seek opportunities to reduce hospitalization and readmission risk for patients. CNMs can play a leadership role in creating these opportunities in their organizations. The opportunities for RDNs to obtain reimbursement from private and government payers for MNT have expanded. The intricacies of reimbursement for MNT are complex and diverse, and extensive resources have become widely available through the efforts of the dietetics profession. The aim of this section is to provide tools and practical tips for identifying ways to implement revenue-generating services within the ambulatory setting of a hospital nutrition department, including through traditional billing of third-party payers for MNT, as well as nontraditional means such as charging a fee for community nutrition classes.

Payment Models in the Ambulatory Setting

The organizational structures of the hospital and community markets are important factors to understand when assessing the potential for revenue-generating services. Within the hospital outpatient setting, RDNs may provide MNT and bill services to insurance providers, including Medicare and private insurance payers. Detailed guidelines on billing requirements, covered services, and steps to becoming a credentialed insurance provider are well established and available from the Academy of Nutrition and Dietetics as well as CMS.[51,53] In order to accurately interpret these guidelines, it is essential to understand the setting and population in which the RDN will be providing services to establish an effective payment model.

Three primary methods of generating revenue within the ambulatory setting include making direct charges to insurance providers for MNT; charging another department, provider, or organization for RDN services; and establishing a flat customer fee for a service provided. In the event that the cost of the RDN labor is transferred to another responsible party, it is worth exploring the feasibility of the patient's insurance still being billed for services rendered by a supervising provider. For example, additional Current Procedural Terminology (CPT) codes may provide opportunities for reimbursement when billed as "incident to" the physician. Additional information on eligible incident to services and CPT code definitions are available on the coding and billing website of the Academy of Nutrition and Dietetics.[54,55] In the event the service is not reimbursable by insurance, a flat fee may be determined to cover the service being provided. Examples of various payment models to consider are shown in Box 4.5.

BOX 4.5 Examples of Payment Models in Ambulatory Settings

Payment model	Responsible billing provider	Current procedural terminology code
Bill to Insurance		
Nutrition counseling and medical nutrition therapy (MNT)	Registered dietitian nutritionist (RDN) as facility provider	97802-97804
RDN providing diabetes self-management training within an accredited program (individual or group)	RDN as facility provider	G0108, G0709
Transfer of RDN Labor Cost		
RDN providing MNT within hospital cardiac rehabilitation clinic	Cardiac rehabilitation program	93798
RDN teaching preoperative bariatric nutrition education class	Bariatric surgery clinic	97802
RDN providing intensive behavioral counseling for obesity to patients enrolled in Medicare within a physician's clinic	Supervising physician (incident to service)	G0447, G0473
Fee for Service		
RDN providing grocery store tours	Nutrition department	Not applicable
RDN providing virtual cooking demonstration	Nutrition department	Not applicable
Clinical nutrition department establishes an advanced practice training program for other RDNs	Nutrition department	Not applicable

When the RDN bills the insurance provider directly within the ambulatory hospital setting, the RDN will typically bill under the organization rather than as an individual provider. This is a result of the revenue belonging to the organization rather than the individual provider. It is still essential for the RDN to obtain a

National Provider Identifier (NPI) number.[56] When filing for reimbursement, hospitals often use their own NPI numbers rather than the NPI of the RDN who provided the service, but the NPI number of the RDN may still be listed as the rendering provider. In addition, final regulations for Medicare Part B MNT benefits state the following[53]:

Medicare will pay RDNs who enroll to obtain provider status in the Medicare program regardless of whether they provide the MNT services in an independent practice setting, hospital outpatient department or any other setting, except for services provided to patients in an inpatient stay in a hospital or skilled nursing facility. The Medicare Part B MNT benefit is not available to hospitalized Medicare patients (inpatients) since nutrition is bundled into hospital charges and billed under Medicare Part A.

Many organizations use a combination of these payment models. However, to ensure compliance with CMS standards and private insurance providers, charges should be related consistently to the cost of the services and uniformly applied to all patients.[53] Additional payment models are available depending on the organizational structure of the institution and reporting structure of the RDN.

Identify and Assess Revenue Opportunities

To determine the best payment model (or models) for an organization, the CNM must first assess how the following internal and external factors affect their current market:

> referring providers

> patient population

> hospital and insurance market

> competition

> resources

The goal in this assessment is to identify what services are currently provided, what services are available from the competition, and how the organization's services compare with those offered by its competitors. It is important to think broadly and not limit services to the traditional ones RDNs have provided in the past. As CNMs look for revenue-generating opportunities in their organizations, they should begin by identifying the interests and needs of key stakeholders in their market and referring providers, including physicians and licensed independent practitioners such as nurse practitioners and physician assistants. In addition, the patient population in need of services, as well as the hospital and insurance market, must be examined to design revenue-generating services that will also meet the needs of the community. Box 4.6 provides a list of important factors to consider and investigate to better evaluate opportunities for providing revenue-generating services.[57-60]

BOX 4.6 Considerations to Evaluate Revenue-Generating Services[57-60]

Referring Provider Considerations

» Identify whether providers are currently referring patients to registered dietitian nutritionists (RDNs) for medical nutrition therapy (MNT) within the private practice market or to another local competitor.

» Identify which providers do not currently refer to RDNs for any service and evaluate educational opportunities about the improved outcomes of MNT. Refer to the Academy of Nutrition and Dietetics MNTWorks Kit for published MNT outcome data.[58]

» Determine if a referral is required from a physician for the service to be reimbursed. This is dependent on the service being provided, insurance plan, hospital policy for outpatient services, and state licensure regulations. Medicare requires a physician order for reimbursement of MNT.[59]

» Locate large physician and provider groups near the hospital-based service. Assess ease of access to services and the types of services to offer (eg, telehealth, in-person services, satellite clinics).

» Identify physician leaders and evaluate current referral patterns. Look for physicians with formal leadership positions as well as those who lead informally by reputation.

» Collaborate with provider networks already integrated in the existing organizational structure as well as with offices that may be a part of an accountable care organization (ACO) that incentivizes improved patient outcomes.

Patient population

» Are there any disease-specific outpatient clinics associated with the organization? What are the high-volume diagnoses with nutritional implications? Evaluate opportunities to collaborate and demonstrate added value of the RDN within these populations.

» Evaluate the population's age range. For example, if the patient population is young, the clinical nutrition manager (CNM) might focus on maternal and pediatric nutrition services rather than on MNT for chronic diseases associated with an aging population.

» What is the general demographic profile of the patient population? For example, you might gather information about patients' access to transportation, the ratio of working individuals to retirees, and the percentages of military and nonmilitary patients. Such data can help the CNM figure out the types of insurance coverage their population may have and evaluate their ability to keep multiple face-to-face appointments.

» Evaluate the health insurance plans offered by large local employers. This information can assist in determining the potential for worksite wellness programs and whether the employers' insurance plans cover MNT.

Hospital and insurance market

» Evaluate the organization's payer mix of insurance providers including Medicare, Medicaid, and private insurance. This information should be available from the admissions or finance department.

» Review the insurance plan of the hospital itself and determine which diagnoses are covered for medical reimbursement and potential coverage of MNT as a preventive benefit.[60]

» Determine the contractual rates agreed upon by the hospital and the insurance provider. For example, Medicare will only pay an established rate of reimbursement for MNT, based on physician fee schedules, and is dependent on where the service is being provided. Private insurance payors also have agreed-upon contractual rates for services to determine the maximum rate to reimburse for MNT.

Assess the Competition

The second component of the assessment of revenue-generating opportunities involves analyzing the competition. Who else in the community is delivering nutrition programs? Potential competition could be the outpatient departments of other hospitals, physician clinics, RDNs in private practice, or commercial weight management programs. Once the CNM has identified their competitors, they need to find out what specific services the competitors provide, what their fees are, and how their services and fees compare with the offerings provided by the CNM's organization.

Assess Resources

An assessment of current resources including staffing, equipment, technology, and physical facilities will determine what additional resources and action items will be needed to implement services. The following questions should be part of this assessment:

> **Which departments can support essential outpatient workflows in the organization?** For example, explore support services (including scheduling, billing, registration, and so on) that reduce nonbillable activities from the RDN's daily tasks.

> **Is a dedicated physical space needed to provide the service?** Consider a location with quick access to support services and easy access for patients. Explore opportunities for the RDN to provide MNT within a clinic setting where a team of staff can collaborate for outpatient services.

> **What support will the marketing department provide?** Many health care institutions employ physician liaisons to reach out to physicians in the community with the aim of increasing referrals to the hospital.

> **Is there a unified EHR that supports easy referrals between providers? If not, what referral process is used in the absence of an EHR?**

> **What technology will be required?** Evaluate software that may enhance the patient's experience or outcomes, such as programs for nutrition analysis, meal planning, tools for communication between clients and professionals, and documentation. There are many such programs on the market, some of which can be integrated into an existing EHR. If you plan to provide telehealth services, evaluate audio and video capabilities and facility-compliant platforms for conducting virtual sessions.

> **Does the RDN team have any special competencies or skills the CNM could use to generate revenue?** These might include skills in motivational interviewing, public speaking, media outreach, preceptorship, culinary presentation, marketing, teaching, writing, or advanced practice clinical skills.

> **What unique credentials does the RDN team have that will enable the CNM to effectively fulfill the service?** Explore opportunities for staff to develop in focus areas and obtain certifications such a CSOWM, Certified Diabetes Care and Education Specialist (CDCES), CSP, coaching certifications, or culinary-school diplomas.

Evaluate Services to Offer

Once the CNM has completed a basic market assessment and evaluated existing resources, they are ready to consider what types of services to offer. For example, suppose the CNM determines that their patient population is predominately composed of Medicare beneficiaries, and identifies a large nephrology group that provides inpatient services at the organization with offices in the local area. Based on this assessment of the market and recognizing that Medicare covers MNT for kidney disease, the CNM may plan to focus efforts on increasing revenue from nutrition services for patients with stage 3 kidney disease.

As CNMs consider potential products or service lines, they must stay abreast of current trends in food and nutrition. With the burgeoning interest in health and wellness, there is tremendous potential to expand outpatient services. Potential business lines to explore for revenue generation can be divided into two categories: traditional and nontraditional; examples of both are listed in Box 4.7.

BOX 4.7 Traditional and Nontraditional Nutrition Services

Traditional nutrition services

» Individual medical nutrition therapy

» Group weight management classes

» Diabetes self-management training

» Worksite wellness classes

» Presentations to community and corporate groups

» Bariatric education

» Telehealth: counseling by phone or video

Nontraditional nutrition services

» Restaurant consultation and nutrient analyses for local restaurants

» Cooking demonstrations

» Cookbooks

» Health coaching by a licensed wellness coach

» Virtual trainings

» Video demonstrations

» Advanced practice training programs

» Grocery store consulting

» Consultations about food codes and regulations related to locally grown foods, gardening, farmers markets, or purchases made directly from farmers

» Chef–registered dietitian nutritionist partnerships

» Training and supervision of nutrition and dietetics technicians, registered or noncredentialed health professionals (eg, community health workers) providing nutrition and wellness education

» Consultations or menu development for day-care facilities or social service organizations, such as the Salvation Army

» Sales of collateral products (eg, spices, cookbooks, or small wares)

» Mobile applications for smartphones and tablets

» Healthy grab-and-go take-home meals

» Partnerships with culinary schools to teach nutrition topics

Business Plan Development

After the CNM has completed the analysis and determined services to be offered, they will need to develop a business plan. Organizations usually require such plans for proposals for new services, especially if the initiative will require funding for staff and equipment. The goal is to demonstrate how this business will solve a problem or meet a need. Creating a business plan is not as difficult as one may think. There are a variety of formats, including a traditional business plan or a lean business start-up plan, which may work well for a new service. Numerous print, online, and software resources are available to assist in this process. Advisors and sample templates can be accessed from the US Small Business Administration and the Business Model Canvas.[61,62] Refer to the Appendix for more information about developing a business plan as well as a sample plan detailing the expansion of a hospital outpatient program to include telehealth visits.

Extensive resources are available that detail unique factors for the individual components of these business plans for revenue-generating services within the field of nutrition. Many of these are listed in the payment section of the member site of the Academy of Nutrition and Dietetics (www.eatrightPRO.org), as highlighted in Box 4.8.[54] A close examination of these resources is essential as the CNM develops a business plan.

BOX 4.8 Payment Resources From the Academy of Nutrition and Dietetics[54]

- » Coding and billing
- » Diagnosis and procedure codes
- » Referral requirements for coverage of nutrition services
- » HIPAA (Health Insurance Portability and Accountability Act) and other regulations
- » Services, fees, and management resources
- » Guidance on insurance requirements, including Medicare, Medicaid, and private payers
- » Ideas on promoting nutrition services

As the CNM creates financial projections, they should not underestimate possible expenses and should be conservative about revenue expectations. Staff will not generate revenue during every hour of the workday. Projections must include realistic assessments of the time required for nonrevenue activities and how much time is left for revenue generation. For example, consider the typical patient no-show rate for the organization or type of service provided. Also consider how much time is spent in indirect, nonbillable activities, such as preparation and documentation for outpatient MNT. Refer to the staffing and productivity section of this chapter for additional guidance.

Assessment of Effectiveness

The effectiveness of all revenue-generating services needs to be measured using valid methods. Outcomes assessment is particularly important for MNT programs. To demonstrate the effectiveness of MNT, the outcome must be a measurable, positive change—such as improvement in the patient's clinical or functional status, demonstrable financial benefits, or a shortened time period for treatment or care—that is a direct result of the MNT provided. The implementation of the Nutrition Care Process (NCP) and creation of the standardized NCPT have greatly enhanced the ability of RDNs to capture outcomes in data directly related to the care they provide.[63] Documentation should show whether the nutrition diagnosis was resolved, note changes in the signs and symptoms identified in the PES (problem, etiology, and signs and symptoms) statement, and detail improvement in overall nutrition-related health outcomes such as weight, blood pressure, lipid levels, or reduced medication requirements.[60]

Documenting MNT outcomes is essential for the following reasons:

> Managed care demands positive outcomes. Insurance will reimburse only those health care services that are proven to produce positive outcomes in a cost-effective manner.

> Consumers and referring providers also demand outcomes information. Patients expect to see results and may ask about the program's track record before they schedule and come to an appointment or other service.

> Outcomes are the basis for standardized MNT protocols.

> Positive outcomes demonstrate the effectiveness of RDNs to physicians, which in turn generates referrals that can produce revenue for your facility.

> Emerging reimbursement models, such as medical homes and bundled services, will also put outcomes data under enhanced scrutiny to ensure programs are cost-effective and benefit patients.

CNMs should have a plan in place to collect outcomes data at the initial patient visit and then at regularly timed intervals thereafter and should be prepared to report and market positive outcomes to insurers, hospital administrators, and physicians as well as the community, colleagues, and prospective patients. With continued advancements of the EHR, there is ample opportunity to collaborate with informatics specialists to develop reports and automated methods for collecting and reporting outcomes. In addition, resources such as *MNT Providing Return on Investment*[64] and the Academy of Nutrition and Dietetics Evidence Analysis Library (www.andeal.org) may be helpful in identifying key outcomes of interest.

Summary

The CNM's range of responsibilities is extensive and may include both inpatient and outpatient nutrition services. CNMs, especially those new to their position, should seek the guidance of leaders within and outside their department, other CNMs in their hospital system, and CNMs at other hospitals. A network of individuals who can share real-world experiences, as well as advice based on those experiences, is priceless. The Academy of Nutrition and Dietetics has abundant resources of value to the CNM, including the Clinical Nutrition Management Dietetic Practice Group, the Quality Management Committee, and extensive information related to payment and leadership. CNM is a challenging and fulfilling role for RDN leaders, and one that impacts patient care as well as patient and organizational outcomes.

REFERENCES

1   Phillips W, Janowski M, Brennan H, Leger G. Analyzing registered dietitian nutritionist productivity benchmarks for acute care hospitals. *J Acad Nutr Diet*. 2019;119(12):1985-1991.

2   The Joint Commission. Standards FAQs. Joint Commission website. December 21, 2017. Accessed June 19, 2020. www.jointcommission.org/standards/standard-faqs/hospital-and -hospital-clinics/provision-of-care-treatment-and-services-pc/000001652

3   The Joint Commission. EP Review Project: The Joint Commission deletes 225 hospital requirements. Joint Commission website. Accessed December 28, 2020. www.jointcommission .org/-/media/enterprise/tjc/imported-resource-assets/documents/joint_commission_deletes _hospital_requirementspdf.pdf?db=web&hash=5B84CE93904D4CFE1E9194A6AA8DADB1

4   Skipper A, Coltman A, Tomesko J, et al. Adult malnutrition (undernutrition) screening: an evidence analysis center systematic review. *J Acad Nutr Diet*. 2020;120(4):669-708.

5   Skipper A, Coltman A, Tomesko J, et al. Position of the Academy of Nutrition and Dietetics: malnutrition (undernutrition) screening tools for all adults. *J Acad Nutr Diet*. 2020;120(4):709-713.

6   Hand RK, Jordan B, DeHoog S, Pavlinac J, Abram JK, Parrott JS. Inpatient staffing needs for registered dietitian nutritionists in 21st century acute care facilities. *J Acad Nutr Diet*. 2015;115(6):985-1000.

7   Academy of Nutrition and Dietetics. Practice Tips: What is meant by "Under the supervision of the registered dietitian nutritionist"? eatrightSTORE website. Accessed December 30, 2020. www.eatrightSTORE.org/product-type/case-studies-and-practice-tips/practice-tips-what-is -meant-under-supervision-rd?_ga=2.185517871.744631511.1612041334-617299676.1610649025

8   Phillips W. Clinical nutrition staffing benchmarks for acute care hospitals. *J Acad Nutr Diet*. 2015;115(7):1054-1056.

9   Academy of Nutrition and Dietetics. Definition of terms list. eatrightPRO website. Accessed December 30, 2020. www.eatrightPRO.org/-/media/eatrightPRO-files/practice /scope-standards-of-practice/academy-definition-oftermslist.pdf?la=en&hash =397C681EFB1CD79FE03FB60C8D2BC008FC5BC530

10 Academy Quality Management Committee, Academy of Nutrition and Dietetics. Revised 2017 scope of practice for the registered dietitian nutritionist. *J Acad Nutr Diet*. 2018;118(1):141-165.

11 Academy Quality Management Committee, Academy of Nutrition and Dietetics. Revised 2017 scope of practice for the nutrition and dietetics technician, registered. *J Acad Nutr Diet*. 2018;118(2):327-342.

12 Office of Personnel Management. Assessment & Selection. Office of Personnel Management website. Office of Personnel Management website . Accessed January 10, 2021. www.opm.gov /policy-data-oversight/assessment-and-selection/competencies

13 Academy of Nutrition and Dietetics. Standards of practice. eatrightPRO website. Accessed December 30, 2020. www.eatrightPRO.org/practice/quality-management/standards-of -practice

14 Macris PC, Schilling K, Palko R; Academy of Nutrition and Dietetics. Revised 2017 standards of practice and standards of professional performance for registered dietitian nutritionists (competent, proficient, and expert) in oncology nutrition. *J Acad Nutr Diet*. 2018;118(4):736-748.

15 Guenter P, Boullata JI, Ayers P, et al; Parenteral Nutrition Safety Task Force. American Society for Parenteral and Enteral Nutrition (ASPEN) standardized competencies for parenteral nutrition prescribing: the American Society for Parenteral and Enteral Nutrition Model. *Nutr Clin Pract*. 2015;30(4):570-576.

16 Roberts SR. Improving patient outcomes through registered dietitian order writing. *Nutr Clin Pract*. 2013;28(5):556-565.

17 Practice facilitation handbook, module 7: measuring and benchmarking clinical performance. Agency for Healthcare Research and Quality website. May 2013. Accessed June 1, 2020. www.ahrq.gov/ncepcr/tools/pf-handbook/mod7.html

18 Gregoire MB, Theis ML. Practice paper of the Academy of Nutrition and Dietetics: principles of productivity in food and nutrition services: applications in the 21st century health care reform era. *J Acad Nutr Diet*. 2015;115(7):1141-1147.

19 Phillips W, Doley J. Granting order-writing privileges to registered dietitian nutritionists can decrease costs in acute care hospitals. *J Acad Nutr Diet*. 2017;117(6):840-847.

20 Heckathorne J, Roberts S. RDN parenteral nutrition order writing: improving electrolyte and glucose management. *J Acad Nutr Diet*. 2019;119(10):A107.

21 Peterson SJ, Chen Y, Sullivan CA, et al. Assessing the influence of registered dietitian order-writing privileges on parenteral nutrition use. *J Am Diet Assoc*. 2010;110(11):1703-1711.

22 Elliott KL, Kandiah J, Walroth TA. Interdisciplinary discrepancies between parenteral nutrition macronutrient prescribing and recommendations: is body mass index a factor? *JPEN J Parenter Enteral Nutr*. 2017;41(5):759-765.

23 Martin K, DeLegge M, Nichols M, Chapman E, Sollid R, Grych C. Assessing appropriate parenteral nutrition ordering practices in tertiary care medical centers. *JPEN J Parenter Enteral Nutr*. 2011;35(1):122-130.

24 Arney BD, Senter SA, Schwartz AC, Meily T, Pelekhaty S. Effect of registered dietitian nutritionist order-writing privileges on enteral nutrition administration in selected intensive care units. *Nutr Clin Pract*. 2019;34(6):899-905.

25 Centers for Medicare & Medicaid Programs; Department of Health and Human Services. Medicare & Medicaid programs; regulatory provisions to promote program efficiency, transparency, and burden reduction; Part II. *Fed Regist*. 2014;79:27105-27157. Updated May 12, 2014. Accessed December 28, 2020. www.federalregister.gov/articles/2014/05/12/2014-10687/medicare-and-medicaid-programsregulatory-provisions-to-promote-programefficiency-transparency-and#h-22

26 Centers for Medicare & Medicaid Services; Department of Health and Human Services. Medicare & Medicaid Programs; reform of requirements for long term care facilities. *Fed Regist*. 2016;81:68688-68872. Published October 4, 2016. Accessed December 28, 2020. www.federalregister.gov/documents/2016/10/04/2016-23503/medicare-and-medicaid-programs-reformofrequirements-for-long-term-care-facilities

27 Boyce B. CMS final rule on therapeutic diet orders means new opportunities for RDNs. *J Acad Nutr Diet*. 2014;114(9):1326-1328.

28 Academy of Nutrition and Dietetics. Licensure statutes and information by state. eatrightPRO website. Published October 4, 2016. Accessed January 10, 2021. www.eatrightPRO.org/advocacy/licensure/licensure-map

29 Peterson S, Dobak S, Phillips W, et al. Enteral and parenteral order writing survey—a collaborative evaluation between the Academy of Nutrition and Dietetics' Dietitians in Nutrition Support Dietetics Practice Group and the American Society for Parenteral and Enteral Nutrition (ASPEN) Dietetics Practice Section. *J Acad Nutr Diet*. 2020;120(10):1745-1753.

30 American Society for Parenteral and Enteral Nutrition, Board of Directors. Standards of practice for nutrition support dietitians. *Nutr Clin Pract*. 2000;15(1):53-59.

31 Cresci G, Martindale R. Bedside placement of small bowel feeding tubes in hospitalized patients: a new role for the dietitian. *Nutrition*. 2003;19(10):843-846.

32 Jimenez LL, Ramage JE Jr. Benefits of postpyloric enteral access placement by a nutrition support dietitian. *Nutr Clin Pract*. 2004;19(5):518-522.

33 Gray R, Tynan C, Reed L, et al. Bedside electromagnetic-guided feeding tube placement: an improvement over traditional placement technique? *Nutr Clin Pract*. 2007;22(4):436-444.

34 Taylor B, Schallom L. Bedside small bowel feeding tube placement in critically ill patients utilizing a dietitian/nurse team approach. *Nutr Clin Pract*. 2001;16(4):258-262.

35 Small bowel feeding tube insertion by registered dietitian nutritionists: a toolkit for success. Dietitians in Nutrition Support website. Accessed December 29, 2020. www.dnsdpg.org/store.cfm

36 Rollins C, Bailey E, Gregoire J, Milner T. Clinical simulation learning for small-bowel feeding tube insertion. *Nutr Clin Pract*. 2018;33(2):185-190.

37 Yandell R, Chapman M, O'Connor S, Shanks A, Lange K, Deane A. Post-pyloric feeding tube placement in critically ill patients: extending the scope of practice for Australian dietitians. *Nutr Diet*. 2018;75(1):30-34.

38 Carter M, Roberts S, Carson JA. Small-bowel feeding tube placement at bedside: electronic medical device placement and x-ray agreement. *Nutr Clin Pract*. 2018;33(2):274-280.

39 Brown BD, Hoffman SR, Johnson SJ, Nielsen WR, Greenwaldt HJ. Developing and maintaining an RDN-led bedside feeding tube placement program. *Nutr Clin Pract*. 2019;34(6):858-868.

40 Rollins CM. Blind bedside placement of postpyloric feeding tubes by registered dietitians: success rates, outcomes, and cost effectiveness. *Nutr Clin Pract*. 2013;28(4):506-509.

41 Heyland DK, Cahill NE, Dhaliwal R, et al. Enhanced protein-energy provision via the enteral route in critically ill patients: a single center feasibility trial of the PEP uP protocol. *Crit Care*. 2010;14(2):R78.

42 Roberts S, Brody R, Rawal S, Byham-Gray L. Volume-based vs rate-based enteral nutrition in the intensive care unit: impact on nutrition delivery and glycemic control. *JPEN J Parenter Enteral Nutr*. 2019;43(3):365-375.

43 Bharal M, Morgan S, Husain T, et al. Volume based versus rate based feeding in the critically ill: a UK study. *J Intensive Care Soc*. 2019;20(4):299-308.

44 Sachdev G, Backes K, Thomas BW, Sing RF, Huynh T. Volume-based protocol improves delivery of enteral nutrition in critically ill trauma patients. *JPEN J Parenter Enteral Nutr*. 2020;44(5):874-879.

45 Brierley-Hobson S, Clarke G, O'Keefe V. Safety and efficacy of volume-based feeding in critically ill, mechanically ventilated adults using the "Protein & Energy Requirements Fed for Every Critically ill patient every Time" (PERFECT) protocol: a before-and-after study. *Crit Care*. 2019;23(1):105. doi:10.1186/s13054-019-2388-7

46 Taylor B, Brody R, Denmark R, Southard R, Byham-Gray L. Improving enteral delivery through the adoption of the "Feed Early Enteral Diet adequately for Maximum Effect (FEED ME)" protocol in a surgical trauma ICU: a quality improvement review. *Nutr Clin Pract*. 2014;29(5):639-648.

47 Rice TW. Gastric residual volume: end of an era. *JAMA*. 2013;309(3)283-284.

48 Westphal M. Science and fiction in critical care: established concepts with or without evidence? *Crit Care*. 2019;23(suppl 1):125.

49 Reignier J, Mercier E, Le Gouge A, et al. Effect of not monitoring residual gastric volume on risk of ventilator-associated pneumonia in adults receiving mechanical ventilation and early enteral feeding: a randomized control trial. *JAMA*. 2013;309(3):249-256.

50 Wiese AN, Rogers MJ, Way M, Ballard E. The impact of removing gastric residual volume monitoring and enteral nutrition rate titration in adults receiving mechanical ventilation. *Aust Crit Care*. 2020;33(2):155-161.

51 Ozen N, Tosen N, Yamanel L, Altintas ND, Kilciler G, Ozen V. Evaluation of the effect on patient parameters of not monitoring gastric residual volume in intensive care patients on a mechanical ventilator receiving enteral feeding: a randomized clinical trial. *J Crit Care*. 2016;33:137-144.

52 Grim J. *The Clinical Nutrition Manager's Handbook: Solutions for the Busy Professional*. Academy of Nutrition and Dietetics; 2014.

53 Centers for Medicare & Medicaid Services. Medicare benefit policy manual. Centers for Medicare & Medicaid Services website. December 2019, July. Accessed May 16, 2020. www.cms .gov/Regulations-and-Guidance/Guidance/Manuals/downloads/bp102c15.pdf

54 Academy of Nutrition and Dietetics. Payment. eatrightPRO website. Accessed May 16, 2020. www.eatrightPRO.org/payment

55 Academy of Nutrition and Dietetics. Diagnosis and procedure codes. eatrightPRO website. Accessed May 16, 2020. www.eatrightPRO.org/payment/coding-and-billing/diagnosis-and -procedure-codes

56 Academy of Nutrition and Dietetics. Incidents to services for RDNs. eatrightPRO website. Accessed May 16, 2020. www.eatrightPRO.org/payment/coding-and-billing/billing-resources /incidents-to-services

57 Academy of Nutrition and Dietetics. Medicare provider enrollment. eatrightPRO website. Accessed May 17, 2020. www.eatrightPRO.org/payment/medicare/medicare-provider-enrollment

58 Academy of Nutrition and Dietetics. MNTWorks Kit. eatrightPRO website. Accessed May 25, 2020. www.eatrightPRO.org/payment/nutrition-services/promoting-nutrition-services/resources-for-promoting-nutrition-services

59 Academy of Nutrition and Dietetics. Referral requirements for coverage for nutrition services. eatrightPRO website. Accessed May 17, 2020. www.eatrightPRO.org/payment/coding-and-billing/referral-requirements-for-coverage-for-nutrition-services

60 Academy of Nutrition and Dietetics. Practice settings FAQs. eatrightPRO website. Accessed May 25, 2020. www.eatrightPRO.org/payment/medicare/mnt/practice-settings---faqs

61 US Small Business Administration. Write your business plan. US Small Business Administration website. Accessed May 20, 2020. www.sba.gov/business-guide/plan-your-business/write-your-business-plan

62 Business model canvas. Strategyzer website. Accessed May 20, 2020. www.strategyzer.com/canvas/business-model-canvas

63 Academy of Nutrition and Dietetics. *International Nutrition and Dietetics Terminology Reference Manual*. 4th ed. Academy of Nutrition and Dietetics; 2013.

64 Academy of Nutrition and Dietetics. MNT providing return on investment. eatrightPRO website. Accessed December 29, 2020. www.eatrightPRO.org/-/media/eatrightPRO-files/practice/coding-coverage-compliance/11-2011_mnt_providing_return_on_investment_final.pdf?la=en&hash=BF7895277BFC5D8E7D8192E695C3513307A6BE57

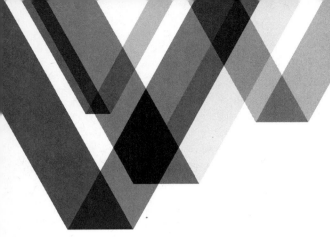

CHAPTER 5

Foodservice Management & Leadership

Kim Brenkus, MBA, RDN, LD, FAND

Introduction

The role of the foodservice registered dietitian nutritionist (RDN) is evolving and expanding. To be an effective foodservice manager, the dietitian must possess both management and leadership skills. As health and wellness trends continue to generate demand, RDNs are developing these important skills. A foodservice manager must be able to manage the resources at their disposal and also communicate, inspire, supervise, and mentor.[1] This chapter will explore the leadership traits, skills, and tools needed to deliver in your role in foodservice management. Additional information can be found in the Academy of Nutrition and Dietetics standards of professional performance (SOPP) in management of food and nutrition systems.[2]

Communication

Some managers may seem to be more naturally gifted with leadership abilities than others, but anyone can become a leader by learning and implementing particular skills. Effective communication is a critical skill that should never be underestimated. If managers and teams do not communicate effectively, employees may lose trust. There is a deep connection between trust and communication. Trust is the foundation of communication, and communication is essential to building trust. Once trust is lost, communication and leadership soon follow. Great communicators engage their audience; they include them by asking their opinions, using their suggestions, and responding to their feedback.[3] Refer to Chapter 1 for more on communication skills for leaders. To quote George Bernard Shaw, "The single biggest problem in communication is the illusion that it has taken place." Often a manager will deliver communication and assume the content was clear but does not verify whether the communication has been received and understood. For example, communicating with employees about the practices necessary to prevent cross-contamination for patients with food allergies is critical to patient safety. In this situation, verbal or written communication should be delivered, and a manager should check to see if the other party has full understanding. Effective communication helps teams work together. Today, we have more ways than ever to communicate, but these myriad technologies can also compete for attention. Effective communication methods will help improve your internal communication strategy and decrease turnover.[4]

Elements of Communication

Essential elements in communication include authenticity, visibility, active listening, and follow-up or feedback. Start with authenticity: be honest and sincere. Employees want genuine leaders, and employees follow people who are "real." Be visible: if you want to communicate well, do not be out of sight. Employees need to feel connected to their work and their leadership, so find ways to interact with all of your employees. Use active listening: good communicators are also good listeners. When you listen, you gain a clear understanding of your employees' perspectives. Listening promotes trust, respect, and openness.[5] Active listening involves more than just hearing someone speak; it is the ability to paraphrase and reflect back what was said, making the other person feel heard and valued. Following up keeps the lines of communication open, which helps employees feel more comfortable opening up about issues when they arise. Making a habit of following up will help you to continue to identify areas for improvement.

Try the following five ways to improve your communication[5]:

> **Communicate continuously.** Use different communications modes and methods, such as meetings, email, huddles, and social media. It is not possible to overcommunicate. Another visible way to communicate is by using a "stoplight" report or communication board posted in a visible area. Red items are items that cannot be done, and they are accompanied by an explanation of why. Yellow items are considered in progress (keep updating these), and green items have been completed. Develop a routine and be adaptive.

> **Simplify your communications.** Say what you mean in a direct manner. Do not hide behind complexity or mountains of information. Simple communication can be smart communication.

> **Listen to and encourage input.** Encourage employees to offer ideas and solutions before you give yours. Listen 80% of the time and talk 20% of the time.

> **Use stories to make your point.** Employees find it easier to repeat a story or refer to an image or quote than to talk about a vision statement, strategy, or project plan. The book *Made to Stick: Why Some Ideas Survive and Others Die* by Chip Heath and Dan Heath offers helpful insights about using stories to communicate your message.

> **Confirm with actions.** Employees need to trust you. Your behavior and actions communicate in a big way. Be clear on the messages you send, even when you are not speaking a word.

Two-Way Communication

It is important that communication runs freely both ways between leaders and employees. This gives leaders a chance to impact employee perceptions and employees an opportunity to be heard. This type of communication can be created through the use of tools such as employee surveys, group meetings, one-on-one meetings, regular check-ins with team members, and communication boards. If leaders use these communication tools properly, they have the power to drive employee engagement. Traditional drivers of engagement have included increased compensation or career advancement. Recent research has shown that perception of leadership is one of the top drivers of engagment.[6] Even a traditional driver such as career advancement opportunities can be positively impacted by improved communication between leaders and employees. Listening to employee feedback and responding with a plan of action can demonstrate good leadership. While the action taken will have the greatest impact on this perception, leadership communication will drive the change.[7]

When communication does not occur freely, it can create fear and doubt among employees. If leaders do not take the time to communicate regularly with employees, employees may create their own versions of what is occurring. Regular interactions between employees and leadership can improve employee morale and engagement. Acknowledge the efforts of your team regularly. Some forms of recognition cost only a small amount of time and have a large return on investment.[7]

Interdepartmental Communication

Leaders can use effective communication to drive meaningful organizational change and help strengthen employees' levels of comfort and confidence.[7] For example, when a change is made to the menu, you should develop a communication strategy. Did you communicate the change to your staff as well as other departments? One useful tool for communicating menu changes is to invite all departments to a taste sampling and let them try the new offerings for themselves. This will provide feedback and build confidence with foodservice staff as well as nursing in a hospital setting. If a patient comments on the new menu item and the nurse has had a chance to taste it, the nurse can be supportive by relaying how much they enjoyed the item to the patient.

Leaders can encourage buy-in and encourage other departments to support each other in *managing up*—a process in which one member of the team puts another member at an advantage in the eyes of the patient or customer. For example, a nurse may introduce a foodservice worker to a patient by stating, "One of our finest hosts, Jordan, will be serving you your breakfast today, Mr. Everett."

Engagement

Employee engagement is based on trust, integrity, mutual commitment, and communication between an organization and its employees. Engagement measures an employee's emotional attachment to their job, colleagues, and organization, which in turn influences their willingness to learn and perform at work. Engagement is not the same as employee satisfaction; being satisfied does not necessarily mean you are engaged in your role. Engagement can be measured, and it varies from poor to great. Engaged employees are involved in and enthusiastic about their work and, therefore, will act in a way that furthers their organization's goals and mission.[8]

Measuring Employee Engagement

There are not many options when it comes to measuring employee engagement. The simplest and most straightforward way to take the employees' pulse is through employee surveys. Your organization might send out an annual employee survey. While this gives you great data, it may not give you a real-time look at engagement.

Consider doing regular check-in surveys, even informal ones. These will give you insights into how employees are feeling in real time, giving you ample time to act before they reach the point of resigning from their position.[8] Some best practices to keep in mind when using a survey are as follows:

> Keep surveys anonymous.
> Keep surveys short.
> Keep the questions simple and straightforward.
> Plan to share the feedback and act on it.

Measuring feedback is the first step, but acting on that feedback is critical for positive results. Engagement isn't a "program of the day" to get your employees to work harder. True employee engagement is the result of care and attention; it is the right thing to do. Employee engagement increases dramatically when their daily experiences include positive relationships with their direct supervisors or managers.

Increasing Employee Engagement

The most engaged employees are more likely to give their best efforts and consider the interests of the team in addition to themselves. Engagement starts with managers. Encouraging an open, two-way line of communication between employees and their supervisors is the first step of engagement and helps the employees feel like a valued part of a team.[8] When employees feel like the processes in their organization are working against them rather than for or with them, they are more likely to withdraw from the organization and turn to a mindset where they simply work their assigned hours with very little engagement.

Employee engagement improves when the manager clearly defines each job description and reinforces this in the onboarding and training process. Many times, the real cause of an employee's underperformance is undefined roles and goals. As part of your routine communication with each employee, ask them whether they feel they have been trained in all aspects of the job to be able to perform at a high level. If you are not communicating responsibilities up front, it is difficult to hold an individual accountable for doing the work.

After sharing job expectations, set regular meetings to enhance employee communication. This is your chance to connect with your employees. Research by Gallup states that when employees have regular meetings with their managers, they are three times as likely to be happier in their work.[9]

Everyone wants to feel valued. Mutual respect is best fostered through praise, support, and encouragement. Positive work environments naturally create a more engaged workforce. When managers and leaders communicate praise instead of negativity, employees feel empowered, feel supported, and will work their hardest to do the best possible job.

Additional insights and advice on this topic can be found in the resource section of the Management in Food and Nutrition Systems (MFNS) Dietetic Practice Group website.[10] An example of communication and employee engagement is outlined in the Stories From the Field box on page 108.

> **STORIES FROM THE FIELD:** Communication and Employee Engagement
>
> A manager in a hospital requested to have a third party hold meetings with the employees to determine the staff's current pulse. Each meeting had four to five employees who were asked the same questions. Meetings were held over multiple days. The data gathered were entered in a mobile application and used to identify the most important areas to the employees. One of the most important considerations in this research was to gather employee input on solutions to specific, ongoing problems in the hospital.
>
> From the data, the manager identified four major categories for improvement, assigned a supervisor and a lead employee to each category, and assigned target dates for completion of the task. The manager enlarged the action plan and hung it in a visible area in the department. Each supervisor updated their assigned area by using the stoplight communication board. In daily huddles, key issues were highlighted to reinforce communication. To keep the process fluid, a manager or supervisor met with a different employee at least weekly, asked the same questions, and recorded the responses in the mobile application. This allowed the action plan to be communicated and updated in real time, as issues were resolved or new ones identified.

Human Resources Challenges

Many nutrition practitioners enter into the foodservice business because they are passionate about using great food to deliver an excellent customer or patient experience. Keeping employees motivated and engaged and providing them with the training they need and the benefits they desire are constant challenges. In foodservice management, oversight of multiple employees is common, requiring ongoing time and attention to human resources issues (see Chapter 11, Human Resources 101). Some top human resources issues are decreasing absenteeism, motivating employees, improving customer service, and providing training on a budget.

Employee Absenteeism

Employee absenteeism can be difficult to address once it has become a habit or an accepted behavior by your team. After all, you cannot force employees to show up on time, or at all. The following are some ways to help reduce absenteeism[4]:

> An employee wellness program can help lower absenteeism and demonstrate sustainable practices. Proactively preventing absenteeism can be done through educating employees on health and wellness concerns. This will give your employees the best tools to make healthy behavioral changes, which can result in less absenteeism.

> An employee could be stressed because of workload, difficulties with coworkers, or feeling overwhelmed. Stress can cause unplanned absences; take a proactive approach, investigating areas of stress for employees and determining what resources you might need to minimize the stressors' impacts.

> Employees can be affected by their personal lives, and there may be a genuine reason an employee fails to show up for work. Workplaces should create a supportive environment in which employees feel comfortable talking to frontline managers or supervisors about stressors outside of the workplace.

> Remember to reward good behavior. If someone does not show up to do their job, it puts a strain on the entire team. Be sure to acknowledge the employees who do show up on time every day to keep the operation running.

Fending Off Challenges: Employee Recognition

The importance of recognizing good behavior should not be overlooked. One recent survey found that employees who do not feel recognized at work are *twice as likely to say they intend to quit in the next year*, and employees who are recognized are more loyal and engaged.[11] The same study reports that up to 76% of Millennials *say they would leave a job if they did not feel appreciated*. Consider these statistics in light of another finding of the same study: only one in three workers in the United States "strongly agree" that they *received recognition or praise for doing good work in the past 7 days*.[11]

Recognizing employees for good attendance and performance can be one of the lowest-cost, highest-impact strategies available. While you may want to focus on disciplining the employees with poor performance, you do not want to lose the great employees you already have. If you are in a union environment, the union contract will need to be reviewed for what has been negotiated. Motivate employees to do their best work by offering rewards they will not want to miss, like an extra day off or a chance to choose their own schedule for a week. There is no quick solution when it comes to managing employee absenteeism, but key elements include having a fair attendance policy, documenting and tracking attendance patterns, addressing absences when they occur, and recognizing good attendance.[11] Remember, recognition can be one of your most affordable and effective tools for addressing attendance and absenteeism.

Employee Onboarding

The first 90 days on the job are the most important for any employee. Hourly workers have a relatively high turnover rate, and effective onboarding is especially crucial for their retention. Turnover is typically high during the early phase of employment; it is not unusual for 50% of an organization's hourly employees to leave within 120 days of hire. Well-planned onboarding has been found to have a strong positive effect on adjustment and work outcomes for new hires with limited prior work experience, which is often the case with the individuals being hired into entry-level hourly positions.[12]

Appropriate and comprehensive onboarding can reduce turnover and associated costs such as recruitment costs and overtime for other employees needing to pick up additional shifts and hours. Turnover and its related costs drain the organization of time, energy, and resources. Standardized onboarding gives you a competitive edge. When employees are not scrambling to fill positions and juggle multiple roles, they can focus entirely on the work in front of them. The result is happier, more productive employees.[12]

Onboarding provides new hires with the information they need to do their jobs. Virtually no one walks into a new job knowing exactly what to do and how to do it. The onboarding process should start even before you begin hiring. Start by developing an onboarding checklist to ensure all essential steps for new hires are completed in a timely way. The checklist should include administrative tasks, such as setting up a new hire's email address, granting them timeclock access, and ensuring they have access to all the tools and information they need to perform their duties.

Before the new employee's first day arrives, send a welcome email or call them to discuss the start time, dress code, where to park, and their schedule. This can help the employee feel well prepared and less nervous on the first day. If possible, employee benefit documents and forms should also be provided in advance, giving employees the opportunity to review and complete them prior to their start date.[13]

Another way to make new employees feel comfortable prior to the first day of work could be to allow for an unpaid "shadowing" experience as part of the interview process. This also allows you to engage current staff and provides feedback on the "fit" between the interviewee and the team.

Make sure that your current employees and supervisors are aware that a new team member is starting and the role the new employee will be assigned. It's a good idea to designate a champion or mentor for the new employee. This person might eat lunch with the new hire and remain available to answer questions as the new team member gets acclimated to the organization and their role.[13]

Incorporate some fun into the onboarding process; skip the standard organizational chart in favor of one that includes photos and hobbies of staff members. A visual representation of the organization not only makes it easier for the new hire to learn names but can reduce the anxiety of approaching someone they have never met. Get to know your new employee by asking their favorite food or beverage, restaurant, hobby, and whether they prefer to be recognized publicly or in private.

An onboarding checklist can be an effective tool in managing the onboarding process. The checklist should include key areas of knowledge that would be most beneficial for the new employee to learn right away to function in their new role. Consider the following steps when developing an onboarding checklist:

1. Start by surveying both the management team and staff. They will have valuable feedback about what is important for a new employee to learn in the first 4 weeks of employment.

2. Include your organization's strategic focus in the materials you provide the new employee. Add modules, videos, or recorded webinars to be reviewed with sign off. Provide hyperlinks for each item for ease of locating the information.

3. Send a welcome email to each new employee with an assigned champion, along with a copy of the onboarding checklist. The champion can be an employee currently working in the role who can help develop skills, answer questions, and offer guidance. The champion should set up weekly meetings or calls with the new employee to provide support and monitor progress.

4. At 30, 60, and 90 days after completing the onboarding checklist, meet or schedule follow-up calls with the new employee. Ask a series of questions in each of these conversations to determine how the team member is acclimating to your department.

At the 30-day follow-up, questions might include the following:

- What do you like about the job and organization?

- Have you faced any surprises since joining us?

At the 60-day follow-up, questions might include the following:

- Do you have access to the appropriate tools and resources?

- Comparing what we explained you would be doing during your interview with what you've experienced since you started here, have you experienced any specific challenges?

At the 90-day follow-up, questions might include the following:

- Which coworkers have been helpful to you since you arrived? (You can then recognize those individuals with an email or letter.)
- Do you believe your ideas and suggestions are valued? Can you share an example?

Having a formal onboarding follow-up will help the new employee feel supported, and you will also gain valuable information to make your program stronger.

Training New Employees

You can hire the best talent, but without the proper training, your employees cannot do their jobs properly and reach their full potential. Training is an investment that employers make in their work force. When organizations offer training and education to their employees, they indicate that they value their people and the contributions they make. By now, you know that people are the most important asset of any organization. Simply stated, providing training is one of the most impactful actions a manager can take. The prime motivator for employee training is to improve productivity and performance. The best place to start is with the topic that is most important to your employees: the knowledge, skills, and motivation they need to do their job. On-the-job training is vital to your employees' success and requires a process to track development, provide feedback, teach employees how to apply what they have learned, and ensure they understand the impact of their new knowledge.[14]

A training guide for each position in your department is important to effectively communicate the day-to-day functions, tasks, and expectations of a position. This type of structured training not only starts a new employee off on the right path but also allows you to cross-train current employees or develop a path for an employee looking to move to the next role or level. Box 5.1 provides an example of a training program.

BOX 5.1 Example of an Effective Training Program

There are many effective training programs a manager might want to implement. This example is an illustration of one program designed to assess the key tasks and activities associated with a specific role. The goal is to use the information to improve the onboarding process for new employees hired to fill the same position. The following step-by-step plan outlines this process:

1. Managers are asked to collaborate with their direct reports currently working in the role the new employee is being hired to fill.

2. Managers ask one or more team members in that role to record all of the tasks that would be needed to train a new employee to do the job well. This recording is done over a few days, with current team members recording which tasks they did at which time of day or on which day of the week.

3. The manager then compiles the reports to obtain a comprehensive view of what the new hire will need to understand, expect, and be trained to do. (Don't forget daily nonnegotiable items, such as shift huddles!)

4. The training process generally takes between 3 and 10 working days to complete, depending on the complexity of the position and the time available for training. During this period, the manager, designated trainer, and new employee should have a daily sign-off on what training was accomplished.

5. At the end of this training period, the manager creates a document listing any remaining competencies the new employee needs to demonstrate before working on related tasks without supervision. In addition to listing pending competencies, indicate the current status of each and include space in the document for progress reports every 2 weeks until competency has been demonstrated.

Management Training

Another essential component of an organization's training program is management training. Many employees join an organization not just to have a job but to develop a career. Opportunities for advancement and engagement are essential to employee retention and performance. Training helps employees realize their goals by giving them the education they need to do their jobs better and learn about new opportunities and skills they can use in the future. Management training is the best place to start setting expectations for your management team. Training should be the most basic requirement for all managers in your organization. Among the most useful skills that can be addressed in training are manager communication, employee motivation, and employee recognition. Having a solid employee development program can be seen as a benefit, build loyalty, and keep employees engaged at work. An employee development program will increase employees' skills, help identify employees' strengths and weaknesses, and train current employees for possible future promotions.[14]

When training managers, have them spend time doing hands-on training in a variety of positions to better understand the role and responsibilities. For additional information on professional staff development, see Chapter 7.

Benchmarking and Performance Improvement

Key Performance Indicators

Benchmarking and key performance indicators (KPIs) are excellent tools and strategies for monitoring and improving a department's performance. A KPI is a performance measurement that is used to evaluate how effectively your organization is achieving its key objectives. KPIs are equally effective for foodservice operations in hospitals, retirement homes, rehabilitation facilities, residential treatment centers, and schools. They allow you to measure, evaluate, and make adjustments within your department for growth and success. Performance of any foodservice department cannot improve unless it is measured. KPIs should provide the answers to the most important questions on the goals set for improvement. Remember the adage: "What matters gets measured!"[15]

The first step in benchmarking is to select KPIs. All selected KPIs must reflect the goals of the organization and measure the performance of the foodservice department. KPIs should be quantifiable and measurable. Every foodservice department should have KPIs to monitor, evaluate, and improve. Beyond being useful, simple measurement tools, KPIs can also detect potential problems.[16]

Dashboards such as the one shown in Figure 5.1 enable the foodservice leader to track key metrics and make changes to business operations as needed.

Monitoring KPIs can also help you control the major expenses of labor, food, equipment, and supplies. Often, the first reaction to controlling labor cost might be to schedule fewer hours, avoid filling open positions, or reduce staffing. All of these steps would have a direct negative impact on customer satisfaction. In food service as elsewhere, one effective way to control labor costs without compromising service

FIGURE 5.1 Sample Foodservice Department Dashboard

Chelsea Shores Foodservice Department Dashboard

Current Month: June   **Fiscal Year Ends:** December 31

Category	Key Performance Indicator (KPI)	Last Month	Current Month	Target
Safety	Number of accidents	1	0	0 = Target 1 or more = Below Target
Operations	Overtime hours worked	400	290	250 or less = Exceeds Target 251-300 = Meets Target 301 or more = Below Target
	Food cost per meal served	2.22	1.90	1.85 and below = Exceeds Target 1.86-1.95 = Meets Target 1.95 and above = Below Target
	Labor cost per meal served	5.20	4.98	4.99 or less = Exceeds Target 5.00-5.15 = Meets Target 5.16 and above = Below Target
Finance	Net revenue	86% of budget	90% of budget	105% of budget or greater = Exceeds Target 100% of budget = Target 99% of budget or less = Below Target
Patient Satisfaction	Rating on quality of food question (5-point scale)	4.22	4.36	4.50 or higher = Exceeds Target 4.30-4.49 = Meets Target 4.29 or lower = Below Target

Legend: Below Target   Target   Exceeds Target

is to train employees. Proper training improves efficiency, which means you can have a leaner workforce without sacrificing customer service. Improving employee retention is important to controlling labor costs. It is well documented that replacing existing employees costs more in the long run than retaining them. Training new hires is an investment of time, resources, and money. Recognizing and rewarding employees improves retention and providing growth opportunities also helps reduce turnover.[16,17]

Analyze all of your processes such as inventory control and scheduling to see if you can identify improvements. To increase efficiency, use a SWOT (strengths, weaknesses, opportunities, and threats) analysis or other quality improvement tools.

Optimized Scheduling

An optimized schedule can save time, improve workforce efficiency, and reduce labor costs. Create a schedule that balances both employee and departmental needs. For example, if you focus mainly on the department needs without considering employees' needs, employee morale, performance, and absenteeism will suffer. Use industry benchmarks to help determine the staffing needed, and regularly analyze your schedule and scheduling processes to identify problems and find solutions. Some scheduling options to consider include the following:

> Change shifts to 10 or 12 hours rather than 8 hours.
> Stagger start times to increase shift coverage.
> Hire more part-time employees rather than full-time employees, or use a pro re nata (PRN) staff person for coverage on an as-needed basis.

Effective employee scheduling can be an ongoing and tricky process. Using industry benchmarks to support the required changes will be your most effective strategy.[18]

Practical Performance Improvement Strategies

It is important to encourage your employees to focus on and improve their performance every day. Some managers think that if they write a memo about service concerns and post it on the employee bulletin board, they have communicated effectively. Covering a topic once in a huddle meeting or putting it in a memo does not mean that the issue will be resolved immediately—or ever. Hospitality requires daily attention and coaching. When you work to improve a particular area, expect the change to be slow. Even after that area has improved, it will need to be revisited and monitored. If you stop focusing on that particular area, within a few months you may find that the problem has returned.[19,20] You may need to reinforce the change until the change becomes a habit.

Getting employees to connect their work with the bigger picture has become an important topic of conversation and research. Your employees are internal stakeholders who deserve to know the work they do matters.[19] One way to accomplish this is to share customer stories, such as the one in following the Stories From the Field box.

> **STORIES FROM THE FIELD:** Sharing a Customer Story

It is important for any foodservice department to identify and comply with allergies and food intolerances. A food and nutrition department director received an email from an employee working in a different department. The employee stated that they had recently been diagnosed with irritable bowel syndrome, and certain foods and ingredients could trigger a strong reaction from which recovery could take multiple days. The email went on to say that the employee would need to ask questions about food items and how they were prepared in the cafeteria to be an advocate for their health.

The purpose of sharing this information was to help the food and nutrition staff understand the motivation behind the questions; the employee was not being difficult, just demonstrating reasonable concern for their health.

A real-life story is a powerful tool. The director invited this employee to the next department meeting to share this story in person. This had a great impact on the employees attending the meeting, as it allowed them to connect compassion and empathy to those they serve. In their willingness to share their story in person, the employee who wrote the email made the impact of the situation far greater and enduring than had the manager simply shared the email with the team.

Employee Empowerment and Recognition

Empower your employees to speak up. *Empowerment* means valuing employees and giving them the information and tools they need to achieve results. Create a culture where opinions matter and are taken seriously. Employees who understand the "why" behind customer service are far more likely to provide great experiences to the people they serve.[20] Empowerment will change the role of the manager from "boss" to "coach."

Recognition matters. Just like with KPIs, what matters gets measured, and what you reward gets repeated. Recognition is absolutely essential in a great organization, and it does not need to be complicated or expensive. Ask your employees what type of recognition is most meaningful to them. You may be surprised to find how simple, genuine expressions of gratitude inspire people to do their best.[19]

While it is crucial to recognize major accomplishments, an everyday expression of thanks can motivate employees just as much. Recognition helps employees see that their organization values them. Celebrating National Foodservice Workers Week is another way to recognize your team. If you have limited funds, write a letter to each employee, recognizing them for the specific work they do, and mail the letter to their home. What a surprise to receive a thank-you letter from the boss at home! Recognition is something all employees appreciate and respond to. Frequent and visible recognition reminds everyone that they are all working toward a shared goal. Offer recognition as close as possible to when the event took place. When an employee performs positively, provide recognition immediately. It's likely the employee is already feeling good about their performance; your timely recognition of the employee will enhance the positive feelings. This positively affects the employee's confidence in their ability to perform well in their position.[20]

Why Company Culture Matters

How would you describe your organization's culture? Culture is less about a written policy and more about people, especially in a service-oriented business like food service. Culture matters because *culture is what sets you apart.* After all, if you are not different, how can you be the best?

Hiring for Fit

To create a hospitality culture, it is important to have a defined mission and values. Your mission and values must be more than just words, and they need to relate back directly to the goals of the organization. Hire people who are committed to these same values. Then, train to your values, measure employees against your values, and reward and recognize based on your values.[21] An interview guide based on your values is a helpful tool to hiring for culture. (Remember that skills can always be trained.) Interview questions can be categorized by your company values. Ask the candidate at least one question related to each value. For example, an interview question for hospitality might be, "We all have our ups and downs. When your mood is not the best, how do you ensure you will still provide excellent customer service?" Use a rating scale to rate the answer (eg, 1 might mean "unacceptable" and 5 might mean "exceptional"). Based on the total score, the determination can be made about whether to move the candidate to the next step in the hiring process.[21]

When you hire people who fit well with your culture, you are more likely to secure a long-term commitment from them. The following Stories From the Field box provides an example of a manager who engaged employees to change the culture of the department with stunning results.

> **STORIES FROM THE FIELD: An Example of Hospitality Culture Change**
>
> Changing the culture of an organization can be very challenging. Culture cannot be mandated. One manager who needed to change the hospitality and service culture in their department decided the best way would be through new experiences. These included:
>
> » inviting employees to hospital meetings to help demonstrate what professional behavior looked like;
>
> » taking frontline employees out to a restaurant so they could experience hospitality;
>
> » planning celebrations, such as bowling parties or ordering pizza or chicken wings; and
>
> » offering verbal recognition sincerely and frequently.
>
> When this manager started, the patient satisfaction was in the first percentile. Nine months later, patient satisfaction scores had soared to above the 60th percentile.

Managing Hospitality Culture

Managing your hospitality culture for success is more about a feeling you create than putting specific programs in place. The concept of a service culture can be defined as having a shared purpose under which everyone is focused on creating value for others in the organization and those they serve. A service culture exists when you motivate the employees in your organization to take a customer-centric approach to their regular work duties.

When employees know what is expected of them, have the tools to do their jobs, and believe their managers support them, employees will commit to accomplishing the goals of the department. A culture of hospitality flourishes in a workplace where the employees are appreciated and supported.[21] Achieving culture change can take time, but with active leadership commitment, positive results can be seen early in the process. Once employees become aware that the culture is changing for the better, they will be more willing to adapt and change.

Empathy

An important aspect of having a hospitality culture is empathy. Simply put, *empathy* means putting yourself in the shoes of another person. An organizational culture that emphasizes empathy is sure to stand out. Empathy is more than just words, and it only works if it is genuinely offered. If empathy comes from having similar experiences, the easiest way to help foodservice employees become more empathetic is to put them in their customers' shoes.[22] An exercise in teaching empathy is outlined in Box 5.2.

BOX 5.2 An Exercise in Teaching Empathy

Many people think empathy is either a trait a person has or doesn't have, but empathy can be taught. This exercise is one way to do just that with your team.

1. Pass out two cotton balls, two foodservice gloves, and two pieces of tape to each employee present.

2. Ask each employee to put on the foodservice gloves, tape two fingers together on one hand and tape a knuckle on the other hand. Then place the cotton balls in their ears.

3. Explain to the employees that these actions just aged them by 20 years. The gloves demonstrate decreased sensitivity, the taped fingers demonstrate arthritis, and the cotton balls demonstrate loss of hearing. Sensory limitations such as sight changes, hearing loss, arthritis, and reduced mobility are common for older patients.

4. Ask your employees to take a critical look at the patient food trays. Begin a discussion with some questions, such as the following:

   › Are fruits cut into bite-sized pieces?

   › Is the lettuce completely chopped?

   › Are packets for condiments or dressings easy to open?

   › Are the team members conscious of acoustic challenges in the department's public spaces, and can they think of ways to minimize the challenges these pose for people with limited hearing?

   › What could team members do to demonstrate empathy for the people they serve?

Making adjustments as needed can help *all* patients feel appreciated and cared for.

Summary

Leadership skills must be learned and practiced. In foodservice management, focusing on developing the right skills to solve problems is critical. Leaders in the food industry need to think beyond the specific area in which they currently work. Approaching food service in an open-minded and cross-disciplinary way will achieve better results for business growth, well-being, food production, and environmental sustainability. Leaders build relationships with employees who help turn a vision into reality. By equipping yourself with critical thinking skills, you will be able to make an impact in your organization and your profession.

REFERENCES

1   The difference between leadership and management. Next Generation website. Accessed February 8, 2020. www.nextgeneration.ie/blog/2018/03/the-difference-between-leadership-and-management

2   Berthelsen RM, Barkley WC, Oliver PM, McLymont V, Pukett R. Academy of Nutrition and Dietetics: Revised 2014 standards of professional performance for registered dietitian nutritionists in management of food and nutrition systems. *J Acad Nutr Diet.* 2014;11(7):P1104-1112. E21. doi.10.1016/j.jand.2014.03.017

3   Bell R. Effective communication in leadership. West Bend website. Accessed February 8, 2020. www.thesilverlining.com/resources/blog/effective-communication-in-leadership

4   Reducing absenteeism in the workplace. Employee Benefits website. Accessed February 9, 2020. https://employeebenefits.co.uk/reducing-absenteeism-workplace

5   Center for Creative Leadership. Why communication is so important for leaders. Accessed February 9, 2020. Center for Creative Leadership website. www.ccl.org/articles/leading-effectively-articles/communication-1-idea-3-facts-5-tips

6   Four steps to improve employee engagement. Gallup website. Accessed April 7, 2022. www.quantumworkplace.com/future-of-work/employee-engagement-trends

7   Barrett Q. Benefits of effective leadership communication. People Element website. Accessed February 9, 2020. https://peopleelement.com/benefits-effective-leadership-communication

8   Harrison K. Good communication can hugely lift employee engagement. Accessed February 9, 2020. https://cuttingedgepr.com/good-communication-can-hugely-lift-employee-engagement

9   Employee engagement and leader approachability: new Gallup research. Approachable Leadership website. Accessed February 9, 2020. https://approachableleadership.com/employee-engagement-approachability

10 Resources. Management in Food and Nutrition Systems website. 2022. Accessed April 7, 2022. www.rdmanager.org/page/resources

11 Mann A, Dvorak N. Employee recognition: low cost, high impact. Gallup website. June 28, 2016. Accessed April 3, 2022. www.gallup.com/workplace/236441/employee-recognition-low-cost-high-impact.aspx%22%20/t%20%22_blank

12 Krauss AD. Starting them off on the right foot: why onboarding is important. TLNT Talent Management & HR website. Accessed February 15, 2020. www.tlnt.com/starting-them-off-on-the-right-foot-why-onboarding-is-important

13 Reinhart C. Organizational culture in the hospitality industry. CHRON website. Accessed February 16, 2020. https://smallbusiness.chron.com/organizational-culture-hospitality-industry-12969.html

14 Horowitz B, Horowitz A. Why it's crucial to train your employees. Insider. Accessed February 16, 2020. www.businessinsider.com/why-its-crucial-to-train-your-employees-2010-5

15 What is a Key Performance Indicator (KPI)? KPI.org website. Accessed April 7, 2022. https://kpi.org/KPI-Basics

16 Pezzini G. The top key performance indicators every restaurant CEO should track. LS Retail website. Accessed February 16, 2020. www.lsretail.com/resources/top-key-performance-indicators-every-restaurant-ceo-track

17 Ramesh S, Manimegalai B, Valsan A. Hospital food service key performance indicators. *IJARIIT*. 2019;5:779-781.

18 Darlington N. Nine steps on how to schedule employees effectively. 7Shifts website. Accessed February 22, 2020. www.7shifts.com/blog/how-to-schedule-employees-effectively

19 Heathfield SM. How to empower your employees. The Balance Careers website. Accessed March 1, 2020. www.thebalancecareers.com/empowerment-in-action-how-to-empower-your-employees-1918102

20 Zhang K. How to empower your employees to do their best work. Entrepreneur website. Accessed March 1, 2020. www.entrepreneur.com/article/334710

21 Snower S. Culture does matter—big time! Foodservice Equipment & Supplies website. 2020. Accessed February 22, 2020. http://fesmag.com/topics/perspectives/point-of-view/5998-culture-does-matter-%E2%80%93-big-time

22 Goh G. Empathy: the must-have skill for all customer service reps. Catcat website. Accessed April 1, 2022. www.catcat.com/student/activity/440353-empathy-the-must-have-skill-for-all-customer-service-reps

CHAPTER 6

Public Health & Population Health Management & Leadership

Samia Hamdan, MPH, RDN, and Janelle Gunn, MPH, RD

The findings and conclusions in this chapter are those of the authors, written in their personal capacity, and do not necessary reflect the official position of the Centers for Disease Control and Prevention or the US Department of Agriculture.

Introduction

Public health is an evolving profession that can trace its roots back to ancient Rome and Greece. In recent centuries, public health became formalized through the establishment of international, national, state, and local organizations and governmental agencies dedicated to protecting the health of the public. The inception of public health agencies in the United States began at the grassroots levels; in fact, the New York City Health Department, created in 1866, was the first of its kind.[1] Since that time, many leading public health organizations were formed, including the Centers for Disease Control and Prevention (CDC), which was formally created in 1946 as the United States' leading public health agency. Along with the establishment of these new organizations came many public health advancements in the 20th century. According to the CDC, between 1900 and 1999, the average lifespan in the United States increased by 30 years, mostly due to substantial accomplishments in public health.[2]

Public health is defined in different ways by various organizations. It is also used interchangeably with the terms *population health* or *community health*. The American Public Health Association defines it as follows: "Public health promotes and protects the health of people and the communities where they live, learn, work and play."[3] The CDC refers to the popular definition originating with American bacteriologist and public health pioneer Charles-Edward Amory Winslow; Winslow said public health was "the science and art of preventing disease, prolonging life, and promoting health through the organized efforts and informed choices of society, organizations, public and private communities, and individuals."[4] The shared aspect of many definitions is that public health is an interdisciplinary profession that takes a societal approach to preventing disease. Policy, epidemiology, education, disaster preparedness and response, research, and community design can all be part of this interdisciplinary approach. While working with communities most in need and addressing that health disparities have been longstanding components of public health nutrition, there are also increasing efforts underway to address social determinants of health and racism. This chapter provides a broad view of nutrition-related public health and population leadership and management as it relates to the registered dietitian nutritionist (RDN). It also offers advice on how to increase skills and experience in this critically important field.

Defining Public Health Nutrition

Improving nutrition is one of the critical components of public health. Not only has it led to historical advancements through the establishment of national standards for food labeling and safety, but science has also demonstrated that improved nutrition is an effective tool in preventing many chronic diseases. The *2020–2025 Dietary Guidelines for Americans* include recommendations for the general public that have been scientifically proven to reduce the risk of cardiovascular disease, type 2 diabetes, some types of cancer, overweight and obesity, and possibly neurocognitive disorders.[5] With many leading causes of death currently attributed to diet and physical inactivity, the field of nutrition is an integral component of public health.

Public health nutrition is a term that emerged in recent decades to help formally define and establish this important intersection. The Academy of Nutrition and Dietetics defines public health nutrition as "the application of nutrition and public health principles to design programs, systems, policies, and environments that aim to improve or maintain the optimal health of populations and targeted groups."[6] Many public health nutritionists are credentialed as RDNs, and some have a master's degree in public health or another science-related degree. Public health nutritionists work in a wide variety of settings both traditional and nontraditional, including government agencies, nonprofit organizations, local health agencies, food manufacturing industries, research institutions, universities, schools, tribal organizations, food banks, hospitals, relief organizations, and many other settings around the world.

A survey conducted in 2021 by the Academy of Nutrition and Dietetics Public Health/Community Nutrition Dietetic Practice Group (PHCNPG) revealed that its members work in diverse settings and capacities.[7] Areas of nutrition practice included maternal and child health; the Special Supplemental Nutrition Program for Women, Infants, and Children (WIC); contributing to the Dietary Guidelines for Americans; older adult nutrition; the Supplemental Nutrition Assistance Program (SNAP); SNAP Education (SNAP-Ed), child and adult care food programs; school lunch programs; food sustainability; local municipal food policy; food recovery/food waste; international nutrition, and other related areas.[7] In addition, the survey revealed that many members work with populations across the human lifespan. Given the reach that public health nutritionists have through the various populations they serve and the wide variety of settings in which they work, opportunities abound for making decisions, influencing the field, and having an impact at various levels—from individuals to national or global efforts.

Public Health Programs and Services

Many programs and services impact public health nutrition. For example, several federal programs support public health nutrition initiatives nationally and globally. These programs are administered and operated at a multitude of levels, including community, local, state, national, and international, and represent one part of the public health nutrition workforce. For example, the US Department of Agriculture (USDA) administers 15 nutrition assistance programs that reach 1 in 4 Americans. These programs are operated in schools, child and adult day care settings, WIC clinics, food banks, farmers markets, and many other settings. The USDA also issues science-based nutrition guidance and nutrition education, coordinates nutrition policy, and ensures that the supply of meat, poultry, and egg products is safe and properly labeled.[8]

The US Department of Health and Human Services (HHS) is made up of several operating divisions that impact nutrition, including the CDC, Indian Health Service (IHS), National Institutes of Health (NIH), and the US Food and Drug Administration (FDA). The CDC monitors the nutrition status of Americans at the state and national levels, along with the presence of related policies and practices at the state and local levels.[9-11] The CDC also funds states and communities in implementing evidence-based nutrition strategies.[12] The IHS provides direct medical and public health services to American Indian and Alaska Native people, including diabetes treatment and prevention programs.[13] The NIH supports research in the areas of basic science, clinical studies, and innovative research to develop effective strategies for dietary behavior change.

The FDA provides oversight of more than $1.5 trillion of food, cosmetics, and dietary supplements crossing state and country lines to ensure these products are safe. The historical significance of the inception of the FDA is outlined in Upton Sinclair's classic novel, *The Jungle*, which exposes and details the brutal working conditions and contaminated meat resulting from unregulated meat-packing facilities.[14] The FDA has modernized the Nutrition Facts labels found on packaged foods and also implemented menu and vending machine nutrition labeling laws as part of its Nutrition Innovation Strategy launched in 2018.[15] These efforts, aimed at addressing poor nutrition and chronic disease in the United States, help consumers make informed decisions when eating food away from home. These federally funded programs and services offer many opportunities for RDNs to serve as the leading nutrition experts across collaborative, multisector teams aimed at improving public health.

International organizations have also committed services to improve public health nutrition worldwide. In 2016, the United Nations (UN) launched the United Nations Decade of Action on Nutrition, with a goal of providing equitable access to healthy diets across all populations globally. The formal call to action acknowledges that malnutrition exists in three forms across the world, including undernutrition, micronutrient deficiency, and overweight and obesity. The 10-year plan, running from 2016 through 2025, invites countries to submit their individual plans that commit to eliminating malnutrition and preventing noncommunicable diseases. The Food and Agriculture Organization of the United Nations and the World Health Organization (WHO), both subsets of the UN, have taken the lead on this effort.[16]

Public health nutrition has also played a critical role in disaster preparedness and response. Natural disasters and public health emergencies can have a tremendous impact on the infrastructure, delivery, and availability of food. Most recently, the COVID-19 pandemic, which has afflicted millions of people worldwide, caused disruptions in the food supply by shutting down food manufacturing plants, retail food outlets, restaurants, and institutions that serve food to millions of people, such as schools. This public health emergency called for government response to purchase and deliver foods and provide additional services to ensure foods were provided to communities in need. During other disasters—whether naturally occurring, such as hurricanes, or caused by human beings, such as water contamination—similar government responses have been implemented to ensure safe and equitable food access across populations in the United States. This includes broad education focused on food safety, the role of nutrition, and preventive practices.

Leadership Skills and Qualities in Public Health

Public health nutritionists are in a position to provide strong leadership. As addressed in the previous section, their services impact many different human populations. In addition to the leadership skills addressed in Chapters 1 and 2 of this book, Stephen Covey, author of *The 7 Habits of Highly Effective People*, identifies four essential leadership attributes that drive teams into success and can be directly applied by public health nutritionists. Covey asserts that leaders of successful teams must inspire trust, create vision, execute strategy, and coach potential.[17] Inspiring trust among others can be done in a variety of ways. For public health nutrition leaders, it means projecting a strong sense of competence, expertise, and a willingness to work alongside others to create a vision and accomplish a public health goal. Public health nutrition leaders can also exude strong influence by executing strategy and communicating their vision and by negotiating buy-in from stakeholders to help execute this vision. An example of building trust could be bringing a variety of community voices together to collectively discuss issues, solutions, and community needs and following through on prioritized areas. As a subject matter expert in nutrition, public health nutrition leaders can coach potential in others and provide continuous feedback to the team on the progress and outcomes.

Leadership Gaps and Opportunities

There are existing gaps and leadership opportunities for RDNs working in public health and community nutrition. Many of these were identified by nutrition professionals at an open roundtable discussion on public health nutrition leadership facilitated by the PHCNPG at the 2016 Food & Nutrition Conference & Expo (FNCE). Three of the challenges identified were a lack of formalized training about leadership, a lack of promoting RDNs as leaders and subject matter experts, and a lack of upward mobility in many organizations. However, leadership opportunities do exist throughout the career path of an RDN working in public health nutrition. RDNs in public health can serve in leadership positions as directors, managers, team leaders, supervisors, and project coordinators as part of their official work capacity. Public health nutrition professionals can also serve in leadership positions as volunteers and advocates throughout their communities. For example, they can serve on local food policy councils, wellness councils, school district committees, and other community-led committees. Volunteering and increasing visibility through media and marketing opportunities may also help promote leadership for RDNs in public health community nutrition.

Attendees at the 2016 FNCE who participated in the open roundtable discussion on public health leadership were also asked to define what leadership meant to them. The qualities identified were being supportive, being a good listener, and being transparent. Strategies such as mentoring, succession planning, involvement in local and national associations, and formalized teaching were identified as ways to help build leadership skills in the profession. Attendees suggested that the strategies identified at the roundtable be implemented with students and continued across the life of the profession during both the dietetic internship and career phase of a public health RDN. They further suggested promoting and enhancing the management skillset of all RDNs (such as supervisory and budgeting experience), increasing visibility, and utilizing professional organizational resources to provide these opportunities.

There is no "traditional" or "best" career path, and one's path does not necessarily need to include a management position. Management may occur at any stage of your career, and volunteer work may also provide essential leadership experience.

Assessing and Building Public Health Skills

The *Guide for Developing and Enhancing Skills in Public Health and Community Nutrition*, developed by the PHCNPG and the Association of State Public Health Nutritionists (ASPHN), provides a comprehensive self-assessment tool that covers the following six areas of core competency[18]:

1. Food and nutrition
2. Communications, marketing, and cultural sensitivity
3. Advocacy and education
4. Policy, system, and environmental change
5. Research and evaluation
6. Management and leadership

Figure 6.1 presents one example of the self-assessment for management and leadership competency development from the guide.[18]

FIGURE 6.1 Sample self-assessment tool for management and leadership competencies

Self-Assessment Tool

	Knowledge What is your level of knowledge related to...			Confidence How confident are you in your abilities related to...					
	Little or no	General	Thorough	Not at all	Not very	Moderately	Very	Extremely	Guide Knowledge & Skills Reference Number
Management & Leadership									
■ Ensuring adherence to legal and ethical principles	○	○	○	○	○	○	○	○	ML1
■ Identifying visions, missions, and goals of health agencies	○	○	○	○	○	○	○	○	ML2
■ Applying principles of community engagement, assessment, and program development	○	○	○	○	○	○	○	○	ML3
■ Applying management principles	○	○	○	○	○	○	○	○	ML4
■ Enhancing consumer participation in public health nutrition programs and services	○	○	○	○	○	○	○	○	ML5
■ Establishing priorities, goals, and SMART objectives for public health nutrition programs	○	○	○	○	○	○	○	○	ML6
■ Identifying community assets, social capital, and other resources	○	○	○	○	○	○	○	○	ML7

Abbreviation: SMART = specific, measureable, acheivable, relevant, and time bound

Reprinted with permission from Sisk K, Conneally A, Cullinen K. *Guide for Developing and Enhancing Skills in Public Health and Community Nutrition.* 3rd ed. Public Health/Community Nutrition Practice Group of the Academy of Nutrition and Dietetics, and the Association of State Public Health Nutritionist;. 2018. Accessed November 24, 2021. www.phcnpg.org/phcn/resources/2018-3rd-edition-the-guide[18]

After completing the self-assessment, develop a targeted work plan to expand these skills, including dates for completion of key activities. Figure 6.2 illustrates a sample workplan for developing targeted management and leadership skills identified from completing the self-assessment in the guide.[18]

 FIGURE 6.2 Sample work plan for management and leadership competencies

Management & Leadership ■

RDN	NDTR	Suggested Work-Related & Learning Activities	Example Resources
ML5. Public Participation Utilizes community engagement strategies to enhance consumer participation in health, food, and nutrition programs and services, including collaborating with public/private sectors, participating in outreach and referral systems, and working with voluntary and community organizations.	**ML5. Management and Leadership** Recognizes the principles of management in community-based public health nutrition programming, including community engagement, community assessment, planning, marketing, implementation, and evaluation of community-based public health nutrition programs, policies, and services.	■ Describe the Principles of Community Engagement in community health improvement; List examples of their use by an international, federal, state, and/or local public health nutrition organization. ■ Describe the community engagement continuum as an organizing concept for engaging population segments by levels of engagement and participation; List examples of the community engagement continuum utilized by an international, federal, state, and/or local public health nutrition organization. ■ Explain the relationship of community engagement to collaborative decision-making and intervention design. ■ Interview a representative of a local public health organization (e.g., American Heart Association, American Cancer Society) regarding their community engagement practices; Summarize how their practices relate to the 10 Essential Public Essential Public Health Services and performance improvement.	■ Principles of Community Engagement – Second Edition, CDC https://www.atsdr.cdc.gov/communityengagement ■ Mobilizing for Action through Planning and Partnerships (MAPP), NACCHO http://archived.naccho.org/topics/infrastructure/mapp ■ The Public Health System and the 10 Essential Public Health Services, CDC https://www.cdc.gov/stltpublichealth/publichealthservices/essentialhealthservices.html

Abbreviations: NDTR = nutrition and dietetics technician registered | RDN = registered dietitian nutritionist

Reproduced with permission from Sisk K, Conneally A, Cullinen K. *Guide for Developing and Enhancing Skills in Public Health and Community Nutrition.* 3rd ed. Public Health/Community Nutrition Practice Group of the Academy of Nutrition and Dietetics, and the Association of State Public Health Nutritionists; 2018. Accessed November 24, 2021. www.phcnpg.org/phcn/resources/2018-3rd-edition-the-guide[18]

Opportunities for Leadership Development

Public health nutrition professionals can serve in a variety of leadership roles. In a formal capacity, they can serve as directors, supervisors, team leaders, and managers of teams. They can also serve as project coordinators, committee leaders, subject matter experts, advisors, advocates, and other more informal leadership roles. Leaders influence, motivate, inspire, assist, and provide guidance to others. These skillsets can be employed in any type of position. When it comes to being a leader, building and leveraging these skillsets is much more critical than carrying an official leadership title. Public health nutrition professionals can build their leadership skills in several ways.

Building Leadership Skills Within the Workplace or Current Role

Public health nutritionists may want to consider adding skillsets to prepare for critical leadership roles. Dietetic internship programs, leadership training programs for nutrition professionals, and continuing education are key ways of advancing public health leadership for nutrition. Within a current job, RDNs at any level of experience can begin developing themselves as leaders. See the Stories From the Field box on page 126 for an example of building and leveraging leadership skills. A variety of opportunities in current positions may be available.

Team building and collaboration RDNs can seek opportunities to lead a specific work project or ad hoc task force. Sometimes these opportunities must be sought out or requested by the RDN. For example, an RDN may inquire about joining the team to lead or colead a project for a new grant. If a program is implementing community-wide nutrition improvements, there could be an opportunity to lead one of the focused areas, such as activities that relate to young children or older adults. Often, RDNs can use leadership skills even when they are not in an official leadership role. Such circumstances may offer an opportunity for the RDN to practice their "influencing" skills to bring a cross-disciplinary team together to execute a project. There may be situations in which an RDN can negotiate buy-in from colleagues or stakeholders on a project or task. An example of this type of collaboration would be working with a team of individuals to assess whether a workplace offers foods consistent with nationally established foodservice guidelines. This could be an opportunity to bring a variety of stakeholders together to address the needs and challenges of implementing these guidelines. Committee members could include vending machine operators, cafeteria shop owners, employee wellness committee members, and building management. In addition, some worksites offer trainings or continuing education opportunities and team-building sessions. The RDN can explore these opportunities for career development. If leadership training courses are not offered by the employer, RDNs can inquire whether the employer would support taking leadership training elsewhere.

Using expertise as leverage In public health, sometimes having specialized expertise will give you an opportunity to gain leadership skills on a project or become a project leader. Nutrition expertise could strengthen applications for grants or cooperative agreements and could provide a unique angle to an interdisciplinary chronic disease project or initiative. Some examples of these projects are a chronic disease program expanding its work into nutrition; a local health department receiving a nutrition, physical activity, or tobacco cessation grant; or a WIC clinic educating a community about early childhood nutrition. Public health expertise can also be utilized in other settings or in the public health nutrition setting; some of these skillsets include program planning, policy development, grant writing, and evaluation.

Precepting students or interns Sometimes moving into more formal management positions requires previous experience supervising staff members. This can be a challenge if past positions did not provide opportunities for supervisory experience. A good way to gain experience is to start by precepting students or mentoring interns. As a preceptor, you can develop projects and timelines to meet competencies, help a student develop their skills, and provide performance coaching when necessary.

Succession planning Participating in succession planning (the process of passing on skills and knowledge to an individual succeeding you in a position) is another great opportunity to gain leadership skills. RDNs may want to ask themselves the following questions: Does my employer conduct succession planning? Is my employer open to me participating in the planning? What objectives have they laid out? Are there roles I can move into? Am I missing a skillset I need in order to fill a future role of interest?

Demonstrating cultural humility As discussed in Chapter 3, demonstrating cultural humility is critical to becoming a successful public health nutrition leader. The populations that public health nutrition programs serve are diverse. Understanding the community, building an inclusive table for program development, and including the community in planning, execution, and evaluation can improve the acceptance and success of public health strategies and intervention. To gain these types of experiences, you can serve on your organization's diversity and inclusion committee or host an event that builds awareness of underserved or underrepresented populations. You can also attend trainings and sessions on equity and access to public health services. For example, the Michigan State University Center for Regional Food Systems offers a variety of resources online, including papers on how to conduct inclusive meetings and collaborate with diverse local communities (www.canr.msu.edu/foodsystems/resources). You can help recruit members of teams, committees, community coalitions, or events that reflect diversity through race, gender, ethnicity, national origin, sexual orientation, political affiliations, socioeconomic status, age, and opinions and ideologies. Dietetic interns may seek rotations in underserved populations to gain direct service experiences.

> **STORIES FROM THE FIELD:** Building and Leveraging Leadership Skills
>
> A policy analyst on a team in the nutrition branch was interested in becoming a team lead or a deputy branch chief. In conducting a self-assessment of their skills and experience and comparing it to the qualifications for a deputy branch chief, the analyst identified a lack of budgeting experience. The analyst worked with their current team leader to gain some budgeting skills. The analyst was then assigned to oversee two projects that involved forecasting travel and costs for the year. The analyst was responsible for identifying travel needs, travel costs, and the staffing required for those business trips.
>
> By identifying an experience gap and working to build skills in that area, the analyst became better prepared to eventually serve as a team lead or deputy branch chief.

Formalized Leadership Training

Formalized leadership training could be a pathway to enhancing leadership skills, but only a few trainings specific to public health nutrition leadership exist. Leadership trainings are offered in the disciplines of public health, nutrition, and general professional leadership. Institutions such as the CDC, American Public Health Association, and various universities offer public health leadership training courses or programs.[19,20] RDNs can apply the lessons and skills they learn in leadership training in their current roles or in future ones. A comprehensive list of resources for advancing leadership in public health can be found on the Academy of Nutrition and Dietetics website.[21]

Cross-Training Leaders From Other Nutrition and Dietetics Sectors

RDNs who practice in other areas, such as clinical dietetics, may find opportunities to gain public health leadership skills by applying expertise from their own practice area to public health programs, policies, or issues. By training in public health leadership, RDNs from other areas can learn public health principles and approaches to which they may not otherwise be exposed. For example, academic research dietitians could gain experience and be an asset to a local or state health department that needs to analyze data to identify disparities and inequities. Another example could include clinical dietitians assisting in a community health initiative to reduce added sugars or sodium intake among local citizens. Clinical dietitians' knowledge about decreasing the sources of added sugars and sodium among individuals, as well as what motivates individuals and families to make changes, could be an asset to this community project. RDNs from sectors other than public health can be cross-trained to transition into public health roles. The ASPHN and the PHCNPG offer additional trainings on various public health topics.[22]

Finding a Mentor

The vast world of public health could be made smaller through mentoring. Finding and keeping a mentor can provide inroads to new opportunities and, at a minimum, a sounding board for career-related issues and discussions. Connecting with a mentor can happen through an informal or formal process. Many alumni associations, worksites, and professional organizations offer formal mentoring programs. In addition, many of these organizations are exploring new formats, such as speed mentoring and peer and group-based mentoring. A public health nutrition mentor will be able to show you at least some of the many roles a public health nutritionist can play.

Community and Local Leadership Experience

RDNs can gain leadership skills outside of their employment setting through civic engagement. Before undertaking any outside activity, understand whether your current employer has restrictions on who this can be with or how it should be done. Running for a local board position or accepting a volunteer role on a community task force can advance RDNs' leadership skills and enhance their resumes. Board service can increase RDNs' understanding and perspectives on constituent needs and provide experience collaborating with peers to achieve a common goal. These forms of community service can broaden RDNs' understanding of public health principles and expand their professional networks.

Dietetic Internship Programs

Students in dietetic internships can look for opportunities that increase their public health expertise. It may be that a dietetic intern seeks experiences with a strong public health focus or tries to build public health into an internship program. Program directors may be able to leverage relationships for placement in local, state, national, or international public health organizations. Students may also wish to work with a public health nutrition leader to help support their work. The student could identify field experiences related to public health. Even without formal public health rotations, most rotations could be applicable to public health. For example, an outpatient class in a clinic setting could be very much like a nutrition class in a community center.

Becoming a Leader: Challenges and Opportunities

Multiple Pathways to Leadership

If 10 public health nutrition leaders were interviewed, they would tell 10 different stories from 10 unique perspectives on how they paved their career paths. Some may have worked for years in a clinical setting before becoming public health leaders. Some may have become a dietitian as a second career. And some may have begun their path in public health right out of college. The variety of different public health nutrition positions and careers enables unique paths to public health leadership positions. These various and unique pathways all have pros and cons. For example, a position that provides many opportunities to be creative and take on new opportunities could naturally foster advancement—or it could prove extra challenging, since there isn't a clearly defined pathway to leadership.

Profiles of two RDN public health leaders, and their pathways to leadership, are discussed in the following Stories From the Field box.

STORIES FROM THE FIELD: Profiles of Public Health Leaders

Public Health Nutrition Leader Profile: Alice Lenihan, MPH, RD, LDN[a]

What was your path to public health leadership?
I was fortunate to begin my career in public health nutrition in the mid-1970s, a time when there was significant support for the provision of nutrition care and food assistance to at-risk populations. Milestone studies and reports led to expanded career opportunities for dietitians and public health nutritionists.

My entry into public health nutrition was as a [Special Supplemental Nutrition Program for Women, Infants, and Children (WIC)] director in northwest Montana at a county health department. The need to quickly organize and implement the WIC program provided the opportunity and experience in both clinical and management aspects of a public health program. In addition, a 1-year experience with the Indian Health Service as a WIC director enriched my professional experience.

Career opportunities at the state health department in North Carolina, completing my [master's in public health] degree, and increasing responsibilities all contributed to my leadership path. I was fortunate to work in a state health department with a long history and tradition of evidence-based practice and service to the community.

Professional organizations including the Academy of Nutrition and Dietetics, the Public Health and Community Nutrition Dietetic Practice Group, the Pediatric Nutrition Practice Group, and the Association of State Public Health Nutritionists were an essential part of my path. They offered the opportunity to contribute to the practice of dietetics through networking, sharing clinical expertise, and collaborative work, and to advance public policy.

What are some of the challenges you had to overcome during your leadership role(s)?
The rapid growth of the WIC program resulted in the need for workforce development, not only recruitment and retention of public health nutritionists but the need to ensure ongoing continuing education and a career path for advancement.

continued on next page

---

continued from previous page

What do you know now about public health leadership that you wish knew at the beginning of your career?

While I was passionate and committed to my work, there will always be someone or some groups who are not supportive. This may be due to use of government funds, [concerns about] the "Nanny State," alternative nutrition beliefs, distrust of government, and many other reasons. Be prepared to respond with honesty and follow evidence-based practice.

What is the most essential skill to being an effective public health leader?

Bring everyone to the table; we don't own it all. Input and partnership with a wide variety of health professionals, community leaders, consumers, business, academia, and faith communities are just a few. Interprofessional practice and education are key to our success. It is the team or organization that succeeds, not the individual leader.

Public Health Nutrition Leader Profile: Angie Tagtow, MS, RD, LD[b]

What was your path to public health leadership?

Following my undergraduate and graduate work, I knew I wanted to work in the prevention space and my first position as a registered dietitian was with the Iowa Department of Public Health WIC program. This was an amazing introduction to governmental public health, public policy, food and nutrition policy, and politics. Working at the state level offered opportunities to work "upstream" with [US Department of Agriculture (USDA)] regional and headquarter staff and to also work "downstream" in building capacity in local WIC agencies. This experience exposed me to the complex issues of food insecurity and poor health outcomes as well as the paradox of high rates of hunger in a state (Iowa) that dedicates more than 85% of its landscape to agriculture.

It was during this time that I became more engaged in local, state, and national groups that focused on ameliorating food insecurity, and I launched the *Journal of Hunger & Environmental Nutrition*, which focuses on global food and water system issues that impact access, nutrition, human health, and ecological health.

I then established a consulting firm that applied comprehensive solutions to address leading causes of diet-related chronic diseases using coordinated policy, system, and environmental strategies. The central tenet of the company was to use current scientific evidence and theoretical public health models to support the linkages between the health and availability of natural resources (soil, water, air, energy), to the health of the food system, and to the health of populations.

This work led to two dynamic fellowships that further built my tacit knowledge of the interconnections between food, policy, and sustainable agriculture. In 2014, I was appointed by President Barack Obama to serve as the executive director of USDA's Center for Nutrition Policy and Promotion and oversaw the development and launch of the *2015–2020 Dietary Guidelines for Americans*. This amazing opportunity offered a national perspective on population health issues and the impact of national food-based dietary guidance on chronic disease rates and health care expenditures.

Today, I offer strategic management and systems change initiatives to a variety of organizations that aim to improve human, social/cultural, environmental, and economic health. This includes strengthening the leadership capacity of the public health workforce.

What are some of the challenges you had to overcome during your leadership role(s)?

Each career transition was exciting and brought varying degrees of risk as I [ventured into] uncharted areas in dietetics and public health. The challenges that ensued included convincing others that dietitians did have the expertise to work in food and water systems. This required working with nontraditional partners, nurturing relationships, building new partnerships, examining the interconnections between parts of a larger system, and sometimes asking difficult questions. There were missteps along the way, but each failure resulted in profound lessons learned.

continued on next page

continued from previous page

What do you know now about public health leadership that you wish knew at the beginning of your career?
Many things! Public health leaders work in a state of constant change and I rely on three essential tools in my toolbox to navigate challenges. First, I approach nutrition and public health with a systems lens. The art and science of systems thinking builds a better understanding of the numerous moving parts and how making certain decisions results in positive and negative implications. The second tool is critical examination and asking the right questions. This offers contextual dynamics (eg, operational, political) to situations beyond the data. The third, and perhaps the most important, tool is nurturing stakeholder relationships. Tackling complex nutrition and public health problems requires engagement and coordination with stakeholders in order to drive greater impact. All of these tools, when used simultaneously, support better decision making.

What is the most essential skill to being an effective public health leader?
Authenticity. I believe public health leaders should be sincere, with no pretenses. This builds trust with coworkers, stakeholders, and, most importantly, the public.

[a] Email communication with the author January 24, 2020
[b] Email communication with the author February 13, 2020

Shifting Responsibilities

Taking a leadership role in management typically means assuming a higher level of responsibility. This can take nutrition professionals away from their technical work. For example, it may mean that an RDN will have fewer opportunities to write nutrition articles, provide technical nutrition guidance, read the most recent nutrition studies, or work directly with target populations in the field. As a new leader, this may require some picking and choosing of what technical tasks or skills are maintained and which ones are delegated to team members. New leaders might also experience new time management challenges and need to reprioritize their activities from providing technical expertise to staff supervision and development. However, the advantage is that a public health nutrition leader in a management role can apply their skills to higher-level activities. This could include reviewing and clearing technical content, improving and advising on approaches and processes, mentoring nutrition professionals, and improving program outcomes through strategic thinking. They can also use their skills to manage and motivate teams to accomplish goals that improve public health nutrition.

In some cases, traditional management roles can help transition the RDN from technical expert to a new role as manager of the technical experts. This can create new opportunities to utilize skills such as decision making, budgeting, and human resources development.

Keeping Leadership Expertise Up to Date

Public health nutrition leadership roles often require both the maintenance of nutrition expertise and continued leadership and management training. Because public health nutritionists and leaders work in a wide variety of roles, capacities, and settings, it is up to each individual to determine what expertise and training is needed to be successful in their position. Self-assessment should be an ongoing activity to ensure continued competence and identify new skills that need to be strengthened through continuing education or practice. In addition, obtaining and utilizing feedback from peers, mentors, and supervisors can help ensure expertise is kept up to date.[23,24] Chapter 1 addresses tips and resources for obtaining and utilizing feedback to enhance leadership skills.

Leadership Resources in Public Health

Public health nutrition professionals can benefit from developing and building their skills to establish themselves as leaders. This can be applied to any employment setting, volunteer work, or advocacy role. This should begin with a self-assessment and identification of strengths and skill gaps. ASPHN works to develop skilled leaders in the public health nutrition workforce, and the ASPHN website contains a variety of resources that help public health nutrition professionals advance their leadership skills.[25] The National WIC Association offers a Leadership Academy program to help develop leaders who work in WIC by offering training on strategic thinking, critical thinking, and managing results-driven teams.[26] Within the HHS, the Maternal and Child Health Bureau (MCHB) Division on Maternal and Child Health Workforce Development works to address emerging maternal and child health workforce needs by providing support to leaders in a variety of public and private sectors in the field.[27] Part of these efforts include the grant-based Maternal and Child Health Nutrition Training Program that helps prepare graduate nutrition students and RDNs for careers in public health nutrition.[28] The MCHB also links to the Maternal and Child Health (MCH) Navigator, a tool designed to help maternal and child health graduates and established professionals map out and build their career paths.[29] The MCH Navigator includes a self-assessment of knowledge and skills that address the MCH Leadership Competencies.

Summary

Public health nutrition is an evolving profession that offers a wide array of leadership opportunities. Often these roles are in diverse settings and can be self-navigated by RDNs. Leadership may or may not include positions of formal authority or a management title. In fact, RDNs can serve as leaders by being subject matter experts. If they learn to build key relationships with stakeholders, collaborate across disciplines, communicate their expertise, negotiate needs, and seek opportunities where they can be more visible, they can become strong leaders in their field. They can inspire and lead through mentorship, guidance, and technical assistance. RDNs may sometimes mistakenly be valued only for their nutrition expertise in an organization, despite the cross-curricular training required in dietetic internship programs. RDNs can work to change this perception by serving on cross-disciplinary teams, including ones that are not related to nutrition.

Although there are still some gaps and challenges for RDNs in public health who wish to obtain formal leadership positions, the opportunities are diverse and allow for creativity, innovation, and gaining additional expertise in other fields.

RDNs may wish to conduct a self-assessment and explore opportunities to develop leadership skills in their workplace. These may include building leadership skills within their current role or participating in formalized leadership training or cross-training. Consider your own career goals and identify opportunities where you can build these skills. Look for opportunities where you can be more visible, challenge your own expectations of the roles an RDN can play, work across the aisle with other public health professionals, and negotiate your position. The opportunities to build these skills are numerous and can help you create a rewarding career path.

REFERENCES

1   Institute of Medicine Committee for the Study of the Future of Public Health. *The Future of Public Health.* National Academies Press; 1988. doi:10.17226/1091

2   Ten great public health achievements – United States, 1900-1999. *MMWR Morb Mortal Wkly Rep.* 1999;48(12):241-243.

3   American Public Health Association. What is public health? American Public Health Association website. Accessed January 31, 2020. www.apha.org/what-is-public-health

4   Centers for Disease Control and Prevention. PH101 series: Introduction to public health. CDC website 2021. Accessed May 8, 2021. www.cdc.gov/training/publichealth101/public-health.html

5   US Department of Agriculture, US Department of Health and Human Services. *Dietary Guidelines for Americans, 2020–2025.* 9th ed. US Department of Agriculture and US Department of Health and Human Services; 2020. Accessed May 8, 2021. www.dietaryguidelines.gov /resources/2020-2025-dietary-guidelines-online-materials

6   Academy of Nutrition and Dietetics. Public Health and Community. eatrightPRO website. Accessed January 8, 2020. www.eatrightPRO.org/practice/practice-resources/public-health -and-community

7   Academy of Nutrition and Dietetics Public Health/Community Nutrition Practice Group. 2021 *Member Survey Results Membership Profile.* Academy of Nutrition and Dietetics; 2021. Accessed April 1, 2022. https://higherlogicdownload.s3.amazonaws.com/THEACADEMY/c86efab1-021a -4be7-a2ef-300d170419e4/UploadedImages/PHCN/Documents/2021_PHCN_DPG_Member _Profile.pdf

8   US Department of Agriculture. Mission areas. USDA website. Accessed February 3, 2020. www.usda.gov/our-agency/about-usda/mission-areas

9   Centers for Disease Control and Prevention. About the National Health and Nutrition Examination Survey. CDC website Updated September 15, 2017. Accessed February 2, 2020. www.cdc.gov/nchs/nhanes/about_nhanes.htm

10 Centers for Disease Control and Prevention. Using the new BRFSS module. CDC website Accessed February 2, 2020. www.cdc.gov/nutrition/data-statistics/using-the-new-BRFSS -modules.html

11 Centers for Disease Control and Prevention. School Health Policies and Practices Study (SHPPS). CDC website Accessed February 2, 2020. www.cdc.gov/healthyyouth/data/shpps/index.htm

12 Centers for Disease Control and Prevention National Center for Chronic Disease Prevention and Health Promotion. Poor nutrition. CDC website Accessed February 2, 2020. www.cdc.gov /chronicdisease/resources/publications/factsheets/nutrition.htm

13 Indian Health Service. Agency overview. US Department of Health and Human Services website. Accessed February 3, 2020. www.ihs.gov/aboutihs/overview

14 US Food and Drug Administration. When and why was FDA formed? FDA website. Accessed January 12, 2020. www.fda.gov/about-fda/fda-basics/when-and-why-was-fda-formed

15 US Food and Drug Administration. FDA Nutrition Innovation Strategy.FDA website. Accessed January 12, 2020. www.fda.gov/food/food-labeling-nutrition/fda-nutrition-innovation -strategy

16 United Nations Standing Committee on Nutrition. The UN Decade of Action on Nutrition, 2016-2025. United Nations Standing Committee on Nutrition website. Accessed April 9, 2022. www.unscn.org/en/topics/un-decade-of-action-on-nutrition

17 The 4 Essential Roles of Leadership. FranklinCovey course website. Accessed February 3, 2020. www.franklincovey.com/Solutions/4essentialroles.html

18 Sisk K, Conneally A, Cullinen K. *Guide for Developing and Enhancing Skills in Public Health and Community Nutrition.* 3rd ed. Public Health/Community Nutrition Practice Group of the Academy of Nutrition and Dietetics, and the Association of State Public Health Nutritionists; 2018. Accessed November 24, 2021. www.phcnpg.org/phcn/resources/2018-3rd-edition-the-guide

19 Centers for Disease Control and Prevention. National Leadership Academy for the Public's Health. CDC website Accessed February 2, 2020. www.cdc.gov/publichealthgateway/nlaph/index.html

20 American Public Health Association. Learning Institutes. American Public Health Association website. Accessed February 2, 2020. www.apha.org/learning-institutes

21 Academy of Nutrition and Dietetics. Advancing Leadership in Public Health Resources. eatrightPRO website. May 2018. Accessed November 24, 2021. www.eatrightPRO.org/-/media/eatrightPRO-files/leadership/advancingrolesofleadershipinpublichealthresources.pdf?la=en&hash=0D6EADEE8D84C7258F86870BFD9476A752C8BFF6

22 Association of State Public Health Nutritionists. Resources: trainings, webinars & meetings. Association of State Public Health Nutritionists. website. Accessed April 16, 2022. https://asphn.org/trainings-webinars

23 Stone D, Heen S. *Thanks for the Feedback: The Science and Art of Receiving Feedback Well.* Penguin; 2014.

24 Porter J. How leaders can get honest, productive feedback. *Harvard Business Review.* Accessed February 2, 2020. https://hbr.org/2019/01/how-leaders-can-get-honest-productive-feedback

25 Association of State Public Health Nutritionists. ASPHN leadership. Association of State Public Health Nutritionists website. Accessed January 31, 2020. https://asphn.org/leadership

26 National WIC Association. National WIC Association Leadership Academy. National WIC Association website. Accessed January 31, 2020. www.nwica.org/snippet-leadership-academy

27 Health Resources and Services Administration, Maternal and Child Health Bureau. Workforce training and development. HRSA Maternal and Child Health website. Accessed April 9, 2022. https://mchb.hrsa.gov/training/index.asp

28 Health Resources and Services Administration, Maternal and Child Health Bureau. MCH Nutrition. HRSA Maternal and Child Health website. Accessed January 31, 2020. https://mchb.hrsa.gov/training/projects.asp?program=12

29 MCH Navigator. Self-assessment. MCH Navigator website. Accessed January 31, 2020. www.mchnavigator.org/assessment

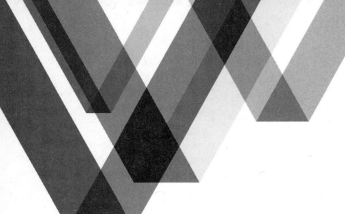

CHAPTER 7

Professional Staff Development

Mandy L. Corrigan, MPH, RD, CNSC, FAND, FASPEN;
Agnieszka Sowa, MS, RD, LD; Bonnie Javurek, MEd, RDN, LD;
Claire Loose, MA, RD, LD; and Cindy Hamilton, MS, RD, LD, FAND

Introduction

Professional development includes growing knowledge and skills that benefit both the employee and the organization. It is far deeper and more complex than simply providing training to grow a skill or technical ability. Professional development enhances knowledge, improves effectiveness, and can enhance commitment to the organization's mission and vision. Furthermore, it can help align goals between the organization and the individual. Although many people associate professional development with job title advancement, it is important to recognize that development within a role is equally important to job satisfaction and engagement. Development needs for individuals change over time, and different strategies are important along the career continuum. The manager's role is to identify strengths and opportunities for growth in their team members.

Identifying the collective needs of the department, partnering with employees to identify personal goals that support department goals, and aligning to the broader institutional goals creates a sense of purpose. This chapter discusses staff development tools and resources including strategic planning, career ladders, individual development planning, professional organization involvement, employee engagement, and employee recognition for managers and leaders to develop individuals, teams, and leadership abilities in their teams. Developing a strategic plan for your department (see Chapter 8, Strategic Planning) with the involvement of employees from all different levels in the department is an important activity that can promote professional growth, inspire employees to achieve new heights, and have a meaningful impact on employees' workflow or work environment.

Strategic Planning

Strategic planning is an important process to the business of dietetics and allows the manager to set a clear purpose for the department, align the department to the institution and professional organization, outline goals, and measure results. Strategic planning is inclusive and should involve employees that represent all the roles in a department—for example, registered dietitian nutritionists (RDNs), nutrition and dietetics technicians registered (NDTRs), support staff, supervisors, managers, and so on. By creating an open environment and providing employees a voice, strategic planning can be one important tool in employee engagement and connect employees to the purpose of the department, organization, and the dietetics profession as a whole.

Employees can have a meaningful role in all phases of strategic planning. See Figure 7.1 for an overview of the strategic planning process. After aligning to the mission of the organization, an excellent next step is to perform a SWOT (strengths, weakness, opportunities, and threats) analysis. A SWOT analysis is important to gain employee perspectives, demonstrate that the managers value employee input, and provide employees an opportunity to be involved with decision making and developing department priorities and goals. After identifying the key issues from the SWOT analysis, the team begins identifying key priorities or focus areas, developing action plans and ways to measure outcomes, implementing action plans, and monitoring progress toward metrics.[1-4] Managers can guide professional growth and development by involving employees in various projects that will assist with achieving the overall strategies.

FIGURE 7.1 Overview of the strategic planning process

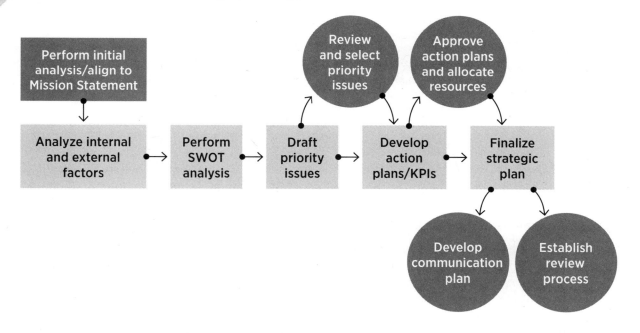

Abbreviations: KPI = key performance indicator | SWOT = strengths, weaknesses, opportunities, and threats

See the Stories From the Field box on page 136 for an overview of a problem identified as part of a strategic planning session at one institution. Therein we outline one example of how involving employees in the strategic planning process was apparent throughout identification of the problem, development of a program, implementation, and measurement of the outcomes.

STORIES FROM THE FIELD: Developing Programs in Response to Strategic Planning

During the strategic planning process at our institution, the focus area of advocacy and advancement was identified with an emphasis on developing individuals, promoting the department, and elevating the dietetics profession. One strategy was developed for the purpose of creating opportunities to enhance employee communication skills for the promotion of professional roles. This was borne from the SWOT (strengths, weaknesses, opportunities, and threats) analysis, one finding of which was that dietitians collectively believed it was common for other disciplines to make nutrition decisions and develop protocols without collaboration. This lack of inclusion and effective collaboration created substantial divides between interprofessional teams and weakened relationships. There were varying abilities of self-empowerment behaviors among department members, some of whom lacked the confidence to collaborate with other teams. In addition, the SWOT analysis identified the need to enhance leadership and effectively mentor others. It became evident that although the clinical skill sets of dietitians were typically strong, they were only part of the equation for successful work performance and acceptable clinical outcomes.

A project team of nine volunteers included registered dietitian nutritionists (RDNs), nutrition and dietetics technicians, registered (NDTRs), and a nutrition manager. Recognizing the need for improvement in the areas of communication, leadership, and empowerment, the team quickly realized it had an opportunity to develop an innovative grassroots program using untapped problem-solving techniques and creative skills.

In an effort to measure the program's impact and understand employees' needs, an electronic survey was created that included 23 statements using a 5-point Likert scale with responses ranging from "strongly agree" to "strongly disagree." The intent was to measure preprogram attitudes and beliefs and compare these to postprogram results using the same survey.

Statements on the scale were categorized into five domains: Leadership, Communication, Mentoring and Development, Empowerment/Sense of Self, and Building Relationships. The majority of responses (more than 75%) were favorable. The team then focused on the statements having mostly responses of "neutral," "disagree," or "strongly disagree" within the domains of Communication, Leadership, and Empowerment; the team developed content to address these areas. The team of volunteers evaluated the existing resources within the organization and determined that a unique program to meet the needs of the nutrition department was necessary.

The team created three mandatory training sessions customized for the specific needs of RDNs and NDTRs. Cohorts of 12 to 25 attendees were assigned to attend training classes together to enhance networking opportunities. Attendees were required to complete surveys before and after the sessions and participated in various learning activities that were both didactic (such as short lectures, storytelling, and deductive reasoning) and Socratic (such as those that took a problem-centered approach, involved class dialogues, or used inductive reasoning) in nature. Short homework, including readings and journaling, was also assigned and completed outside of class sessions. The course culminated in a case study and incorporated all three aspects of the course for group discussion.

The training program was created to align with the department's strategic plan initiative to meet the needs identified by clinical nutrition professionals. By empowering one another to fulfill an initiative, program creators enhanced their own professional abilities, including teamwork, communication, and presentation skills. In turn, program attendees participated in assessing their own strengths and learned various strategies to capitalize on them.

Comparison of pretraining and posttraining survey results showed the following notable positive changes in employee attitudes after completion of the program:

» I feel I can comfortably voice my opinion to a member of another department (increased by 10%).

» I am confident I can positively influence and lead others (increased by 12%).

» I feel empowered to make changes within my department (increased by 14%).

» I believe it is more important to focus on developing people's strengths than to fix their weaknesses (increased by 24%).

Based on postprogram survey results, department members improved communication skills, are stronger self-leaders and leaders of others, and are empowered to be more inspired and motivated clinicians.

Individual Employee Goals

Every employee should have both opportunity and encouragement for professional development. Cultivating employees' skills or abilities can help them achieve their career and personal goals, improve their competencies, and increase work morale and job satisfaction. It can empower and motivate individuals to produce and grow and to serve the organization while building their careers. Discussing employees' professional needs and aspirations for growth enables managers to help those employees establish professional goals and identify the learning activities needed to reach them. It can also lead to change in, or addition of, assignments to enable employees to develop different competencies. It is the responsibility of the nutrition leader or manager to recognize employees are the organization's greatest assets and to help develop them.

While there are many ways to derive goals and make plans to achieve them, the process must begin with identifying where the employee is in relation to their main objective. Many health care institutions have adapted the individual development plan (IDP) process as a guide for identifying and setting goals and pinpointing the steps needed to achieve each goal's components. An IDP can help employees identify their strengths, interests, and areas needing improvement so they can meet job expectations and identify and reach their career goals. Although there are no formal rules for developing and documenting this and the IDP, the process usually includes five sequential steps: preplanning, employee-supervisor meeting, IDP preparation, IDP implementation, and evaluation.[5]

The IDP process begins with the employee and is completed in partnership with the manager. Employees are the main drivers in leading their own professional growth, and managers are key partners to provide coaching and support to assist employees in reaching the employees' goals. Employees begin the IDP process by drafting their individual plan and completing any required paperwork. In this draft of the plan, employees identify their strengths and areas that need to be improved, their professional goals and aspirations, and the possible steps needed to achieve those goals.[6]

Meeting with the manager to discuss the drafted plan is the second step in the process. The employee and manager should work together to make sure the IDP is realistic, attainable, and agreeable to both parties. Managers act on behalf of the institution to ensure the development of skills or realization of goals identified in the IDP is needed by the organization, while the employees act on their own behalf to ensure the attained expertise and objectives will result in greater satisfaction with their work and enhanced potential for career progression.

A good time to establish the initial IDP with the employee is during an annual performance review. It is important to note that the IDP is not an evaluation or appraisal tool but a tool that focuses exclusively on the employee's growth and development. The IDP belongs to the employee and should not be a reflection of what the manager or employer is expecting. Its primary purpose is to help employees reach short- and long-term career goals, as well as improve current job performance by obtaining and improving on the skills required for their current position.[5]

The third step is to prepare the IDP (see Figure 7.2 on page 138). In this step, the employee and supervisor complete a written plan of goals, outline steps needed to reach those goals, and set completion dates for those steps. The written plan places ownership of career development and professional growth on the employee and makes them accountable for completing the objectives. The IDP can align with the employee's continuing education or professional development portfolio, as appropriate, but it should also be consistent with the needs of the employer. The manager must keep the organization's current and future needs and objectives in mind while providing direction for each goal that can ultimately lead to the employee's success.

Once the plan is set and approved by both sides, the employee begins the fourth step in the process: pursuing training and completing tasks as outlined in the IDP. Although the ultimate responsibility of meeting the defined objectives lies with the employee, the manager's role is to offer support by providing the employee with agreed-upon educational opportunities, trainings, assignments, and time. External trainings or resources to achieve a goal may be needed; in the absence of a department professional development budget, these are often obtained at the employee's expense. After they finalize the IDP, the employee and manager should also plan to meet to assess progress, identify problems, and make any necessary changes to the plan. Encouragement and coaching should also be provided at each check-in. Check-ins can be done informally, but they should occur on a regular basis to track progress and make changes as needed.

The evaluation of the IDP is the fifth and final step in the process. In this step, the manager and employee meet again to discuss and appraise the training and development experiences that helped or hindered the employee.[5]

Setting a development plan and assisting employees in growing their careers can help them keep abreast of today's workplace demands. While there are no regulatory requirements that mandate the use of IDPs, it is considered a good management practice.[5] The manager should provide direction for the IDP that can ultimately lead to the employee's success.

FIGURE 7.2 Sample individual development plan

Individualized Career Development Plan

Name:	Job Title: Registered Dietitian Nutritionist		Date:
Professional goal: To meet department criteria to become an Advance Practice I Dietitian by July 2023			
Strengths:		**Areas for improvement:**	
	Objective 1	**Objective 2**	
Development goal	Publish review article in peer-reviewed professional journal.	Obtain specialty credential: Certified Nutrition Support Clinician (CNSC).	
Action plan *(Work that must be done to reach goal)*	Determine subject matter; identify potential journal. Determine and collaborate with authors (coworkers). Review literature, establish outline, draft manuscript, and submit.	Study for certification exam. Submit application to take exam. Take exam.	
Resources needed *(Identify tools or support required)*	Guidance from manager	Department study resources. Financial reimbursement after passing the exam.	
Time frame *(Completion date)*	December 31, 2022	June 6, 2023	
Measure *(Define success: How will you know you achieved your goal?)*	Acceptance of article in a peer-reviewed journal	Passed examination and awarded CNSC	
Employee signature:	Date:	**Manager signature:**	Date:

Team Goals

Setting goals with your team is a crucial step in management. Establishing clear objectives can inspire and motivate your team to make positive changes, increase engagement, steer your group, and help team members focus on pertinent tasks. Like individual goals, team goals present a challenge that allows your team to flourish and serve the organization.

The key to creating effective team goals is to align them with those of the institution. In order to develop team goals that will support the organization's goals, it is important that you and your group have a clear understanding of the institution's needs and objectives. A good place to start is by reviewing the mission and modeling your group's goals to support the achievement of that mission. The manager's role is directing and advising the group, but goals should originate from within the team. Allowing your team to identify their own goals increases buy-in and follow through, and in addition promotes accountability. Assigning ownership of goals to team members lets them be responsible for pursuing goal completion. It also enhances engagement and increases investment in the team's interests.

An ideal time for group goal setting is at the beginning of the calendar or fiscal year. The team should meet and decide on one to three goals they find most important to the team and on which they will collaborate throughout the year. It is imperative that each person in the group have a voice. Ideas for goals can be solicited either in a group or in one-on-one meetings with each person on your team. Group meetings should be set up in a conversation-friendly way, with chairs or tables arranged in a circle or "U" shape. All ideas should be written down. Goal suggestions can be identified by probing each team member for recommendations or by having each person write down their idea and then sharing all ideas with the team. Ideas that cannot be addressed immediately should not be dismissed. Instead, the manager should explain why these ideas cannot be addressed right away and document them so they can be tackled in the future.

While businesses have different ways of ascertaining goals, all successful goals hinge on SMART (specific, measurable, achievable, realistic, and time bound) components. Specific goals are defined as being clear and concise, without room for misinterpretation. Measurability also adds to the specificity of the goal, as having a measure removes ambiguity and enables success to be assessed in objective ways. While determining the measure, the group also needs to define whether the goal as envisioned is both achievable and realistic. The goals set by your team must be achievable in order to be fruitful. Setting unrealistic and unachievable goals can lead to your team feeling discouraged and disengaged and can have a detrimental effect on your team's overall performance. Finally, goals need to be time bound. Having due dates sets the pace for the completion of various steps that need to be finished in order to achieve the main goal. Once the team's goals are determined, the nutrition manager should share them with the department director or institution leadership for guidance and help with removing barriers to success.

It is essential that your group set a schedule for regular discussion regarding progress toward, needs for, and hindrances to goal completion. Work accomplished on each goal should be reported by the individual or individuals who were responsible for completion. This report can be made during formal meetings, informal huddles, or during one-on-one conversations. Your team can also use visuals to monitor goal progress (for example, a dashboard, tracking spreadsheet, Gantt chart, and so on); a sample visual is shown in Figure 7.3. These visual displays can be exhibited during meetings or even available on a shared electronic platform for goal owners to update. Regular discussion and goal progress checks reinforce the accountability of team members and ensure work required for success is not forgotten or delayed.

FIGURE 7.3 Dashboard for goal tracking

Strategy to Meet Focus Area Goal	Target Measure	Report Out Owner	Fiscal Year Action Plans	Q1 Progress	Q1 Status	Q2 Progress	Q2 Status
FOCUS AREA: Outpatient Nutrition Access							
Strategy 3.1 **Increase use of virtual visits as a service of the nutrition department**	**Objective:** Increase the number of virtual visits and nutrition consults from outpatient areas to improve access to medical nutrition therapy. **Key Result:** Increase the number of virtual visits as a service.	Manager	Investigate options for increasing virtual visits	Virtual visit equipment installed in all sites and registered dietitian nutritionists trained	On track	50% of outpatient nutrition appointments are done with virtual visits May 2020—1,092 virtual visits completed June 2020—872 virtual visits completed	Strategy met

Finally, it is vital to celebrate successes. If your team has achieved a goal, you should recognize the accomplishment and reiterate how this impacts the team and the department.[7] Commending the successful completion of goals can set the stage for further goal planning and improvement. Teams that feel recognized and appreciated will be motivated to continue working, advancing, and striving to improve their processes. It is your responsibility as a nutrition manager to guide effective team goal development and achievement that will result in boosting team morale and engagement while substantially contributing to the achievement of the institution's goals and mission.

Employee Engagement

Employee engagement is a measure of commitment, motivation, and emotional attachment to a place of employment.[8] A variety of surveys, such as Press Ganey or Gallup, can be used to measure engagement. Key engagement themes are typically happiness, belongingness, purpose, and trust. The concept of employee engagement has been in the workforce for many years and is a strong component of having a successful team. Employees who are engaged in their work are typically more productive or perform work of a higher quality, stay with the organization longer, and have less absenteeism. Employees who believe they have a voice in their organization will work to improve and advance the organization and attract other high-performing team members. The manager's role is no longer simply to tell staff what to do and how to do it (a "command and control" management style). The manager acts as a "servant leader" who nurtures employees' individualism and the diverse ideas that can come from a working team. The manager guides the team forward and provides coaching to meet goals.

A survey of workers in health care and other fields conducted by TINYPulse in 2019 found decreasing loyalty, decreased feelings of recognition by employers, and a sense of culture in their workplace as being weak.[9] A 2018 Gallup poll of employees across various professions found employees want better work-life balance and better personal well-being; in fact, 91% of employees report the last job change they undertook was in order to meet this need.[10] Given the desire to enhance engagement and provide the positive culture and environment for retention and growth of employees, managers should investigate different initiatives and tools that can help, and ways to show recognition that employees will appreciate.

Managers have various means to improve engagement. How a manager helps improve employee engagement will depend on the results of measuring engagement. After the manager shares the results of an engagement survey, it's important to involve employees in interpreting the results. This includes looking at the themes of what is working well, identifying areas for improvement, generating ideas of what could be done to improve the situation (from the employees' perspectives), providing a supportive environment where all team members have a chance to provide input, and formulating a plan together. For example, if a particular workflow or process is identified as problematic, the manager can partner with employees to better understand the current challenges, form interdisciplinary workgroups if the process is dependent on work streams from other departments, facilitate shared problem solving, set a timeline, and determine how improvement will be measured after implementing changes.

At the core of engagement are four essential needs: the need to build trust, exhibit active listening, be honest, and be supportive in your responses and actions. Guide your employees to utilize their individual strengths and talents so they can believe they are part of the outcome. Their trust in you will grow when they believe you trust them to perform in this capacity.[11] Consistency in your actions will also help strengthen trust.

The performance evaluation process is an area that can be adjusted to meet business and employee engagement needs. A change from traditional, formal delivery of an annual performance evaluation to more frequent and informal evaluations may prove to be more useful and meaningful. An informal evaluation may include a note to file for your tracking purposes if your business does not have a formal midyear or quarterly evaluation plan in place. Plan on more frequent meetings with your staff throughout the year to provide opportunities for open dialogue during which the employee can update you on any issues or concerns as well as any desired roles or activities. These meetings represent a prime opportunity to demonstrate your ability to listen, coach, and recognize employees' input. Having more frequent opportunities for direct communication will help build mutual trust and enable stronger work relationships with employees.

Employee Recognition

Human resources (HR) professionals note one reason employees leave their jobs is lack of recognition from employers. Recognition of employees (whether peer to peer, manager to employee, or department to department) helps engage employees and reinforce behavior consistent with a department or institution's mission and values. There are many ways recognition can be presented, and it should be customized to the employee. For example, some employees want to be recognized in front of their peers, whereas others will prefer to be recognized out of the spotlight. Following are some options for recognizing employees:

> Employee awards system with established criteria

> Nutrition manager nomination of employees for recognition in organization-wide or HR-based programs for recognition

> Handwritten thank-you note

> Positive verbal feedback

> Recognition in a staff meeting

> Recognition in a newsletter

> Appreciation treat, meal, coffee break, or team potluck

> Saying thank you in person, including the specific reason

> Peer recognition fund (for example, staff contribute an agreed-upon amount such as $1 a month, and funds are used to purchase a gift card or meal ticket when the group wants to reward someone for their extraordinary support or contributions to the team)

> Department sponsoring the registration fee for a seminar or conference

> Pay raise or recognition in annual performance review rating

Career Management and Clinical Ladders

Not all employees aspire to management or leadership roles, yet many still have the potential to grow within their roles or focus areas of dietetics. As such, it is important for managers to support career growth of RDN and NDTR team members within their roles and help employees recognize their potential for career advancement in new roles when opportunities arise.

The Academy of Nutrition and Dietetics standards of practice (SOP) and standards of professional performance (SOPP) are tools for RDNs, NDTRs, and nutrition managers that can be used for many purposes, including professional development.[12] The SOP and SOPP documents outline minimum competence levels and provide guidance for self-assessment with measurable indicators. The three levels of practice are *competent*, *proficient*, and *expert*. A *competent* RDN is a novice who is able to perform the basic skills required for entry-level practice. RDNs at the next level are considered *proficient* because they have developed a deeper understanding and are better able to apply evidence-based principles in practice and modify their practice in unique situations. Advanced practice RDNs are considered *experts* who demonstrate their superior clinical skills and ability to make complex decisions. Managers can review the SOP and SOPP documents with employees, compare with self-assessment, assist employees in developing individual goals, and provide coaching and support of professional development. The manager can also use the documents for management as a tool for self-development.[12]

Clinical Ladders

Managers can create more formal pathways of career development within the institution by partnering with administrators and HR staff to create a clinical ladder. Clinical ladders have been in place for decades in many health care institutions and are widely utilized in the nursing profession. Ladder programs are tools to promote professional development within the employee's current work role and thereby retain employees within the role. Ladders are used to differentiate levels of expertise, provide recognition for accomplishments, and increase job satisfaction or engagement and are designed to promote the vision for practice within the profession.

The concept of a clinical or career ladder is easily transferrable to dietetics. If a clinical ladder is not in place, managers can engage in discussions with administrators and HR to obtain buy-in. These discussions may include outlining benefits to the organization, reviewing proposed criteria, evaluating existing career ladders within the institution for other disciplines, and exploring ladders external to the institution. Collaborating with HR on adjusting job descriptions for ladder levels, updating job titles or grades, establishing compensation incentives, and developing a policy for the ladder process are all important.

For career ladders and plans to be effective, managers must establish procedures to continually evaluate whether employees are progressing as expected and determine whether they meet the criteria for higher-level positions. See Box 7.1 on page 144 for an example of activities that can be included on an institution's RDN clinical ladder. Managers provide employees the opportunities to meet criteria on career ladders through various activities throughout the year, such as leading department committees, being involved in projects related to the department's strategic plan, contributing to publications or research, and taking part in speaking engagements.

Succession Planning

Managers can utilize succession planning for preparation as well as to fill critical positions or future leadership role openings. The premise of succession planning is to leverage existing talent within the organization, identify skill gaps, and provide an individualized development plan to help potential candidates strengthen their skills so they be ready when positions become available in the future.[13,14] Succession planning is not preselection but rather an investment in expanding skills of employees with high potential, promoting retention of these employees, and shortening the time required to fill critical positions when needed.[13,14]

The first step in succession planning is for managers to identify roles within the department that are difficult to replace (such as managers, supervisors, internship director, lead dietitian, specialty areas of RDN practice, and others) and identify which current employees are most likely to be ready to fill these key positions in the future. Once key positions are outlined, succession planning is more than just making a list of great potential future candidates. Review the list of employees with

BOX 7.1 Dietitian Career Ladder Activities

Activity	Examples
Attend a local, regional, state, or national nutrition-related conference	Academy of Nutrition and Dietetics Food & Nutrition Conference & Expo (FNCE), American Society for Parenteral and Enteral Nutrition (ASPEN) Nutrition Science and Practice Conference, dietetic practice group symposium, district or affiliate Academy of Nutrition and Dietetics organization, etc
Seek out, learn, and apply new clinical skills or improve existing skills	Placing enteral feeding tubes, learning to use a metabolic cart, or providing nutrition to critical-care patients
Actively participate in the development, implementation, analysis, or publication of a quality improvement (QI) project or institutional review board (IRB)–approved study	Serve as principal or coinvestigator on an IRB-approved study or as a project leader or team member on a QI project; coauthor of a poster accepted at a national nutrition conference
Obtain or renew certification in a specialty area	Commission on Dietetic Registration Certifications (Specialist in Renal Nutrition, Gerontological Nutrition, Oncology, Pediatric, etc), Certified Diabetes Care and Education Specialist, Certified Nutrition Support Clinician, etc
Author or coauthor a book chapter or review article published in a national peer-reviewed publication	Any peer-reviewed publication
Review a professional abstract, poster, article, or textbook chapter	Review FNCE or ASPEN Nutrition Science and Practice Conference abstracts; review textbook chapter for national publisher
Actively participate in a committee, work group, or task force at the departmental, institutional, state, or national level, including being involved in the following types of work: » reviewing, revising, or developing and implementing clinical guidelines or care pathways » developing and implementing educational projects or programs	Academy of Nutrition and Dietetics Evidence Analysis Library work group, ASPEN clinical standards, institution committees (examples: enteral nutrition committee, diabetes committee, pharmacy and therapeutics committee)
Obtain a leadership position in local, state, or national professional organization	Elected or volunteer leadership roles in nutrition organizations such as the Academy of Nutrition and Dietetics, dietetic practice groups, ASPEN, etc
Teach a college-level class	Adjunct professor

the highest potential in order to identify their strengths, past experiences (including roles external to the institution), and skills that need development and estimate the amount of time they would need to grow skills in order to be well prepared for the new role.[13,14] It is critical that managers understand the long-term career aspirations of their employees and discuss future growth plans at least annually with them. Developing an IDP for these potential successors can include addressing gaps in skills, coaching, mentoring, assigning new work or special projects, and recommending leadership classes or coursework. The Stories From the Field boxes on page 145 offer examples of succession planning.

> **STORIES FROM THE FIELD:** Creating a Lead Dietitian Role

Our institution has had a career ladder in place for many years to grow clinical skills; however, there was a gap in a formal pathway for growing future department leaders.

The need for a lead dietitian role was identified and our team worked with the human resources department staff and hospital administration on a job analysis to develop the lead role. Components of the job analysis included a business justification, proposed lead duties of operational support (scheduling, onboarding schedules and training, competencies, quality projects, and serving as a team liaison to the manager), evaluation of whether these key duties could be done with an existing role, key job specifications (leadership attributes, organizational skills, and communication and confidence skills), proposed minimum qualifications (master's degree, 3 to 5 years of registered dietitian nutritionist experience), and budget considerations.

While completing the job analysis, managers also evaluated the development needs of the potential lead role. An orientation development plan was created for key skills and utilized instructor-led courses, self-study learning modules, and mentoring.

The development of the lead role as a succession planning tool helped grow candidates for when a manager position became available, offered internal candidates the skillset they needed to apply for a manager role, and decreased the time to hire by promoting from within the organization.

> **STORIES FROM THE FIELD:** Developing a Registered Dietitian Nutritionist Leader in the Community Health Setting

In our community health setting, one of the registered dietitian nutritionists (RDNs) who reported to me was interested in leadership, but there were not a lot of opportunities for advancement in our current setting. When we did this RDN's annual performance review, we discussed her interest areas and the competencies she could potentially develop while in her current role to be ready for management opportunities when they arose. I encouraged the RDN to look at the standards of practice and standards of professional performance, the Commission on Dietetic Registration practice competencies, and the *Guide for Developing and Enhancing Skills in Public Health and Community Nutrition* and identify three or four competencies she most needed to develop.

Once those tasks were completed, we discussed them and together developed a plan that included self-led education outside of work hours and key activities in the work setting that would help develop those competencies. This plan had clear target dates and dates that the two of us would check in on her progress.

There were a few bumps in the road, but I am proud to say that as a result of this development plan, the RDN expanded her motivational interviewing skills and group facilitation skills and was able to take a leadership role, working with several other community health team members to develop a program plan for a grant we were submitting for a diabetes prevention program. I am happy to report that we received the grant and the RDN was able to step into the role of program manager for our new diabetes initiative.

Professional Organization Involvement

Volunteer opportunities, including committee work, volunteer leadership, or advocacy effort, are offered by various organizations, groups, and professional societies. These can include national organizations, dietetic practice groups, and chapters of organizations at the local, state, or national level. Managers serve as role models to their employees by being involved in these organizations. Fostering employee involvement in these organizations is an important strategy for managers to help employees support their development outside the institution's walls and in the profession at large. It is important for managers to connect their employees to opportunities in professional organizations matching the employee's interests. Once employees are involved in a professional organization or society, they can continue to develop their skills on a specific project or committee and then seamlessly transfer these skills back to the department and institution. Growing leadership, delegation, or communication skills by taking on larger roles within a professional organization can benefit the employee and institution alike. Fostering employee involvement in professional societies also helps grow the institution's brand, supports professional networking, and allows the department to stay abreast of trends in the profession. Activities or involvement in professional organizations can also be incorporated into clinical ladder criteria to incentivize employees.

Summary

Staff development is continuous and ultimately serves to improve employee performance and the quality of care delivered to patients. Managers ensure employees have the knowledge and skills to perform their roles and keep abreast of changes in dietetics practice where staff will need education and training to fill practice gaps. Developing employees is an investment not only for the future of the department but also for our profession. Staff development is a top priority for managers and allows us to evaluate the skills and knowledge of teams and individual employees frequently as well as to develop successors for future roles. By providing employees growth opportunities, mentoring, and involvement in department goal setting, managers can offer both a supportive work environment and professional development.

REFERENCES

1   Melnick L, Hamilton C. Developing a strategic plan to position your team for success. *Future Dimensions in Clinical Practice*. 2019;(Fall):1-6.

2   Jordan BI. Strategic planning: positioning clinical dietitians to be proactive in today's healthcare arena. *Top Clin Nutr.* 2007;22(1):37-44.

3   Harvard Business Publishing. Harvard ManageMentor: strategy planning and execution. Harvard Business Publishing Education course. August 27, 2019. Accessed December 20, 2019. https://hbsp.harvard.edu/product/7183-HTM-ENG?itemFindingMethod=LandingPage

4   Figliuolo M. Strategic planning foundations: understanding the principles of strategic planning. LinkedIn Learning website. 2020. Accessed April 9, 2020. www.linkedin.com/learning/strategic-planning-foundations/understanding-the-principles-of-strategic-planning-2

5   US Government Office of Personnel Management. Training and development policy wiki: individual development plan. OPM website. Accessed September 23, 2019. www.opm.gov/WIKI/training/Individual-Development-Plans.ashx

6   Yale University. Individual development planning: achieving higher performance. Yale University website. Accessed September 23, 2019. https://your.yale.edu/sites/default/files/idp-guide-to-getting-started_0.pdf

7   Pyecha J, Versteeg A, Davies S, Yount S. *Leading Your Business Forward: Aligning Goals, People, and Systems for Sustainable Success.* McGraw Hill; 2013. O'Reilly Online Learning Platform: Academic Edition. Accessed December 12, 2019. https://learning.oreilly.com/library/view/leading-your-business/9780071817134

8 Phin D. Employee engagement. LinkedIn Learning website. Updated 2021. Accessed March 8, 2022. www.linkedin.com/learning/employee-engagement

9 McGugan C, Forbes Technology Council. Three strategies for transforming employee engagement. Forbes website, November 20, 2019. Accessed March 31, 2020. www.forbes.com/sites/forbestechcouncil/2019/11/20/three-strategies-for-transforming-employee-engagement/#208e8d3f1485

10 Gallup's perspective on designing your organization's employee experience. Gallup website. 2018. Accessed March 31, 2020. www.gallup.com/workplace/355601/employee-experience-paper.aspx

11 Desimone R. Employees want work that matters—managers can help. Gallup website. January 8, 2020. Accessed March 31, 2020. www.gallup.com/workplace/275417/employees-work-matters-managers-help.aspx

12 Doley J, Clark K, Roper S. Academy of Nutrition and Dietetics: revised 2019 standards of professional performance for registered dietitian nutritionists (competent, proficient, and expert) in clinical nutrition management. *J Acad Nutr Diet*. 2019;119(9):1545-1560.

13 Hagemann B. Succession planning. LinkedIn Learning website. May 2018. Accessed April 9, 2020. www.linkedin.com/learning/succession-planning/welcome?u=74687194

14 Sharon K. Talent management. LinkedIn Learning website. February 2017. Accessed April 9, 2020. www.linkedin.com/learning/talent-management/build-a-successful-plan?u=74687194

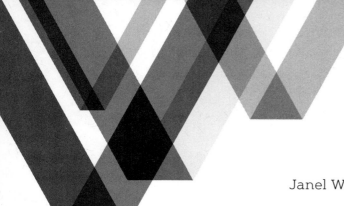

Strategic Planning

Janel Welch, MS, MPA, RDN, CDN, FAND, CPHQ, QCP, OHCC, and Marsha Schofield, MS, RD, LD, FAND

Introduction

Consider the following two scenarios:

Scenario 1: Mateo is the clinical nutrition manager (CNM) for a 300-bed local community hospital. He has been in this position for 3 years and feels like he spends most of his time putting out fires: rearranging staffing to cover maternity and medical leaves, responding to demands from his director to increase patient satisfaction scores, obtaining formulas for nonformulary requests, trying to figure out whether or not a staff member might be available to speak to a community group on nutrition, and doing last-minute preparations for Joint Commission surveys. Every year when it is time to prepare his annual budget, he just quickly takes last year's budget and adjusts it for inflation.

Scenario 2: Tatyana is the CNM for a regional home infusion company. After 7 years in the position, she has expanded the staff from three to five registered dietitian nutritionists (RDNs) with board specialist credentials. She has expanded contracts with health care systems in the region and has achieved a 100% referral rate for nutrition consults for all patients receiving home infusion services. These successes are partially attributed to the fact that her staff is actively engaged in collecting outcomes data on all their clients. Eighty percent of Tatyana's time is spent overseeing implementation and regular evaluation of her unit's strategic plan. While she often faces unanticipated requests and demands from the company's administration, she feels comfortable using the strategic plan to guide her responses and courses of action.

Why is Mateo enmeshed in solving daily crises, whereas Tatyana can focus on the future? Is Mateo simply a less experienced manager than Tatyana? Do Tatyana's challenges stem from the size or type of facility in which she practices? Would their stories change if their roles were reversed?

The key distinguishing feature between these two scenarios is the presence or absence of strategic planning. No matter the size of the facility, the type of practice setting, or the years of experience a leader has in the role, success depends on a leader's ability to plan strategically. The importance of strategic planning skills is highlighted in a 2008 study conducted by the Center for Creative Leadership (CCL).[1] In the CCL's survey of 2,200 leaders from 15 organizations in three countries, strategic planning was identified as one of seven critical leadership skills. Nutrition leaders must develop strong strategic planning skills to be successful.

Whether you are an experienced nutrition leader or new to the role, this chapter provides a framework for understanding what strategic planning is, why it is important, and how to do it. The following information applies to nutrition leaders working in all types and sizes of organizations.

What Is Strategic Planning?

Strategic planning has been defined as "the process for assessing a changing environment to create a vision of the future, determining how the organization fits into the anticipated environment based on its institutional mission, strengths and weaknesses, and then setting in motion a plan of action to position the organization accordingly."[2] It is a process that enables an organization or a unit within an organization to chart where it is going over the next 3 to 5 years, how it is going to get there, what resources it will take to get there, and how outcomes and success will be measured. Strategic planning is an attempt to shape the future. A strategic plan serves as a means of communicating a company's mission, vision, values, and long-term goals and engages employees, customers and stakeholders. There are several resources and tools available to RDN leaders through the Academy of Nutrition and Dietetics professional website (www.eatrightPRO.org). Some of these tools will be discussed or provided in this chapter.

Businesses have used strategic planning since the late 1940s and early 1950s. The concept first took hold in the health care industry in the 1970s and has become more prominent as the industry has adopted more of a business mindset.[3] Strategic planning prepares you to move into the broader world of strategic management. Creating a plan is not enough; you must also implement and manage the plan to ensure the intended results are achieved. The world continues to change during implementation. Therefore, you will inevitably face difficulties and need to adjust strategies along the way.

Why Do Strategic Planning?

"To be in hell is to drift; to be in heaven is to steer." —George Bernard Shaw

Strategic planning results in a documented process called a strategic plan. The plan will specifically outline the path the organization will take in order to guide its mission, vision, and goals. A strategic plan helps create clarity and improve communication within an organization, department, or team. John M. Bryson defines strategic planning as "a deliberative, disciplined approach to producing fundamental decisions and actions that shape and guide what an organization is, what it does and why."[4] Strategic planning, when done well, allows you to steer and have control over your future. Strategic plans enable you to:

> create organizational focus;

> motivate the workforce;

> build stakeholder support;

> identify how to allocate resources;

- set priorities;
- make short-term decisions based on long-term implications;
- be proactive, not reactive; and
- make your organization competitive.

A strategic plan helps you shape your entity into the organization you want it to become. According to Barksdale and Lund, "if done correctly, the strategic plan should be a document that motivates employees to achieve the plan's stated goals and tactics."[5] And, as Collins points out in his landmark book, *Good to Great*, there are three essential elements in becoming a great company: disciplined people, disciplined thought, and disciplined action.[6]

Strategic planning is not any one thing but, instead, an adaptable set of concepts, procedures, tools, and practices intended to help determine what an organization should be doing, how it should be doing it, and why.[5] Strategic planning is not reactively fixing a problem; you can do that through process improvement techniques such as those discussed in Chapter 13. Instead, strategic planning is determining how best to attempt to shape the future.

Organizations can benefit from both the actual strategic plan and the planning process itself. While the plan provides a roadmap to success, the planning process can help unite the organization, facilitate communication, and forge bonds among stakeholders. In addition, by going through the process, people learn how to think strategically and make strategic decisions on a continuing basis moving forward.

Strategic Planning in Health Care

The health care environment is continuously changing, which can make it tricky to navigate. Changes in economic trends, government policies, federal laws, technology, and medical advances have a substantial impact on hospitals' and health care organizations' strategic plans.[5] Planning for the future with so many unknown quantities and variables can be challenging.

The health care market has changed dramatically since the Patient Protection and Affordable Care Act (ACA) was passed in 2010. Under the ACA, hospitals and other health care organizations must provide more services for more insured patients. As the financial model in health care changes, pay-for-performance models require strategy for programming. As a result, relationships between medical providers and hospitals are evolving and hospital systems are becoming increasingly complex. These are all reasons that strategic planning is more important than ever before.

How to Facilitate Strategic Planning

There are 10 steps to facilitate strategic planning.[5]

Step 1: Choosing the Process

Many models exist for strategic planning, and most models are similar in nature. Your choice of models is not as important as due diligence to the process and implementation, so don't agonize over which model to pick. Recognize that both simple and complex models can result in good or bad strategic plans.

If your organization already conducts strategic planning, it makes sense to use the model adopted by leadership and look to experienced colleagues within your organization for mentoring. If your organization does not do strategic planning, select a model that makes sense to you. Choose a process that you understand; that is appropriate and feasible in terms of sophistication, complexity, and your organizational culture; and that supports the types of outcomes you and your organization aim to achieve. If this is your first attempt at strategic planning, a simple model may be best. Your planning efforts can evolve into a more sophisticated process as your experience and expertise grow.

Step 2: Planning to Plan

Initially, it is important to assess the readiness of the organization to evaluate its current state and determine where it would like to be in the next 3 to 5 years.[7] Without stakeholder buy-in, any strategic plan is bound to fail. The most effective strategic planning processes involve careful planning up front. Following that, it is ideal to time all strategic decisions, operational plans, and budgets to align with the beginning of the organization's fiscal year. Some key questions to consider during the planning process are discussed in the following paragraphs.

What is the scope of the strategic plan, and what are the desired outcomes? Defining the scope of the plan as early as possible is essential. What are the desired outcomes of this plan? What results do you want to achieve? When do you want to achieve these outcomes? What metrics will demonstrate successful outcomes? Determine a time frame for developing the plan. This may be adjusted along the way; however, the time frame is important, as it relies on the availability and accessibility of resources dedicated to the plan. Although the desired outcomes of the plan may seem obvious to you, it is important for everyone to understand what you are trying to achieve. You can begin to define the desired outcomes by completing the sentence, "Develop a strategic plan for the next 3 years that will . . ." Some possible desired outcomes include the following:

> position clinical nutrition services as a source of revenue for the organization;

> gain respect from physicians, the administration, or both;

> establish department employees as vital collaborators or leaders in the organization; and

> improve awareness across the organization of the value and offerings of the clinical nutrition services department.

Who should be included in developing the strategic plan? When considering whom to include in developing the strategic plan, ask yourself two questions:

> **Whose support will you need to ensure adoption and execution of the plan?** Stakeholders are those individuals or departments who have the most to gain or lose from your strategic plan. It is critical to identify stakeholders early on in the planning process, as this will direct key components of developing and implementing your strategic plan. The first group to consider is departmental staff. Inclusion of staff in the process helps to build their buy-in and commitment to the plan and contribute their "on the ground" working experience to the plan-

ning process. The next group to consider is organizational leadership (within and beyond your department). Having strong senior leadership advocates for your plan can help immensely with its success. Senior leaders can provide organizational direction, guidance, and support. If your leadership is not supportive or your vision does not align with organization's mission or goals, your strategic plan is unlikely to succeed. Determine how your strategic plan will impact other departments in the organization, and then request input on the plan from the leaders of those departments.

> **Whose perspectives will be valuable to include or will enhance the quality of the plan?** One pitfall to avoid is "group think." Although we often feel more comfortable in a conflict-free situation, your planning group should include individuals who can challenge traditional thinking or play devil's advocate as well as people who hold similar views. Consider including individuals from outside your department and organization (such as administrators, other health care professionals, departmental staff, and patients or customers). Informal leaders can be influential either within or external to your own group. They can help support the plan and vision, so obtain as many different perspectives in the planning process as you can.

How many people should be part of the planning committee? As is true for any committee work, the size of the planning group will have an impact on its effectiveness. Because additional resources and number of individuals on the planning committee have financial implications, you need to consider the budget when creating the planning committee. An optimal size for the strategic planning committee is 5 to 10 people.

How will you orient the strategic planning team? The individuals you invite to participate in the strategic planning process may or may not have experience in this process. Even if they are an experienced group of individuals, they will benefit from a basic orientation that covers your goals for the process, describes the process, introduces participants, and sets expectations for participants. If members of the team have never done strategic planning, you will need to expand the orientation to include an introduction of some basic concepts (discussed later in this chapter). The orientation can be provided in written communications (such as email), a conference call, a webinar, or a face-to-face meeting—whichever is best suited to your group.

Who would be your best facilitator? A good facilitator will help ensure that the traditional and nontraditional thinkers on your committee work together in a constructive manner. Consider whether an internal facilitator (someone from within your organization) or an external one is most advantageous for your situation (see Table 8.1).[8] Ideally, you should not facilitate the process yourself because your staff may feel inhibited about sharing their ideas candidly and challenging your thinking if you direct the committee proceedings. You want everyone in the process to have an equal voice and do not want to do anything that hampers open discussion and creative thinking. Using a facilitator (other than yourself) also frees you up to participate more actively in the planning process.

TABLE 8.1 Choosing an Internal or External Facilitator

	Advantages	Disadvantages
Internal facilitator	» Familiar with the organization, the people, and the issues » May inspire a higher level of comfort in discussions of sensitive issues » Less expensive than hiring an external facilitator	» May lack objectivity » May lack the ability to realign the group if discussion digresses or implodes » May have limited time to keep the process on course
External facilitator	» May have a broad wealth of experience working with other organizations » Able to work with the group throughout the planning process and preparation of the final plan » Perceived as being objective	» Limited knowledge of the group and its specific issues » More expensive than using an internal facilitator

Adapted with permission from *Strategic Planning: The Roadmap to Success. A Guide for Affiliates and Dietetic Practice Groups.* American Dietetic Association; 2006.[8]

How will you implement the planning process? Working with your facilitator, map out an action plan and timeline for your strategic planning process. Your approach and timeline will depend on several factors, including:

> whether you are revising an existing plan or creating one for the first time;

> the complexity of the department or organization;

> your previous experience with strategic planning;

> whether necessary data are readily available; and

> the availability of committee members to participate and complete assignments.

A strategic plan can take from 3 months to 1 year to develop. At a minimum, expect development to take 3 to 6 months. If you try to create and implement a plan too quickly, you risk sacrificing quality. If you stretch out the development process over too long a period of time, interest and momentum may wane. You may also fall prey to "paralysis by analysis."

When setting the timeline, consider whether or not you want to do everything via face-to-face meetings or complete some pieces outside of these meetings (such as by email or virtual meeting platforms). Will you expect participants to do any preparation in advance of meetings? Will you expect participants to complete assignments between meetings? Understand that individuals involved in the strategic planning process will need to take time away from their daily responsibilities to participate in meetings and other activities.

Plan at least one face-to-face meeting that lasts 1 to 2 days. Pick a location away from the worksite so the group can be free of distractions. If committee members are on call, arrange for other staff to take their calls so they are not interrupted. You may have appropriate meeting space within your facility, or you may need or want to find an off-site location. Off-site meetings do not need to be expensive. Many community agencies, churches, and public libraries offer free meeting space. For both face-to-face and virtual meetings (including email exchanges), consider adopting a set of ground rules agreed upon by the group. See Box 8.1 on page 154 for a sample set of ground rules.

One effective approach to the planning process is to divide it into three phases: premeeting, meeting, and postmeeting. See Figure 8.1 for an example of such a staged strategic planning process.

> **FIGURE 8.1** Sample strategic planning process

Nutrition Department 6-Month Planning Process

Phase 1: Premeeting (complete over 3 months)

Action	Desired Outcome	Person(s) Responsible	Deadline
1.0 Conduct orientation session.	Participants will understand basic strategic planning concepts, goals of the project, the process to be used, and expectations of participants.	Facilitator, clinical nutrition manager (CNM), participants	[Indicate deadline date]
2.0 Conduct environmental analysis.		Facilitator, CNM, participants	
2.1 External trends: Provide list of trends culled from research and ask group (electronically) to rate the relevance of each trend.	Identify the top 10 trends affecting the nutrition department or organization.		
2.2 Internal trends: Conduct a SWOT (strengths, weaknesses, opportunities, and threats) analysis electronically.	Provide a clear snapshot of the organization's current position.		
3.0 Identify, collect, and review relevant data and documents.	Strategic planning participants will become familiar with this information to prepare them to fully participate in strategic planning meetings.	Facilitator, CNM, participants	

continued on next page

continued from previous page

Phase 2: Face-to-Face Meeting (1 to 5 meetings depending on length of meeting and time needed to complete each agenda item. Some areas may take longer and require time to work between meetings.)

Session	Session Outcome(s)	Time
1.0 Introduction	Review purpose, plan, desired outcomes, and ground rules.	30 minutes
2.0 Ice-breaker activity	Stimulate creative thinking.	30 minutes
3.0 Results of environmental analysis	Confirm top 10 trends affecting the clinical nutrition unit. Approve or modify results of SWOT analysis.	1 hour
4.0 Vision and mission statements	Review and discuss unit's vision and mission statements; modify if necessary.	30 minutes
5.0 Strategic goals	Develop three strategic goals for the unit in alignment with those of the organization.	1 hour
Lunch		
6.0 Objectives and tactics for each strategic goal *(Conduct first as a small-group activity, then have entire group review and rank options.)*	Identify potential objectives ("what") and tactics ("how") for each strategic goal set in item 5.0.	2 hours
7.0 Measurement system *(Conduct first as small-group activity, then have entire group review and rank options.)*	Identify potential performance measures for each objective.	1 hour
8.0 Summary and next steps	Review accomplishments of meeting. Determine future assignments.	30 minutes
9.0 Adjourn		

Phase 3: Postmeeting (complete over 1 to 2 weeks)

Action	Desired Outcome	Person(s) Responsible	Deadline
1.0 Compile a summary of meeting outcomes and distribute to participants for review.	A draft is approved or modified.	Facilitator, participants	[Indicate deadline date]
2.0 Develop executive summary and final strategic plan document.	Final documents are ready for distribution.	Facilitator, CNM	
3.0 Finalize and launch communications plan.	Strategic plan is communicated to key stakeholders.	CNM	
4.0 Implement plan.	Clinical Nutrition Unit begins to operate under new strategic plan.	CNM	

Step 3: Identifying Your Mission, Vision, and Values

Before you can map out your future, you need to understand what the organization is, why it exists, and its desired future. This information is typically expressed through a mission statement, a vision statement, and a stated set of values. These statements may already exist for your department, the entire organization, or both.

The mission and vision serve as guides in resource-allocation decisions. They should also provide guidance for evaluating opportunities and making decisions about proposals. Therefore, it is imperative that you understand, affirm or modify existing mission and vision statements, or create new statements if none exist. When the organization has a mission and a vision, you may decide to adopt the statements for your department's use or personalize the language to fit your needs.

The *mission statement* answers the question, "Why do we exist?" It describes what the organization does and for whom. A good mission statement is brief (generally one sentence) and to the point. For example, the mission of a clinical nutrition department might be: "To enhance the health and quality of life of our patients through individualized, evidence-based nutrition care." Generally speaking, mission statements remain fundamentally the same over time; therefore, you probably will not need to substantially change one that already exists.

In contrast to the mission statement, the *vision statement* describes the organization's desired future (no more than 10 years out). It should describe how the organization will look when the strategy has been achieved. It is an aspiration and, as such, it should be motivational. The vision is your destination, and the strategic plan is your road map to get there. One approach to creating a vision statement is to ask the group: "Imagine we are 5 years into the future and your most desirable organization has been created. How would you describe what the organization looks like?" One possible answer could be: "Our clinical nutrition services department will be the provider of choice for pediatric nutrition services across the region." If a vision statement already exists for your department, you will likely need to update it as you develop the strategic plan. If one exists for the entire organization, you will want to adapt it to fit your specific department.

Values statements define the organizational culture. They identify traits, behaviors, and qualities that should be displayed through decisions and actions. Values statements are only meaningful if they are translated into organizational policies, activities, and behaviors that make the organization's values readily evident to any observer. If the overall organization has values statements, you should not change them for your department. After all, your department culture should blend in with the larger culture. If the organization does not have values statements, you should develop them for your department to communicate to your staff and others the behaviors that are considered important as you conduct your business.

Step 4: Environmental Analysis

The next step in strategic planning involves understanding the internal and external environments and how they might affect your ability to achieve your desired future. Box 8.2 provides an overview of questions to guide this analysis.[9]

One common way to complete this task is to perform a SWOT analysis (looking at strengths, weaknesses, opportunities, and threats). An environmental SWOT analysis is designed to help the group identify and understand the department's current state so you can determine what actions will be needed to take the department to its desired future. The analysis should form the basis for developing your goals and strategies. Be candid and realistic in your SWOT analysis.

The external environment includes the industry or segment in which the organization competes, its competitors, its markets, and other relevant environmental trends and changes. You need to understand how the relevant environment is changing and how it might change in the future. When analyzing the external environment, consider four important forces as they relate to the health care industry[9]:

> social forces, such as the aging population;

> economic forces, such as a downturn in the economy;

> political forces, such as health care reform; and

> technological innovations, such as electronic care processes (eg, e-prescribing and telehealth).

Many sources of information help you analyze the external environment. For example, the Academy of Nutrition and Dietetics Council on Future Practice conducts and publishes ongoing environmental scanning and visioning work,[10] as does the American Hospital Association.[11] Professional and industry journals and other publications may also provide useful information, and your organization may conduct market research that would aid your analysis. You can also gather your own data by conducting personal interviews with key industry leaders within and outside your organization.

Your analysis of the internal environment should examine the following items:

> financial performance and condition

> organizational and departmental capabilities, including facilities, technologies, staff competencies, and processes

> organizational culture

> management and leadership capabilities

> strengths and weaknesses (referring to resources or capabilities that help the organization accomplish its mission, and deficiencies in resources and capabilities that hinder the organization's ability to accomplish its mission)

> opportunities and threats (referring to forces and events in the external environment that create new markets or need for services, or might limit or interfere with the organization's efforts to accomplish its mission)

A strong internal analysis will consider both quantitative and qualitative data. Some possible sources of information include accreditation surveys, patient satisfaction surveys, employee satisfaction surveys, performance improvement data, financial reports (including billing and revenue data), benchmarking data, staffing patterns, productivity data, patient acuity data, personal interviews (eg, feedback from physicians, other health professionals, and leadership staff), focus groups (eg, feedback from clients), and data from organization-wide strategic planning efforts. Asking others within your organization for input during this stage of the process may showcase your leadership skills to key decision makers and set the stage for needed support when it comes time to ask for resources and execute your strategic plan.

As you do your internal assessment, try to not get bogged down analyzing the past. Don't make historical performance a point of major focus; instead, look at the past just enough to learn for the future.[3] Take a look at overall trends to gain understanding and inform future direction. Also keep in mind that the effectiveness of your strategic plan depends on the quality, and not necessarily the quantity, of data used to establish tactics. Before you spend too much time collecting data you don't need, ask yourself why you need the information and how you will use it.

The following questions about internal and external environments can help guide your SWOT analysis:

> Who are your stakeholders and what are their expectations?
> What are the current and future requirements and opportunities of the health care market?
> What are the opportunities for innovation?
> What are your unit's core competencies?
> How does your unit's performance compare to that of competitors and similar organizations?
> What innovations or changes might affect your health care services and how you operate? For example, how is technology likely to affect future operations?
> What are your workforce development and hiring needs?
> What are the potential financial, societal, ethical, regulatory, technological, and security risks and opportunities?
> What is the current state of the local, national, or global economy? What economic trends seem likely in the future?
> What changes are taking place in your parent organization?

Step 5: Establishing Goals

The strategic planning committee should determine a set of goals for the organization. Goals are general statements about what the organization needs to accomplish to fulfill the mission and vision. The number of goals should be reflective of the organization's capability and services. Each goal should be accompanied by one or more objectives that define the projects created to support the goal. Objectives (or strategies) break goals into specific activities that need to be completed to help you reach your goals. They are your game plan. Objectives should answer the questions of *what* you want to achieve and *how* you will go about achieving it. The results of your SWOT analysis should drive development of your goals and objectives.

One technique for developing objectives is the TOWS matrix. This tool integrates the SWOT analysis to come up with objectives that take advantage of strengths and opportunities, minimize or downplay weaknesses, and counter threats.[12] The TOWS matrix divides strategies into four types:

> SO strategies allow you to pursue *opportunities* that capitalize on the department's *strengths*.

> WO strategies are ways to overcome the department's *weaknesses* and pursue *opportunities*.

> ST strategies are ways the department can use its *strengths* to minimize its vulnerability to external *threats*.

> WT strategies prevent the department's *weaknesses* from making it susceptible to external *threats*.

You do not need to develop objectives to fit all four quadrants. Rather, use the matrix as a guide for brainstorming. Figure 8.2 presents the TOWS matrix in a graphic format.

FIGURE 8.2 TOWS Matrix

	Strengths	Weaknesses
Opportunities	SO strategies	WO strategies
Threats	ST strategies	WT strategies

Since virtually every organization has resource limitations, you will need to prioritize your objectives and determine which ones have the greatest impact for the cost. Typical priorities include the following[5]:

> revenue generation

> competitive advantage

> customer satisfaction

> public perception or reputation

> safety

> regulatory compliance

> labor and resource allocation and availability

> employee satisfaction

> being at the leading edge in the marketplace

> technological development

> operational efficiencies

The objectives should include a scope that sets the parameters of the project. Use the process of developing SMART goals as a guide when setting objectives and establishing tactics. SMART goals are specific, measurable, attainable, relevant, and time bound. Additional information regarding goal setting can be found in Chapter 13, Quality Management and Improvement.

Step 6: Establishing Tactics

Tactics are the specific steps or short-term activities needed to meet the objectives. Tactics should answer the question, "*Who* is going to do *what*, and (by) *when?*"

Tactics should be the most flexible part of the plan. Based on new information, changes in the internal or external environment, or the outcomes achieved, tactics may be added, revised, or abandoned. You will gain nothing by clinging to tactics that do not support objectives. As you define your tactics, be sure to specify the resources needed to complete the activity. Figure 8.3 provides a sample form to help your group develop tactics for each objective.[8] The following are examples of tactics:

> The nutrition informaticist will work with the software vendor to map out an electronic health record implementation timeline by the end of the first quarter.

> The CNM will meet with the marketing department by June 1 to design a marketing brochure.

> Pat Smith, RDN, will attend the Commission on Dietetic Registration Certificate of Training in Childhood and Adolescent Weight Management workshop in March.

FIGURE 8.3 Tactics planning worksheet

Tactics Plan

Goal: _____

Objective: _____

Instructions: Use this form as a template to develop a plan of action for each objective. Keep copies handy to update regularly and bring to meetings for review. You may decide to develop new or revised action plans over time. This worksheet can be used in the development of tactics and to review progress of each tactic throughout the strategic planning process. This worksheet can also be used as a tool to update and modify tactics for annual program planning.

Tactics/Action Steps *What will be done?*	Resources *What funding, time, people, and materials are needed?*	Responsibilities *Who will do it?*	Timeline *What is the deadline (date)?*	Progress
1.				
2.				
3.				
4.				
5.				
6.				
7.				
8.				
9.				
10.				

Adapted with permission from *Strategic Planning: The Roadmap to Success. A Guide for Affiliates and Dietetic Practice Groups.* American Dietetic Association; 2006.[8]

Before finalizing the objective and tactics, see how well they meet some agreed-upon criteria, such as the following:

> Do the objective and tactics help us fulfill our mission?

> Is this tactic related to our goals and objectives?

> Do we have, or can we obtain, the resources needed to meet our objective?

> Is the strategy measurable, and are its results meaningful to the organization?

Step 7: Measuring Success

The final developmental component of the strategic plan is the measurement system. You need to know whether your strategy is working and whether you are achieving your goals. Define indicators that will be monitored to measure progress. Good performance measures focus employees' attention on the factors most critical to success. The indicators should focus on outcomes (accomplishments), not processes (the work that was done). In other words, the measurement system should not simply evaluate whether a tactic was completed; it must also tell you whether the tactic achieved the desired goal. For example, if the goal is to use technology to enhance the efficiency and cost-effectiveness of clinical nutrition services, use of technology is a tactic and efficiency and cost-effectiveness are outcomes. In this situation, you could use a combination of productivity data, quality measures, and financial data (expenses) as indicators. The measurement system should define the indicators, target values, how the information will be collected, who will collect it, and how often the indicators will be evaluated. Figure 8.4 provides a template for your measurement system.

FIGURE 8.4 Measurement system worksheet

Strategic Plan Measurement System

GOAL:				
Indicator	**Target Value**	**Data Collection**		**Frequency**
		Who?	**How?**	

GOAL:				
Indicator	**Target Value**	**Data Collection**		**Frequency**
		Who?	**How?**	

Step 8: Communicating the Plan

Your strategic plan can be a strong marketing tool for your organization. It can let internal and external stakeholders know who you are and what you are striving to achieve. As such, a strategic plan can be used to build commitment, support, and potentially even funding for your efforts. It also can help you achieve recognition and respect. But it cannot do any of these things if it is not shared.

Before you can share the plan, it needs to be captured in writing. The final strategic plan document should include the following items:

> executive summary of the plan (rationale for preparation of the plan, background on process used, major findings, and major recommendations);

> mission, vision, and values;

> outcomes, goals, and objectives;

> tactics and resources; and

> commitment or authorization from upper management.

The communication plan should not be an afterthought. Instead, start developing it at the beginning of the strategic planning process, taking care to define what types of information are going to be shared, the audience(s) for this information, and the methods and timing of communications. The communications plan should span the life of the strategic plan. In addition to announcing the plan's launch, share your progress and results when you reach milestones or key points in time. At a minimum, you should communicate results annually. Tailor what you share and how you share it to each target audience, including stakeholders you identified at the beginning of the process. Put yourself in their shoes and ask, "What's in it for me?" For each part of the plan, develop a few key talking points that you and your staff can use when communicating with stakeholders. Develop an elevator pitch you could deliver during the course of a short elevator ride, keeping your message both compelling and concise. See Figure 8.5 for a worksheet you can use to develop your communication plan.[8]

Step 9: Monitoring the Plan

Your strategic plan will go nowhere if you fail to develop a monitoring plan that defines both scheduled and unscheduled times for evaluating progress and making course corrections or changing tactics. As you create your monitoring schedule, consider your measurement indicators and how frequently information will be available for review. If you have access to real-time information, it will be very useful. It is important to communicate the status of the plan in order to keep stakeholders engaged. If you wait too long to report information, there is no time to discuss how to modify the plan to make it successful.

Scheduled reviews should occur at least once a year and include a limited update about the environmental assessment, modification of goals, new or revised objectives and tactics, and assessment of progress. For the annual review, ask the team the following questions:

> What are we trying to achieve?

FIGURE 8.5 Communication plan worksheet

Communication Plan

Directions: Use the template to create a communication plan that answers the following questions:

- » *With whom* do you want to communicate?
- » *Why* do you want to communicate?
- » *What* do you want to communicate?
- » *How* do you want to communicate?
- » *When* do you want to communicate?
- » *Who* will be responsible for the communication?

Stakeholders for Communication	Objectives to Be Communicated	Content of Communication	Method of Communication	Timeline	Responsibility for Communication
Identify groups and individuals who need communication updates.	Identify what you plan to accomplish with the communication.	Identify what general types of information you need to communicate.	Identify how you will communicate (written reports, videos, emails, group presentations, etc).	Identify how frequently or at what milestones you will communicate.	Identify the person or group responsible for communication.

Adapted with permission from *Strategic Planning: The Roadmap to Success. A Guide for Affiliates and Dietetic Practice Groups.* American Dietetic Association; 2006.[8]

> Are the objectives still relevant given the current environment, or do they need to be altered?

> Do we need to add or delete any objectives?

> What is needed to execute the plan successfully?

Keep in mind that a strategy could be working even if the objectives have not been met. Consider the following possibilities:

> Were the tactics executed appropriately?

> Did we underestimate how long the strategy would take?

> Were our objectives too ambitious or otherwise unreasonable?

During the strategic planning process, the team should identify triggers for revisiting the plan at times other than the scheduled reviews. Triggers are events or results that, if they occur, lead you and your team to discuss whether course corrections are indicated. For example, an organizational merger or a change in the facility's software might trigger a review. Another approach to consider is contingency planning in which the team anticipates key factors that could change in the future and proactively identifies ways to address those changes should they occur.

Step 10: Recognizing the Team's Success

As a leader, it is important to recognize the hard work of the team that developed the strategic plan. Take time to acknowledge and thank your team. More information on ways to celebrate success is shared in Chapter 7, Professional Staff Development.

Implementing the Plan

"Vision without execution is hallucination." –Thomas Edison

The strategic planning process does not end once the plan is written; the real work has just begun. The best plan is worthless if it is not executed.[13] Your job now is to inspire and lead your team toward realization of the defined future.

The best way to ensure the plan gets implemented is to integrate it directly into departmental operations. The strategic plan should drive all aspects of department management, forming the basis of an ongoing cycle of implementation, assessment, refinement, implementation, reassessment, and so on. The department's infrastructure needs to be aligned with the plan in terms of staffing and daily operations. For example, measurement indicators should be part of your performance improvement system. Include periodic monitoring of the strategic plan as a standard agenda item for staff meetings. Require staff to set goals related to the strategic plan as part of their annual performance reviews (and do so for yourself, as well: hold yourself accountable for implementation of the plan). Use the strategic plan annually to design the department budget. The strategic plan should provide a framework for daily decision making. Also remember to celebrate achieving specific milestones along the way; such commemorations help keep staff engaged in the plan and motivated. Figure 8.6 provides a sample tool that you can use to monitor progress.

FIGURE 8.6 Strategic plan monitoring tool

Annual Progress Report for Strategic Plan

Goal: _____

Objectives	Tactics for Current Year	Responsible Party or Parties	Resources Needed (Funding, Time, People, Materials, and Equipment)	Status	Completion Date

Tips for Success

As you embark on strategic planning for your department, there are several key steps you can take to increase the likelihood of success in achieving your vision. Some of these ideas have already been mentioned but bear repeating.

> **Devote adequate time to the process.** A good strategic plan is not developed overnight. The carpenter's adage, "measure twice and cut once," also applies to strategic planning. You want to make sure you take the time to both plan the process and conduct it. Doing so will enhance the quality of the end product.

> **Be sure to involve the right people in the process.** It is important to include key constituencies so they will support the strategic plan. Consider asking constituents for their input through interviews, surveys, or focus groups. Involve your staff early in the process so they become committed to the plan. By doing so, you can help them think strategically, place their roles in a broader context, and build skills in decision making.

> **Coordinate strategic planning with financial planning.** Time the strategic planning process so the plan is written prior to the start of the budget development cycle. In that way, the budget can be built based on the priorities and needs set forth in the strategic plan. In subsequent years, plan to complete an annual review and update the strategic plan prior to submitting your annual budget request. (See Chapter 9 for more information on the budgeting process.)

> **Develop consensus about the organization's internal and external environments.** The environmental analysis drives the development of the entire strategic plan. If the parties involved in planning do not agree on the analysis, the final plan will lack focus and direction.

> **Don't fall prey to "paralysis by analysis."** While understanding the past is important, do not spend too much time analyzing historical data at the expense of thinking about the future. People sometimes focus too much on data analysis because thinking creatively about the future takes them out of their comfort zone. A skilled facilitator can help the group avoid this common pitfall.

> **Don't be afraid to confront critical issues.** While it may be uncomfortable, the planning team must identify and face critical issues in order to create an effective plan. You will never be able to reach your vision if you pretend certain environmental issues do not exist or if you omit key tactics necessary for success from the plan.

> **Don't assume the objectives will take care of themselves.** Your goals will not be achieved without conscious action. To keep the momentum going, identify a champion for each goal. Plan periodic progress reviews (quarterly, annually, or when a triggering event occurs).

> **Be disciplined but flexible.** On one hand, you need to be prepared to stick with a plan for as long as several years before you can tell whether your strategy has been successful. On the other hand, staying locked into your plan can do more harm than good if you overlook a critical course correction. As your plan progresses, keep an eye open for emergent strategies and be prepared to make adjustments and respond creatively to unexpected events.

Summary

While you may consider strategic planning a daunting task, it needn't be so. The time invested up front will pay dividends later when you realize that you are spending less time in crisis-management mode and more time building on the successes achieved by an engaged and high-performing team. Food and nutrition leaders who have never done strategic planning may want to begin with a simple version of the process to get their feet wet; as you build experience with the concept, you can advance to a more sophisticated planning process.

Your decision to do strategic planning should not depend on whether your department or organization has a strategic plan or on the size of your department or organization. While strategic planning is often a top-down process that originates with top leadership in an organization and cascades down to the department level, it does not need to happen that way. In the spirit of managing up, a clinical nutrition unit can take the lead in developing a process and strategic plan that serves as a model for the rest of the department and organization.

Finally, make strategic planning an ongoing process similar to performance improvement. Create a culture of strategic thinking where you and your staff continually analyze the environment, evaluate progress, and revise tactics as needed to achieve your vision. Figure 8.7 illustrates this ongoing and cyclical nature of strategic planning management.

FIGURE 8.7 Strategic planning cycle

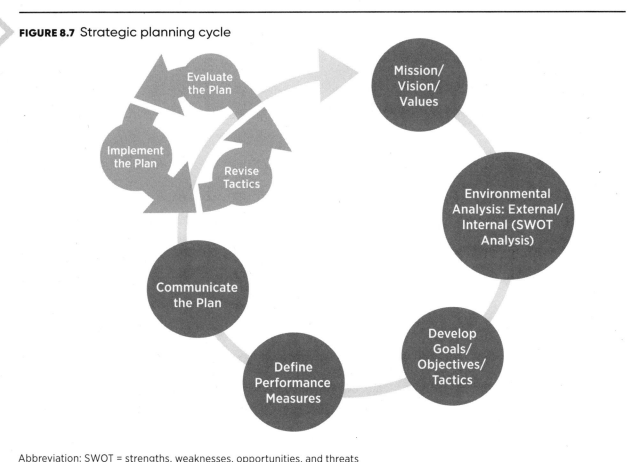

Abbreviation: SWOT = strengths, weaknesses, opportunities, and threats

REFERENCES

1   Leslie JB. *The Leadership Gap: What You Need, and Still Don't Have, When It Comes to Leadership Talent.* Center for Creative Leadership; 2009. Updated 2015. Accessed March 3, 2022. https://cclinnovation.org/wp-content/uploads/2020/03/leadership-gap-what-you-need.pdf

2   Zuckerman AM. *Healthcare Strategic Planning: Approaches for the 21st Century.* Health Administration Press; 1998.

3   Abraham SC. *Strategic Planning: A Practical Guide for Competitive Success.* Thompson South-Western; 2006.

4   Bryson JM. *Strategic Planning for Public and Nonprofit Organizations: A Guide to Strengthening and Sustaining Organizational Achievement.* Wiley; 2011.

5   Barksdale S, Lund T. *10 Steps to Successful Strategic Planning.* ASTD Press; 2006.

6   Collins J. *Good to Great: Why Some Companies Make the Leap… and Others Don't.* HarperCollins; 2001.

7   Combe M. Change readiness: focusing change management where it counts. July 2014. Accessed March 10, 2023. www.pmi.org/learning/library/change-readiness-11126

8   *Strategic Planning: The Roadmap to Success. A Guide for Affiliates and Dietetic Practice Groups.* American Dietetic Association; 2006.

9   Harrison JS, St. John CH. *Foundations in Strategic Management.* Thompson South-Western; 2008.

10 Kicklighter JR, Dorner B, Hunter AM, et al. Visioning Report 2017: a preferred path forward for the nutrition and dietetics profession. *J Acad Nutr Diet.* 2017;117(1):110-127. doi:10.1016/j.jand.2016.09.027

11 American Hospital Association. 2022 Environmental scan. American Hospital Association website. Updated 2022. Accessed May 18, 2022. www.aha.org/environmentalscan

12 Weihrich H. The TOWS matrix: a tool for situational analysis. *Long Range Plan.* 1982;15(2):54–66.

13 Bossidy L, Charan R, Burck C. *Execution: The Discipline of Getting Things Done.* Crown Business; 2002.

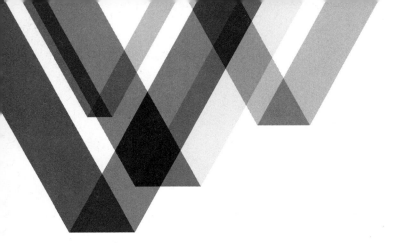

CHAPTER 9

Budgeting & Managing Finances

John A. Papazoglou, MPA/HCA, and
Julie Grim, MPH, RDN, LD

Introduction

Budgeting provides a method for organizing, communicating, and controlling a health care facility's operational progress toward a budget plan stated in dollar terms. It also provides a mechanism for evaluating financial performance and controlling operations in accordance with the objectives, policies, and plans of the institution.[1,2]

Food and nutrition managers should approach the budgeting process as a tool for managing their operations throughout the year rather than an annual accounting exercise. As a management tool, it can serve as a very efficient way to communicate operational and financial expectations within the organization. It helps managers obtain information they need to assess and improve performance. Successful managers work hard to meet their budget targets; therefore, it is important for them to put effort into developing budget targets that are realistic as well as achievable.

New nutrition managers often find budgeting and other financial management processes to be daunting tasks. In fact, some clinicians do not pursue or accept promotions into management positions because they have a fear of managing budgets and other financial responsibilities. Registered dietitian nutritionists (RDNs) are more than qualified to handle the basic financial calculations involved in budgeting. If you plan effectively, define your work processes, and understand the costs and cost drivers in your department, you can project an attainable and realistic budget. The key to taking the mystery out of the budgeting process is to become familiar with the timeline, the language, the electronic or printed forms used, and the methods used at your particular facility. This chapter reviews basic budget vocabulary, types of budgets, common areas of budgetary responsibility for the clinical nutrition manager (CNM), common financial tools, and tips for securing approval for the financial resources needed to accomplish the work required in your department.

The Language of Budgeting and Finance

Health care finances seem to have a language of their own. Following are some of the most common terms you will hear in relation to health care finances.

Payer The entity that pays for an individual's health care. Payers in the health care industry are both public and private. Public payers include federal and state governments—which fund Medicare & Medicaid—and, to a lesser degree, local governments. Private payers are insurance companies. Both public and private payers are often referred to as *third-party payers*.

Payer mix The various types of monies (eg, payments from Medicaid, Medicare, indemnity insurance, or managed care) received by a medical practice or health care institution for patient care.

Operating revenue The direct income from the provision of patient services, revenue from other operating sources (eg, sales and services to guests), and revenue from miscellaneous sources (eg, rental of hospital space, sale of cafeteria meals, gift shop sales) (total operating revenue). Operating revenue is the primary way hospitals make money.

Gross patient revenue Total charges billed by the health care facility for patient care delivery. For example, gross patient revenue for outpatient nutrition counseling is the charges sent by the RDN to the insurance provider for the service provided.

Net patient revenue The revenue from patient care delivery remaining after deductions for contractual adjustments, charity, and indigent care are subtracted from gross patient revenue. Net patient revenue is often reported as the estimated net collectable amounts from patients, third-party payers, and others for services rendered, including estimated retroactive adjustments under reimbursement agreements with third-party payers.[1-3] For example, net patient revenue for outpatient nutrition counseling is the amount of money actually received by a hospital for this service after any discounts or contractual allowances.

Fixed costs Costs that do not vary with the level of patient activity. Typical examples of fixed costs in health care include capital expenditures, most employee salaries and benefits, building maintenance, utilities, and information systems. However, as institutions become more adept at anticipating the number of patient days and the patient census, some costs that have been traditionally defined as fixed, such as the staffing budget, may be understood as varying with patient activity.

Variable costs Costs that vary with the level of patient activity. Examples include health care worker supplies, patient care supplies, diagnostic and therapeutic supplies, and medications. Some salaries, such as those paid to part-time and call-in staff, are based on the volume of activity and are included in variable costs. Salaries for managers or supervisory staff are not typically defined as variable costs because their salaries are the same regardless of total hours worked. For example, the number of hosts you need to deliver trays may vary based on the patient census, so the hourly wages will vary. The salary cost for your tray-line supervisor will remain constant (fixed) because this position is necessary regardless of total patient volume. Other examples of variable costs include food, the cost for RDNs to attend continuing education programs, and membership dues for professional organizations.

Semifixed (or semivariable) costs These are costs that have both fixed and variable components. Examples would be costs where there is a minimum cost to maintain the service or equipment and the cost fluctuates in proportion to its use. Some specific examples are telephone charges and certain utilities. Some labor and repair service contracts may also have minimums in place in order to retain the service.

Fiscal year The 12-month period for which financial results and statements are prepared for a business and reported. Many hospitals use a fiscal year that is different from the calendar year, such as July 1 to June 30 or October 1 to September 30.

Fixed budget Expenses and revenue targets that do not vary with activity levels.

Flexible budget Projected expenses and revenues that vary as a function of activity level, such as patient census or number of patient days.

Productive time Hours worked on the job.

Nonproductive time Hours paid but not worked, such as vacation, time for education, sick days, and holidays.

Income statement (also commonly referred to as a *profit-and-loss statement* or *responsibility report*) A monthly financial report that shows how actual revenues and expenses compare to budget projections.

Inpatient day of care (also commonly referred to as a *patient day* or a *census day* or by some federal hospitals as an *occupied bed day*) The period of service between the census-taking hours on two successive calendar days; the day of discharge is counted as a day of care only when the patient was admitted and discharged on the same day.[2,3]

Patient days The number of adult and pediatric inpatient days of care rendered in a particular time period. This number does not count as patients newborn infants born in the hospital, but it does count days of care for their mothers as well as days of care for infants born in the hospital who are transferred to a neonatal care unit. Patient days count inpatient days for swing beds (beds approved for both acute care and skilled nursing care).

Adjusted patient days A ratio used to calculate occupancy rates, staff workload, and operating costs per patient. To calculate adjusted patient days, first determine the gross revenue and the number of inpatient days.

$$\text{Adjusted patient days} = (\text{Inpatient days} \times \text{gross revenue})/(\text{inpatient revenue})$$

Fixed asset An asset that is not consumed or sold during the normal course of business, such as land, buildings, equipment, machinery, vehicles, and other such items. Any asset expected to last or be in use for more than 1 year is considered a fixed asset.

Depreciation The process of budgeting for the expense of a fixed asset over its expected length of use, rather than charging the entire cost against one budget period. For example, if a hospital bought new tray-line hot-steam wells for $30,000 and expected them to last 10 years, the hospital might use the straight-line depreciation method (depreciation per year equals the total value of the fixed asset divided by the years of anticipated service or use) to record the expense of the steam wells at $3,000 per year for 10 years.[1] For budgeting purposes, depreciation is often broken down further into a monthly cost.

Net operating income The health care institution's operating income after operating expenses are deducted but before income taxes and interest are deducted. Also referred to as *the bottom line* or *PBIT* (profit before interest and taxes).

Controllable costs These are expenses that, generally, a manager has some power to change. Examples of this are uniform expenses, technology expenses, and travel expenses.

Accrued expenses (also commonly referred to as *accruals*) In order to account for an expense properly, it needs to be recognized when it is incurred, which may be earlier than when the invoice is received or paid. An accrual is a journal entry that adds the expense in place of the invoice that has not yet been received.

Noncontrollable costs These are expenses generally considered to be beyond a manager's control. Examples would be rent, insurance, leases, and depreciation.

Cost of goods sold These are generally variable costs directly related to sales, such as food cost, nutritionals, paper supplies, and the costs of other products for resale.

Time Considerations

Budget Timing

Every organization will have an annual budget, but it is important for managers to review how their department is performing relative to the projected budget more frequently than once per year. Many organizations spread their budgets over quarters or months, as we will discuss later in this chapter. This means that the budgeted values are subdivided into quarterly or monthly amounts. It is very important for budgets to be spread appropriately in order to interpret actual results in a way that is both timely and accurate, as this enables managers to make adjustments throughout the year to achieve the annual financial goals.

Accounting Period

Before you decide how to spread your budget amounts, you need to know how your organization organizes its accounting periods. Some use the calendar year, which runs from January 1 through December 31. Others use a defined 12-month period known as a *fiscal year*, which is different than the calendar year; for example, a fiscal year might run from July 1 through June 30. The fiscal year may begin in any month of the year (generally, although not always, on the first day of the month) and (generally) ends exactly 12 months later, on the last day of the month; you need to confirm the first and last days of your organization's fiscal months, as these can also differ from the calendar month. If your hospital is part of a university, your fiscal year will likely start in July, when the first semester of the academic year starts. Other health care facilities mirror Medicare's fiscal year, which starts on October 1. Most companies choose a month that would be the start of a 3-month quarter, such as January, April, July, or October. Some organizations use a 4–4–5 calendar. In this scheme, a year is divided into four quarters. Each quarter has two 4-week months and one 5-week month. When done this way, each month will start on the same day of the week, and each quarter will have the same number of days.

Budget Spread

After the annual budget is determined, you will want to spread your budget by month in order to track your monthly actual results vs your budget. Each individual revenue or expense category in the budget, such as outpatient revenue or uniform expense, is called a *line item*. It is important to spread each line item by how you anticipate that line item will trend in different months. For example, revenue related to patient volume, such as cafeteria sales, would be expected to change in proportion to changes in patient volume (also known as patient days or average daily census). Food cost would typically be spread as a consistent percentage of food sales. Other costs, such as leases and rentals, are typically the same amount each month regardless of volume. These are referred to as *fixed costs*.

Some examples of budget spread methods include the following:

> **patient days:** spread by percentage of patient days

> **calendar days:** spread by days in the calendar month

> **fiscal days:** spread by number of days in the fiscal month

> **historical:** spread by prior year percentage of annual amount

> **flat:** spread equally across all months

> **percentage:** spread by an annual percentage of another budget line

Types of Budgets

This section focuses on the types of budgets that health care managers typically use, which include:

> **capital budgets** (the resources to be allocated to construction, renovation, and equipment-acquisition projects, as well as the cash requirements associated with those projects);

> **statistics budget** (hospital-wide volume and resource projections); and

> **operating budgets** (detailed projections of all estimated revenue and expenses based on forecasted patient census trends during a given period, which is usually 1 year).

This section also reviews two operating budget methods: zero-based budgeting and incremental budgeting. The most common food and nutrition expense and revenue categories associated with operating budgets will be discussed.

Capital Budgets

Capital expenditures are typically a commitment of resources that will provide a benefit for a reasonably long period of time (eg, 2 years or longer). Institutions usually set a threshold of a specific dollar amount (eg, $500, $2,500, $5,000) to determine whether a particular purchase is part of the operating budget or part of the capital budget and use the capital budget for items or projects that exceed the specified dollar amount or threshold. Purchases below the threshold are handled in the nonsalary expense part of the operating budget.[2-4]

It is important to find out what the capital threshold is for your facility. Because the capital approval process is time-consuming and involves many approval layers, some hospitals find it cost-effective to set the capital budget threshold at the high end. It is important to understand how your institution determines what is or is not a capital expense.

Capital budgeting typically involves a 3-year cycle. Thus, for any given budget year, managers will be thinking ahead and planning for the next 3 years.[2-4] The capital budgeting process may occur at a different time of the year than the operating budget process, and purchasing capital equipment generally takes longer and requires more layers of approval than purchasing items in the operating budget. If you need to make a capital request, be sure to gather sufficient data to justify the expenditure and plan for the potential of a long approval process. Because the capital budget typically is ranked by priority, take care to indicate the priority of your request when you submit it—for example, note whether the expenditure is critical to continued or future operations (sometimes called emergency capital), necessary if funds are available, or desirable but nonessential.[2-4] Also be ready to justify cost savings or revenue generation that are likely if the capital budget request is approved.

When you purchase capital equipment, you will probably use a bidding or comparison process where you work with the facility's supply chain, materials management, or purchasing department to obtain price estimates. During the estimation process, bear in mind that items that cost more to acquire may be less expensive in the long run if they have a lower operating cost, longer life expectancy, or slower rate of depreciation or are more compatible with other equipment that your department uses. To ensure you get the equipment that best meets your department's needs, be sure to specify to the supply chain department why a particular model or brand of equipment has been selected (eg, compatibility with existing equipment, guaranteed service contracts, availability, durability, ability to handle projected usage, or safety features). If you are purchasing foodservice equipment, you also need to consider the total cost of ownership. Things to consider in the total cost of ownership are the cost of preventive maintenance, repairs, and the cost of service contracts, any or all of which may add costs to your budget.

Statistics Budget

In smaller organizations, the statistics budget may be embedded in the operating budget process. In a large health care system, it's important that all departments use the same assumptions when building their individual unit budgets. The statistics budget sets the base volume and resource assumption that all units within the organization will use in this process. The primary statistic most clinical nutrition managers will use is patient days; outpatient visits may be another.

When looking at the statistics budget, managers should think about how increases or decreases in the number of patient days will affect their operations and how they might be spread over the year. Reviewing previous fiscal years to understand seasonal patterns is important.

Operating Budgets

The operating budget is made up of a revenue budget and expense budget. Each hospital department typically has its own operating budget, which is counted within the institution's total operating budget. Information from the statistics budget drives the assumptions that feed the revenue budget.

The *revenue budget* combines known volume and reimbursement metrics data to develop a revenue forecast. In addition to operating revenue, there are revenues unrelated to volume that should be forecasted with some thought given to when that revenue is expected to occur. For example, your department may receive revenue for outpatient classes that is paid regardless of the number of attendees.

The *expense budget* is also driven by the statistics budget as well as by what you know about the costs of providing goods and services. Operating costs are typically divided into labor (salaries, wages, and fringe benefits), cost of goods sold, controllable expenses, and noncontrollable expenses. Expenses can be fixed, variable, or semifixed.

Two types of budgeting methodologies used in health care to develop operating budgets are zero-based budgeting and incremental budgeting.

Zero-Based Budgeting

Zero-based budgeting is a method of looking at existing programs or services from a cost-benefit perspective. It involves reviewing the entire budget and justifying every expenditure. No existing program or service is entitled to automatic approval or inclusion in the new budget. Instead, each service is evaluated to determine whether it is being administered in an efficient and effective manner. According to leaders in the field, the benefits of zero-based budgeting in health care include the ability to gain a greater understanding of actual costs as well as an improved ability to control those costs through complete analysis and justification of each proposed expenditure.[2,5] Unsurprisingly, this approach is growing in popularity in health care because of the challenging financial climate.

Avoidable cost is a concept central to zero-based budgeting. The parties who create the budget investigate what each particular service costs and what the consequences of not spending that money would be.[5] For example, if you have offered special meals or take-home gifts for new mothers as a service enhancement or marketing gesture for the past 5 years, you may need to quantify the total cost for that service, provide a numerical measure of the impact of the service on patient satisfaction, and work with the marketing department to attempt to quantify the "goodwill" value of this particular service. You would then complete a cost-benefit assessment to determine whether the service should be continued.

Zero-based budgeting allows operating managers to gain in-depth knowledge of their operations and gives senior administrators detailed information about the money needed to achieve desired outcomes. Zero-based budgeting is time-consuming and can be a bit overwhelming to most health care managers, many of whom are clinical specialists with minimal financial training and little familiarity with zero-based methodology. If managers have done any budgeting at all in the past, it was probably the incremental type, which is discussed next.

Incremental Budgeting

Incremental budgeting is the most common form of budgeting in health care. The budget process starts with existing expenditure levels as a base and allows an increase of a certain percentage per budget year. The percentage increase might be tied to inflation, set at a hospital-wide rate, or both.

Under incremental budgeting, the only spending proposals examined during budget creation and justification are those that represent an increase above the base plus an established percentage.[5] Incremental budgeting assumes that all currently funded department operations are essential to the ongoing mission of the hospital, are currently being performed in a cost-effective manner, and must be continued during the next budget year.

Incremental budgets can be either fixed or flexible. A fixed incremental budget, called the *static budget*, remains set for a designated time period, such as a fiscal year. A *flexible budget* will increase or decrease based on a variety of factors related to patient volume. Using a flexible budget enables a department head to use key statistics, such as patient days, to align expenditures to patient volume most efficiently. The static budget and flexible budget can be used together to analyze budget variances (discussed later in this chapter).

Budget Responsibilities for the Nutrition Manager

As a health care nutrition manager, you will mostly likely be involved with budgeting for both expenses and revenue. See Figure 9.1 on page 176 for a sample annual budget and chart of accounts for a food and nutrition department.

Expense Categories

Nutrition managers are typically involved in making budget decisions about the types of expenses described in the following sections. Each of these categories is a line item in the budget.

Salaries and Benefits

Salaries and benefits are often the largest component of the expense budget and require the most time and energy in the justification process. The following list includes information you will need to evaluate your salary budget for the coming year:

> Know your current number of authorized full-time equivalents (FTEs) for the coming year.

> Know how many full-time and how many part-time employees will be on your staff (the distinction between full-time and part-time status affects benefit and overtime costs).

> Know the hire dates and review periods for each employee, noting any who will be eligible for a raise during the upcoming fiscal year.

> For each employee, calculate regular paid hours, worked hours, time-off hours, overtime hours, and total hours.

FIGURE 9.1 Sample nutrition department budget for fiscal year 2020

Nutrition Department Annual Budget		STATIC BUDGET		
Chart of Accounts Category Description		*FY 2020 Budget*		
PATIENT DAYS		50,000		
Revenues		←	divided into	→
Inpatient revenue (guest trays)	volume driven	$2,100	$0.04	per patient day
Outpatient revenue	volume driven	$10,600	$0.21	per patient day
Total patient revenue	volume driven	**$12,700**	$0.25	per patient day
Cafeteria revenue	volume driven	$622,000	$12.44	per patient day
Intercompany revenue/catering/ nourishments	volume driven	$90,500	$1.81	per patient day
Total revenues	volume driven	**$725,200**	$14.50	per patient day
Expenses				
Salaries	variable	$261,000	36.0%	of total revenues
Employee benefits	variable	$52,200	20.0%	of salaries
Total salaries and benefits		**$313,200**		
Nutrition supplements	variable	$300	14.3%	of inpatient revenue
Supplies—raw food dietary	variable	$162,000	26.0%	of inpatient revenue and cafeteria revenue
Supplies—office supplies	variable	$1,100	0.2%	of total revenues
Supplies—other	variable	$1,200	0.2%	of total revenues
Repairs	variable	$1,600	0.2%	of total revenues
Purchased services	variable	$600	0.1%	of total revenues
Equipment rental	fixed cost	$500	0.1%	of total revenues
Minor equipment	fixed cost	$600	0.1%	of total revenues
Utilities	variable	$10,500	1.4%	of total revenues
Intercompany charges	variable	$900	0.1%	of total revenues
Lease	fixed cost	$1,200	0.2%	of total revenues
Depreciation	fixed cost	$12,500	1.7%	of total revenues
Total expenses		**$506,200**	69.8%	of total revenues
Net operating margin		**$219,000**	30.2%	of total revenues

> Be familiar with the productivity standards and benchmarks in place at your facility. Many hospitals have detailed standards for determining productive and nonproductive time by skill level, procedure, or service. It is important to know how your productivity aligns with those benchmarks. (See Chapter 13, Quality Management and Improvement, for more on benchmarking.)

> Understand your institution's approach to budgeting for payroll taxes and fringe benefits. Some hospitals include the cost of payroll taxes and benefits in the average rate of pay. Fringe benefits typically include health insurance, group term life insurance coverage, tuition reimbursement, childcare reimbursement, cafeteria plans, employee discounts, and other similar benefits. Other hospitals define these expenses separately as a direct cost to the department. Still others include benefits as an indirect cost to the department.

> Know the standard salary increase (if any) built into your facility's overall salary budget and its effect on your department's salary expenses. For example, if the hospital budget allows for a 2% to 3% salary increase, how does implementing that increase affect your department's budget?

When you anticipate salary increases beyond the facility's standard range for raises, you will also need to account for that expenditure in your budget and be prepared to justify the variance. If you anticipate no changes to your business, look at your past history and the impact of performance increases to determine your salary expense for the upcoming fiscal year. However, if your business is likely to change in ways that will affect staffing needs, you must make additional calculations. For example, suppose the facility is adding another patient tower. How many and what types of positions will you need to include in your budget to meet the patient and clinical services needs of those units? If the tower is farther away from food services, how will that impact your delivery time? Will you need additional delivery staff to ensure patients receive food in a timely manner? Other factors that could affect staffing include the implementation of a new menu model, such as room service, or the adoption of an electronic health record (EHR) system that will require additional staff training hours and possibly overtime during implementation.

Food or Tray Costs

Food or tray costs may or may not be in your scope of budgetary responsibility. Even if they are not, you should understand how to budget for changes in this category. Tray cost is affected by several factors, including an inflation factor for the cost of food and paper products, and projected patient days for the upcoming fiscal year. Also, remember that fuel costs, environmental conditions, and other factors can substantially affect food cost, as has been the case in recent years for many commodities including meat, milk, corn, and wheat (and the products made from them). Staying abreast of current trends in food cost can help you more accurately estimate costs for the coming fiscal year. Also, many health care systems are part of group purchasing organizations, which can provide data regarding projected percentage increases in ingredients for the coming budget year.

Nourishment Costs

Nourishment costs include the costs for juice, milk, gelatin, and other between-meal snacks for patients. Whether your department incurs nourishment costs or transfers them to the nursing units, you will need to estimate the cost for the next fiscal year's budget. The factors to consider are the same as for food and tray costs: the inflation factor for food; projected patient days; and any factors that could potentially affect labor, such as the relocation of nursing units or facility expansion.

Paper Costs

Paper costs include the costs for tray mats, menus, tray cards, clinical care forms, diet education materials, other disposable paper on patient trays, and so on. This budget line is fairly easy to predict from the anticipated patient volume as well as any potential changes that could increase or decrease costs. Examples of changes that could impact paper costs include new vendor contracts; anticipated increases or decreases in the prices for paper goods; and service changes, such as a transition to an automated diet office system or implementation of a new menu that requires reprinting all your current menus.

Supply Costs

Examples of supply costs include printer cartridges, diet kits, and office supplies. This budget amount is fairly easy to predict if you do not anticipate any big changes to your current business.

Enteral Formulary

Formulary costs are affected by the number of patient days and the types of formulas you use. When evaluating the number of patient days, think about how institutional changes might affect volume in the coming year. For example, is the facility adding beds in the intensive care unit (ICU), where a higher percentage of your patients will be on tube feedings?

For each formula in the formulary, determine the volume of formula used in the previous year and any potential price increases. Also review your formula contract. How long is your pricing good for? Is your pricing based on the volume you purchase or on a percentage of purchases made from a primary vendor? If you anticipate that new products will be added to the formulary, project the anticipated usage and start date for each one and estimate its impact on the total cost of formula. If you have an infant formula room or a donor milk bank, also consider the cost of these products and the type of purchasing agreement you have with suppliers.

Dues and Subscriptions

In the dues and subscriptions category, you will budget for professional organization dues, newsletters, and Nutrition Care Manual subscriptions as well as software maintenance fees for automated diet office systems, diet analysis software, and other ongoing subscription costs. Some institutions also include professional liability insurance for RDNs and nutrition and dietetics technicians, registered (NDTRs) in this line item.

Continuing Education

To budget for continuing education, you should identify training needs for your staff (eg, online or off-site programs), the cost of training, and the cost of associated travel if the training is out of town. If the department pays for certification exams, such as those for Certified Diabetes Care and Education Specialist (CDCES) or Certified Specialist in Pediatric Nutrition (CSP), check whether any of your staff are due for recertification and factor that into your forecast.

Equipment Repair

Even if you are not responsible for the equipment repair budget, your supervisor may ask you to project the repair costs for the equipment used in your area of responsibility, such as printers, fax machines, copiers, tray carts, tray-line equipment, and so on. To make these budget projections, review previous repair costs, the age of your equipment, what equipment is still under warranty, and whether the equipment is fully depreciated.

Employee Uniforms

If your department pays for employee uniforms, you need to forecast replacement costs for the number of uniforms allocated to employees annually. Remember, if you are adjusting staff levels, you will need to account for those adjustments in uniform cost as well.

Technology

For the technology section of the budget, consider the modes of communication your team uses, such as pagers, phones, computers, and software, and estimate the associated support, replacement, and upgrade fees.

Revenue Categories

Revenue forecasting can be challenging because a variety of factors can impact revenue. When forecasting revenue, you will need to make certain assumptions. Try to have as much data as possible to increase accuracy and minimize the variability of those assumptions.

Outpatient Revenue

When forecasting outpatient revenue, factors to consider include the following:
> patient volumes from the previous year;
> standard facility annual price increases;
> anticipated new services or programs;
> potential changes in physician referral volume;
> changes in regulations, Medicare fees, or the payer mix that could affect reimbursement rates;
> potential competition that could result in decreased referrals; and
> changes in the scheduling process, appointment length, or method of service delivery (eg, conversion from face-to-face counseling to telehealth that may alter patient volume and impact revenue).

Charges to Other Departments

Charges to other departments might include charges for patient nourishment, snacks, or catering as well as charges for RDN services, such as cardiac rehabilitation nutrition classes. It is important to find out what your facility includes in this category and whether the budget is in your area of responsibility.

The Budget Justification Process

The budget justification process can be a substantial exercise in strategy. All department leaders in your organization are pursuing the same finite pot of money, and the budget committee is likely considering whether any budget requests can be reduced without substantially affecting services. The key to success in getting the budget dollars you request is being prepared, both financially and politically. You will need to understand who the key decision makers are, the role and impact that your physicians have in this process, and how to use that knowledge to your advantage. For example, if you are requesting additional staff in the neonatal intensive care unit (NICU) and the NICU physician director wields power in hospital politics, ask the NICU physician director to put in a good word for you or, if possible, attend the meeting when you present that portion of your budget.

Take care to understand the goals of your organization and identify how your financial requests can help the institution move forward to meet those goals. Current health care priorities include value-based purchasing, chronic disease management and prevention, patient satisfaction, patient-centered care, patient safety, and regulatory compliance. As relevant, use these priorities to frame your budget requests. For example, if your department does not have enough weekend coverage to meet the facility's nutrition assessment and follow-up policies, the facility is at risk of regulatory noncompliance. Assuming that regulatory compliance is a priority at your facility, be sure to emphasize the potential risk in your budget justification. If you are requesting an increase in budget dollars for enteral products because an expensive new product may be added to the formulary, be sure to adequately articulate why that product is justified (eg, make the case based on peer-reviewed research, the potential for patient safety improvements, or potential hospital cost savings due to improved patient outcomes, such as decreased time on the ventilator).

As you prepare for the budget justification process, investigate what your competition is doing and try to identify community standards for service and staffing. For example, check out your competition before you ask for funds to implement a room-service program. After you review other menu and service programs, you will be prepared to show that you can provide a program that is cheaper, higher quality, and likely to get better patient satisfaction scores.

Be prepared to negotiate. When you enter your budget justification meeting, you should understand exactly how much money you *really* need to accomplish your goals and where you can afford to make concessions. People rarely get everything they ask for in the budget process. What can you really live with? Many things about the next year are uncertain, and many of them are uncontrollable. Successful budgets are those that will be approved, authorize the needed resources, and prepare managers to respond appropriately to inevitable surprises.[6]

Variance Analysis

One key responsibility of your role as a manager is understanding and managing controllable factors of your unit's financial performance. A variance analysis is the primary way for you to understand the difference between what you have budgeted and actual performance. When preparing a variance analysis, you should understand the difference between variances to your *static budget* and variances to your *flexible budget*.

The *static budget* is the annual budget that was created based on assumptions for the entire year. For example, your budgeted revenue might be based on a dollar value multiplied by the number of forecasted annual patient days.

Your *flexible budget* is a budget that has been adjusted to account for the volume of services achieved during the budget period. For example, if actual patient days were notably higher or lower than what was forecasted at the start of the year, you would want to recalculate your static budget to reflect the revised volume. This allows you to better understand how your unit is performing in areas that are controllable by management, and therefore helps you create action steps to improve financial performance as needed. Variances in the areas that are controllable by management are called *management variances*. For example, if the number of patient days realized is substantially lower than projected, you would likely not achieve the revenue in your static budget. You would, however, expect to achieve revenues at the same rate per patient day. Likewise, you would expect cost of goods sold (food cost) to be the same percentage of actual sales as indicated in the static budget. Looking at these budget figures in this way allows you to identify opportunities to improve your financials on operating factors, instead of worrying about factors out of your control.[2] See Figure 9.2 for an example of a variance analysis.

FIGURE 9.2 Example of a variance analysis

	Static Budget	Flexible Budget	Actual Results	Flexible Budget vs Actual Results		
Patient Days	$50,000	$56,000	$56,000			
Revenue	$725,200	$812,224	$918,200	$105,976	Favorable	
Payroll	$313,200	$350,784	$326,672	$(24,112)	Favorable	
Cost of Goods Sold	$162,000	$181,440	$190,000	$8,560	Unfavorable	Management Variance
Variable Costs	$329,400	$368,928	$344,697	$(24,231)	Favorable	
Fixed Costs	$14,800	14,575	14,575	—	—	
Total Expenses	$506,200	$564,943	$549,272	$(15,671)	Favorable	
Net Margin	$219,000	$247,281	$368,928	$121,647	Favorable	

Managing Your Budget

Once your budget is approved, the following tips can help you successfully manage your budget throughout the year.

Manage labor effectively To effectively manage your labor, you must understand and routinely review your productivity measures. Do you know how many assessments, tube feeding evaluations, multidisciplinary rounds, and other tasks your RDNs complete per day? What is the goal or benchmark for these activities? What is your ratio of hosts to patients? Do you know how many patients your outpatient RDNs need to see per day to hit budget targets, and do you have a plan for adjusting staffing to account for variations in volume? Additional examples of labor management methods include having a mix of full-time and part-time staff, adjusting your staff schedules based on known admission and census patterns, scheduling staff to work 37.5-hour weeks to minimize overtime, asking for volunteers to take vacation during periods of low patient census, and cross-training staff to perform multiple roles.

Understand the accrual process In your institution's accrual process, are total costs divided evenly by months or allocated specifically for the month when they are due to occur? Knowing the process can help you explain budget variances.

Understand your facility's fiscal calendar and the budget cycle's timeline Since many budget processes have short turnaround times, it is vital that you determine what your role is, what areas you are responsible for, and what you need to prepare ahead of time. Meet with your supervisor or someone in the finance department to gain an understanding of the type of budgeting used and to seek answers to any questions that you may have about your facility's financial statements. For example, if you have an automated diet office, you will most likely need to pay annual software fees; know where and when this expense hits your budget.

Anticipate budget adjustments throughout the year You are not necessarily "home free" when your annual budget has been approved and your department expenses are in line with monthly targets. Your institution may have a history of cutting a certain percentage from its operating budget at a certain time of the year or when the patient census falls to a certain level. Anticipate this, and prepare a cost-cutting proposal for such circumstances. By identifying potential decreases in services and their associated impact ahead of time, you have the time to act strategically rather than reactively and can be ready to recommend changes that minimize the effect on your staff or service levels. For example, if the census is down and costs need to be controlled, the facility could suspend or cut the continuing education budget. Anticipating these types of cuts, a savvy CNM might schedule continuing education initiatives for early in the fiscal year to decrease the likelihood that this type of budget adjustment would affect the department.

Proposed New Services: Use of Pro Formas and Breakeven Analyses

Pro Forma

A pro forma (see Figure 9.3) is a projected financial statement that helps managers and administrators evaluate the potential costs and benefits of new ventures or new strategic initiatives and quickly produce alternative forecasts for different business scenarios or strategies.[6] Pro formas, like budgets, are based on various projections, which can change based on a variety of internal and external factors; however, pro formas often cannot be based on the kind of historical data that are used in budgeting. Many institutions require a pro forma before approving any new service or product. For example, you might be required to create and submit a pro forma if you propose a new meal service delivery style, a new restaurant on campus, outpatient services, a dietetic internship or other education program, an automated diet office, or a diabetes self-management training program.

FIGURE 9.3 Sample pro forma for a registered dietitian nutritionist advanced practice training program

EXPENSES	Explanation	Year 1	Year 2	Year 3
Clinician salary and 27% benefits fringe rate	Initial program development and annual updates	$2,440	$251	$259
Clinician salary and 27% benefits fringe rate	Program management: 2 hours per participant per day	$3,050	$6,283	$9,699
Administrative assistant salary and 27% benefits fringe rate	Program development and ongoing management	$687	$153	$229
Liability insurance	$20.00 per participant per year	$100	$200	$300
Computer	Allocated laptop for program participants	$1,000	$0	$0
Office supplies	Copier paper, binders, flash drives	$200	$250	$300
Printing		$250	$500	$600
Preceptor continuing education		$900	$1,500	$1,500
Program marketing	Newsletter advertising, flyers, brochures	$500	$500	$500
Parking and meals	All participants receive 1 parking voucher and a $6.00 meal coupon per day	$550	$1,100	$1,650
Total Expenses:		**$9,677**	**$10,737**	**$15,037**
REVENUE				
Tuition	$2,000 per student per year	$10,000	$20,000	$30,000
Total Revenue:		**$10,000**	**$20,000**	**$30,000**
Net Profit:		**$323**	**$9,263**	**$14,963**

Breakeven Analysis

One tool commonly used by managers when evaluating new business opportunities is a breakeven analysis. Situations where a breakeven analysis may be useful include:

> deciding whether or not to start a new service;

> reducing services in order to reduce costs or net losses; and

> determining appropriate pricing strategies (eg, price changes, check averages, billable rates, cost reductions, and so on) to sustain a business model.

A breakeven analysis is an algebraic equation used to calculate the level of revenue (or volume of units sold or labor hours billed) required to achieve a net income of $0. The equation is as follows:

Revenue − Fixed Costs − Variable Costs = Net Income

This can be solved algebraically. *Revenue* is unknown and can be expressed as *x*. *Variable Costs* can be expressed as a percentage of revenue (for example, if food cost or cost of goods sold is expected to be 40% of sales, it would be expressed as 0.40*x*). Breakeven *Net Income* is zero. Breakeven analysis is expressed graphically in Figure 9.4, followed by a step-by-step example in the following Stories From the Field box.

FIGURE 9.4 Example of a breakeven analysis

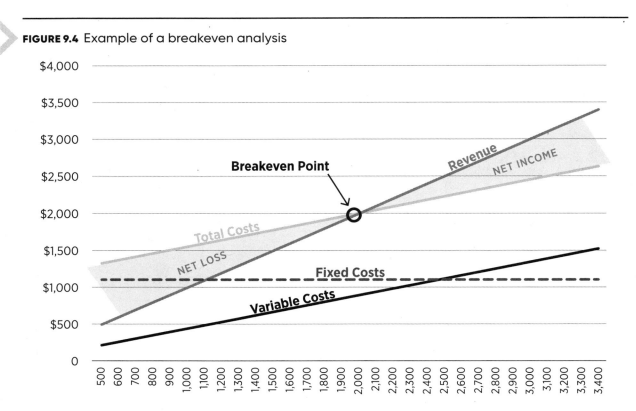

STORIES FROM THE FIELD: Creating a Coffee Kiosk

A food and nutrition manager was asked to consider adding a coffee kiosk operation in the lobby of the hospital. The manager wanted to know what level of revenue would be required to break even if the kiosk were open Monday through Friday, from 7:00 AM to 4:00 PM. Cost of goods sold (food cost) was expected to run at 40% of sales. Minimum staffing required would be 45 hours a week (9 hours × 5 days per week). Average hourly wages would be $15.07 per hour, which included taxes and benefits. If the kiosk is purchased, the depreciation on it will be $100 per week. The breakeven analysis for the coffee kiosk is noted below, the results of which were critical to the decision makers evaluating the project's viability.

Breakeven analysis for coffee kiosk in lobby

Revenue (weekly)	Unknown	x	
Cost of Goods Sold (food cost)	Variable Cost	$0.40x	*Revenue − Fixed Costs − Variable Costs = Net Income*
Payroll (minimum staffing)	Fixed Cost	$678.15	1. $x - \$678.15 - \$100 - \$0.40x = 0$
			2. $x - \$778.15 - \$0.40x = 0$
		($15.07 × 45 hours)	3. $\$0.60x = \$778.15$
			4. $x = \$\frac{778.15}{\$0.60}$
Depreciation	Fixed Cost	$100	5. $x = \$1,296.92$

The analysis determined the coffee kiosk would require $1,296.92 in sales per week in order to break even. If the check average (the amount the average customer spends at the kiosk) was estimated to be $4.04, there would need to be 321 transactions per week to break even. Key stakeholders used this information to determine whether this number of transactions (customers) would be a reasonable expectation as part of their decision-making process.

Financial Management in a University Environment

There are differences between managing in higher education and managing in a health care environment. Many of the management and financial skills you develop while managing in a health care environment are transferable to a university environment, which can be useful if you wish to expand your options when pursuing job opportunities. Although an in-depth exploration of managing foodservice operations in higher education is beyond the scope of this chapter, noting a few key points will be a helpful starting point for further research.

In universities, foodservice operations are considered auxiliary business units, meaning they are services that provide supplementary or additional help to support the mission of the university.[7] Auxiliary units typically operate as self-funded business operations, meaning they do not receive any income from tuition. Revenue comes from other sources, such as meal plans and cafeteria retail sales. Because they do not receive financial support from tuition, these operations are expected to cover all their expenses in full. Any excess margins are typically held in a reserve account, which can be used to reinvest in the unit through repair, maintenance, and capital expenditures. A reserve can also be used to cover losses if expenses exceed revenues for a particular year.

The budget justification process in universities shares some similarities to health care, but there are distinct differences. Because auxiliary budgets are self-funded and separate from academic, tuition-funded budgets, they are typically created independently from one another through separate processes. Because room and board rates are considered student fees, many university bylaws require these to be approved by the university's board of trustees. The budget justification process usually centers around ensuring that meal plan rates can cover projected expenses in the next budget year.[8] Figure 9.5 on page 186 provides an example of a residential dining income statement for a university foodservice operation.

Summary

Like other health care leaders, today's nutrition managers face numerous fiscal challenges related to the national economic climate, reimbursement reforms, and myriad changes to health care. Effective cost management is therefore a critical job requirement for food and nutrition managers. Developing an understanding of your facility's financial language and financial tools is an important step in attaining competence in this area of management. Your annual budget is an important tool for planning and managing the costs in your department and can help you maximize your effectiveness as a leader.

FIGURE 9.5 Sample residential dining income statement

ANNUAL BUDGET

Revenues			
Meal plan revenue	$1,600,000		
Retail sales	$95,000		
Other income	$15,000		
Total revenues	**$1,710,000**		

Expenses			
Salaries	$475,000	27.8%	of total revenues
Employee benefits	$242,250	51.0%	of salaries
Total salaries and benefits	**$717,250**	**41.9%**	
Cost of goods sold	$376,200	22.0%	of total revenues
Supplies	$25,000	1.5%	of total revenues
Repairs	$50,000	2.9%	of total revenues
Purchased services	$22,000	1.3%	of total revenues
Equipment rental	$9,500	0.6%	of total revenues
Equipment	$15,000	0.9%	of total revenues
Utilities	$51,000	3.0%	of total revenues
Intercompany charges	$200	0.0%	of total revenues
Lease	$100	0.0%	of total revenues
Depreciation	$25,000	1.5%	of total revenues
Overhead expenses	$171,000	10.0%	of total revenues
Total expenses	**$1,462,250**	86%	of total revenues
Net operating margin	**$247,750**	14.5%	of total revenues

REFERENCES

1   Lane SG, Longstreth E, Nixon V. *A Community Leader's Guide to Hospital Finance: Evaluating How a Hospital Gets and Spends Its Money.* The Access Project; 2001. Accessed April 20, 2020. www.iihshealth.weebly.com/uploads/8/0/2/4/8024844/hospital_finance_good_paper.pdf

2   Gapenski LC, Reiter KL. *Healthcare Finance: An Introduction to Accounting and Financial Management.* 6th ed. Health Administration Press; 2016.

3   Baker JJ, Baker RW, Dworkin, NR. *Healthcare Finance: Basic Tools for Nonfinancial Managers.* 5th ed. Jones and Bartlett Learning; 2018.

4   Nowicki M. *Financial Management of Hospitals and Healthcare Organizations.* 3rd ed. Health Administration Press; 2004.

5   Wohler R. What is zero based budgeting? TheStreet website. October 2, 2019. Accessed May 23, 2022. www.thestreet.com/personal-finance/what-is-zero-based-budgeting-15109433

6   Joy JA. Preparing financial projections and pro forma statements. Ezine Articles website. July 20, 2016. Accessed April 20, 2020. http://EzineArticles.com/248204

7   National Association of College Auxiliary Services. About NACAS. NACAS website. Accessed November 12, 2019. https://nacas.org/about

8   Goldstein L. Essentials of college and university budgeting. National Association of College and University Business Officers website. Accessed November 12, 2019. www.nacubo.org/-/media/Nacubo/Documents/prof_dev/02_22.ashx

CHAPTER 10
Statutory & Regulatory Issues

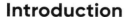

Wendy Phillips, MS, RD, CLE, NWCC, FAND

Introduction

The delivery of safe, high-quality, and cost-effective health care in the 21st century should be a priority for all health care providers, regardless of setting. The myriad legal and regulatory requirements at all governmental and organizational levels can be overwhelming, but every health care provider, including clinical nutrition managers (CNMs), registered dietitian nutritionists (RDNs), and nutrition and dietetics technicians, registered (NDTRs), must nevertheless understand and comply with these requirements. For CNMs who direct and manage personnel engaged in the clinical nutrition or food services components of care, the task of compliance can be immense. A health care facility demonstrates its compliance with health care accreditation and regulatory requirements by providing relevant and acceptable documentation of how each standard is being met. For nutrition care services, it is the CNM's responsibility to ensure that all nutrition care policies, procedures, and processes are consistent with the standards set by the facility, the accreditation organization (eg, the Joint Commission), and state and federal bodies and that any required documentation is prepared in the manner and format approved by the facility. This chapter offers an overview of some of the notable institutions, laws, and regulations related to regulatory compliance for health care facilities and suggests practical steps that CNMs can take to approach legal and regulatory issues of concern for their facility.

Federal Regulation of Health Care Facilities

All CNMs can benefit by becoming familiar with the federal rules, agencies, and organizations most involved in the regulation of US health care facilities (see Figure 10.1 on page 188).

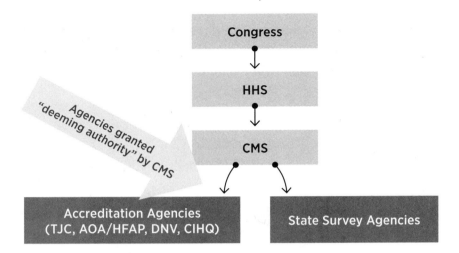

FIGURE 10.1 Illustration of the relationship between governmental entities and survey agencies

Abbreviations: AOA/HFAP = American Osteopathic Association Healthcare Facilities Accreditation Program | CIHQ = Center for Improvement in Healthcare Quality | CMS = Centers for Medicare & Medicaid Services | HHS = US Department of Health and Human Services | DNV = DNV Healthcare Inc | TJC = The Joint Commission

Code of Federal Regulations

The *Federal Register*, published daily in the Code of Federal Regulations (CFR), is the official publication of all federal agencies and executive departments, including the Office of the President of the United States.[1] It contains proposed rules that are open to public comment, finalized rules, and executive orders. It is divided into 50 sections (called *titles*) that represent broad areas subject to federal regulation, including those relevant to health care facilities.[1]

Title 42, Public Health, updated on October 1 each year, is a section of the CFR of notable importance to health care providers and organizations.[2] Of specific importance to CNMs are Chapter IV, Part 482: Conditions of Participation (CoP) for Hospitals, and Chapter IV, Part 483B: Requirements for Long Term Care Facilities.[1] In addition, other parts of Title 42, Chapter IV, may apply to CNMs. For example, Part 484 is relevant to CNMs employed in home health or having oversight of RDNs working in home health, and Part 494 is relevant to CNMs employed in end-stage renal disease facilities or having oversight of RDNs working in end-stage renal disease facilities.

Centers for Medicare & Medicaid Services

The Centers for Medicare & Medicaid Services (CMS), a branch of the US Department of Health and Human Services (HHS), is the federal agency that administers Medicare, Medicaid, and the Children's Health Insurance Program (CHIP) according to the rules and regulations published in the CFR.[1,2] CMS also provides information for health professionals, state and local governments, and consumers about these programs; the Medicare Learning Network provides a wealth of relevant resources.[3]

CMS develops CoP and Conditions for Coverage (CfC) that health care organizations must meet in order to receive payment for services provided to Medicare and Medicaid beneficiaries.[4] These standards are the foundation to ensure that safe, quality health care is provided. CMS also ensures that the standards of accrediting organizations to whom CMS grants "deemed status" (for more, see the next section, Deeming Authority and Accrediting Organizations) meet or exceed the Medicare standards set forth in the relevant CoP or CfC. Unique sets of CoP and CfC apply to the following types of health care organizations[4]:

> ambulatory surgical centers
> community mental health centers
> comprehensive outpatient rehabilitation facilities
> critical access hospitals
> end-stage renal disease facilities
> federally qualified health centers
> home health agencies
> hospices
> hospitals
> hospital swing beds
> intermediate care facilities for individuals with intellectual disabilities
> organ procurement organizations
> portable x-ray suppliers
> programs or organizations for all-inclusive care for older adults
> clinics, rehabilitation agencies, and public health agencies as providers of outpatient physical therapy and speech–language pathology services
> psychiatric hospitals
> religious nonmedical health care institutions
> rural health clinics
> long-term care facilities
> transplant centers

Health care facilities must undergo periodic site surveys and be found compliant with CMS regulations to continue to receive payment from Medicare and Medicaid.[5] They may choose to be surveyed directly by CMS or pay to be a member of one of the accreditation agencies with deemed status from CMS to do the survey.[6] The accreditation agencies are typically collaborative and help health care facilities achieve quality standards, while providing a publicly recognized seal of approval. A small percentage of facilities will still be surveyed by CMS shortly after completing their accrediting survey. This allows CMS the ability to ensure that the accrediting agency is auditing in a manner consistent with CMS requirements.

Deeming Authority and Accrediting Organizations

The Balanced Budget Act of 1997 (BBA) and the Balanced Budget Refinement Act of 1999 (BBRA) authorized CMS to establish and oversee a program that allows private, national accreditation organizations to "deem" whether facilities receiving payments from CMS are compliant with Medicare requirements.[5] Deemable areas include the following:

> quality assessment and improvement

> antidiscrimination

> access to services

> confidentiality and accuracy of enrollee records

> information on advance directives

> provider participation rules

To be approved for deeming authority, an accrediting organization must first demonstrate that its program meets or exceeds the Medicare requirements for which it hopes to be granted deeming authority. These requirements are outlined in the relevant CoP and CfC.[5]

CMS has given deeming authority for hospitals to four national accreditation organizations: the American Osteopathic Association's Healthcare Facilities Accreditation Program (AOA/HFAP), Center for Improvement in Healthcare Quality (CIHQ), DNV Healthcare, Inc (DNV), and The Joint Commission (TJC).[6] Three of these programs have also received deeming authority from CMS for other health care facility types in addition to hospitals: AOA/HFAP accredits ambulatory surgical centers and critical access hospitals (CAHs); DNV accredits CAHs and psychiatric hospitals; and TJC accredits ambulatory surgical centers, CAHs, home health agencies, hospices, and psychiatric hospitals.[6]

These four national accreditation organizations all met the same requirements to attain deeming authority from CMS, but they are not identical in their quality focus and structure. Some provide specialty certifications to health care facilities for care provided to patients with certain diseases, such as TJC's Stroke Certification or Centers for Excellence programs.[6]

Other types of health care facilities, such as dialysis centers, may use other accreditation organizations as approved by CMS.

Centers for Medicare & Medicaid Services State Operations Manual

By reviewing the CMS State Operations Manual (SOM) specific to their type of health care facility, CNMs can more fully comprehend the scope of requirements to maintain regulatory compliance with all applicable CoPs and CfCs.[7] The Interpretive Guidelines and Surveyor Guidance sections of the SOM are the most informative, providing specific instructions to ensure compliance with the regulation as stated in the CoP and CfC. CNMs should also review the standards of the facility's chosen accreditation organization.[6] The facility's quality director or compliance manager can help identify all applicable regulatory agencies, including the accreditation agency, the relevant CMS SOM, and any state-specific regulations. The CNM should partner with the quality committee and other applicable committees to conduct an internal self-audit to identify possible oversights, misunderstandings, or inadequacies in processes or procedures and allow for corrective action before an on-site survey occurs. In fact, many health care facilities hire agencies to conduct mock surveys to ensure they are adequately prepared for the accreditation survey.

At first glance, the SOM is overwhelming in size as well as content. The table of contents of the SOM appendices is a good place to become familiar with the manual as it relates to the CNM's employment setting.[7] CNMs employed in hospitals should review SOM Appendix A: Survey Protocol, Regulations and Interpretive Guidelines for Hospitals Table of Contents.[8] CoP section 482.28: Food and Dietetic Services contains most standards, interpretive guidelines, and survey procedures related to food and nutrition services.

The Academy of Nutrition and Dietetics professional website incudes a page on Quality Management, which features many current practice resources, tools for measuring quality, links to national quality organizations, scope and standards of practice information, and accreditation resources. (www.eatrightPRO.org/practice /dietetics-resources/quality-management)

In addition to the federal regulation of health care facilities discussed in this section, each state can add regulations specific to health care facilities licensed to provide services in their state. An example of these types of regulations is discussed later in this chapter (see Therapeutic Diets and Order Writing).

Common Compliance Challenges

For many years, CNMs have faced a variety of service delivery challenges that are partially shaped by changes in accreditation standards related to food and nutrition services. Some changes are driven by modifications in the CMS SOM content, but others may be caused when enforcement priorities and procedures related to existing SOM content shift.

Professional Scope of Practice

Each RDN and NDTR must proactively take steps to understand regulatory compliance, regardless of employment, practice, or service setting. RDNs and NDTRs must understand how the terms *scope of practice*, *standards of practice*, and *standards of professional performance* apply to them as individual practitioners. Practicing outside of one's individual scope of practice or statutory scope of practice, if applicable, can have serious legal or regulatory ramifications for the dietetics practitioner or employer.

The Academy of Nutrition and Dietetics Definition of Terms List[9] can assist RDNs and NDTRs in the identification and comprehension of their individual and, if applicable, statutory scope of practice. Refer to the Quality Management page of the Academy of Nutrition and Dietetics website for the most updated version of the list, which includes key considerations for applying those terms and concepts to nutrition and dietetics practice.

The Academy of Nutrition and Dietetics publishes and regularly updates several documents that provide credentialed dietetics practitioners (as well as the public, other health care professions, governmental agencies at all levels, and many other entities) guidance in comprehending and using a scope of practice in nutrition and dietetics. Following are guidance offered by the Academy of Nutrition and Dietetics:

> Scope of Practice for RDNs[10] and for NDTRs[11]

> Standards of Practice in Nutrition Care and Standards of Professional Performance (SOP/SOPP) for RDNs[12] and for NDTRs[13]

> Focus Area Standards for RDNs Collection[14]

> Focus Area Standards for CDR Specialist Credentials[15]

The SOP/SOPP document for RDNs[12] provides the framework for self-evaluation and for determining the education and skills needed to advance an individual's level of practice. These are used to further develop the Focus Area Standards specific to an area of dietetic practice, such as nephrology nutrition or sports nutrition.[14,15] The SOP and SOP/SOPP are not regulations themselves but are often used by regulatory agencies such as state dietetic licensure boards to develop statutory scopes of practice that are actual regulations.

CNMs must be familiar with the SOP and SOP/SOPP for RDNs and NDTRs (if NDTRs are employed at their facility). They should also be familiar with the focus area SOP/SOPP for RDNs in clinical nutrition management[16] and any other areas relevant to services provided at their facility. For example, if RDNs are providing nutrition support (enteral and parenteral nutrition) management in the hospital, the CNM should read and apply the focus area SOP/SOPP for RDNs in nutrition support.[17] See Box 10.1 for a practical example of how the SOP and SOP/SOPP for RDNs and the focus area SOP/SOPP for RDNs in Diabetes Care can be used to determine tasks that may be performed by an RDN.[10,12,18] The Academy of Nutrition and Dietetics has also provided a helpful Scope of Practice Decision Algorithm[19] that can assist RDNs and CNMs in performing this analysis.

BOX 10.1 Practical Application of the Registered Dietitian Nutritionist Scope of Practice, and Standards of Practice and Standards of Professional Performance[10,12,18]

As the clinical nutrition manager (CNM), you have been asked to provide registered dietitian nutritionist (RDN) staffing to conduct medical nutrition therapy visits for pregnant patients with gestational diabetes mellitus in the outpatient obstetrics clinic run by the hospital. As part of these visits, the clinic manager wants the RDN to instruct the patients on how to use their glucose monitors. How do you determine if this is within the scope of practice of an RDN?

Step 1. Read the most recent version of the Academy of Nutrition and Dietetics Scope of Practice for RDNs[10] and Revised Standards of Practice in Nutrition Care and Standards of Professional Performance (SOP/SOPP) for RDNs.[12] Both documents refer to tasks that may be performed by RDNs throughout the Nutrition Care Process (NCP), and refers to three tiers of practice: competent, proficient, or expert.

Step 2. Read the most recently published SOP/SOPP for RDNs in *Diabetes Care*.[18] This document states that RDNs who are at the proficient or expert level of diabetes care may do the following activities within the Nutrition Intervention domain of the NCP:

» Plan and review selection and initiation of glucose monitoring equipment (eg, blood glucose meters, continuous glucose monitoring [CGM] systems, and sensor-augmented pumps).

» Provide education and training with required continuous subcutaneous insulin infusion and CGM certification according to institution or organization protocol or approved clinical privileges.

continued on next page

continued from previous page

Step 3. Review federal and state regulations related to the care setting (ambulatory diabetes clinic), the type of provider (RDN), and the payment method (Centers for Medicare & Medicaid Services, private insurances). *In this hypothetical example, there are no federal, state, or payer regulations that prohibit RDNs from providing this service.*

Step 4. As the CNM, your next step is to determine which RDN currently on staff (or whom you will hire for this position) meets the minimum credentialing and competency standards to provide the requested services in the obstetrics clinic as documented in the job description. This can be accomplished by completion of quizzes or exams demonstrating didactic knowledge and performing chart reviews and observations of care provided.

Step 5. The RDN will perform a self-assessment of competency to determine whether they are confident and capable of providing safe, quality services in this clinic.

Step 6. Upon successful completion of steps 1 through 5, the RDN begins providing services. The CNM conducts initial and ongoing competency evaluation and documents the results in the RDN's personnel file at least annually.

Statutory Scope of Practice

Professional scope of practice is established through CDR's credentialing requirements and the Academy of Nutrition and Dietetics SOP and SOP/SOPPs. In addition, RDNs and NDTRs must comply with statutory scopes of practice, which are established through state professional or occupational licensure or certification practice acts. The Academy of Nutrition and Dietetics provides a comprehensive analysis of state scope of practice laws and regulations on its professional website (www.eatright PRO.org/advocacy/licensure/professional-regulation-of-dietitians).

Defining "Qualified Dietitian"

When navigating the maze of what activities can or cannot be undertaken by the RDN or NDTR, CNMs must understand how the term *qualified dietitian* is defined by CMS, which provides the overarching guidance to other federal, state, and private agencies. In the CMS SOM Appendix PP: Guidance to Surveyors for Long Term Care Facilities, a *qualified dietitian* is one who is qualified based on either registration by the Commission on Dietetic Registration (CDR) or as permitted by state law on the basis of education, training, or experience in the identification of dietary needs, planning, and implementation of dietary programs.[20] This definition is also used by the national accreditation organizations that have deeming authority from CMS. Many RDNs contend that people who do not hold the RDN credential through CDR cannot be defined as qualified dietitians. CNMs can work with the human resources department to craft position descriptions to stipulate that the RDN credential is required and whether other certifications that can only be obtained by RDNs are preferred or required. Nevertheless, if there are state regulations (such as professional licensing laws) that supersede such language, those regulations may preempt its inclusion. When writing facility-specific policies and procedures, CNMs should propose and advocate for wording that requires the RDN credential through CDR to provide services within that facility, which would then be enforceable at the facility level.

Therapeutic Diets and Order Writing

Acute Care and Critical Access Hospitals

For CNMs, one of the most contentious compliance challenges in recent history involved a hospital regulation from the CMS SOM: "CFR CoP §482.28(b)—Therapeutic diets must be prescribed by the practitioner or practitioners responsible for the care of the patients."[21] This CoP was issued on October 17, 2008, with a concurrent effective and implementation date, and was of relevance in both long-term and acute care settings.

The definition of the *practitioner responsible for the patient's care* was found in the CMS SOM Appendix A—Survey Protocol, Regulations, and Interpretive Guidelines for Hospitals. The Interpretive Guidelines for §482.28(b)(1) state that "In accordance with State law and hospital policy, a dietitian may assess a patient's nutritional needs and provide recommendations or consultations for patients, but the patient's diet must be prescribed by the practitioner responsible for the patient's care." The practitioner responsible is most often an doctor of medicine (MD) or doctor of osteopathic medicine (DO). However, depending on state law and regulations and the rules of the facility's governing body (eg, the medical executive committee), certain other health care practitioners—including doctors of dental surgery or dental medicine, doctors of podiatric medicine, doctors of optometry, chiropractors, and other non-MD/DO practitioners who meet the definition of physician—are eligible for appointment to the medical staff. Also, the facility's governing body has the authority, in accordance with state law, to appoint some types of nonphysician practitioners (NPPs)—such as nurse practitioners, physician assistants, certified registered nurse anesthetists, and midwives—to the medical staff. Furthermore, the governing body may grant a physician or NPP who has not been appointed a member of the medical staff privileges to practice at the hospital, as long as those privileges are limited to specific practice activities authorized within the practitioner's state scope of practice.[21]

Emphasizing the fact that CMS already allowed NPPs to obtain privileges specific to their scope of practice, the Academy of Nutrition and Dietetics responded to President Barack Obama's executive order in January 2011 to advocate for an expansion of RDN order-writing privileges. The executive order was for all federal agencies, including the HHS and CMS, to reduce unnecessary and burdensome regulations.[22] In response, the Academy of Nutrition and Dietetics Policy Initiatives and Advocacy staff submitted public comments that eventually led to a final rule from CMS enabling RDNs in acute care and critical access hospitals to become privileged to independently order therapeutic diets, effective July 11, 2014.[23] When consistent with state laws and approved by a facility-specific policy and procedure, this rule change enhances the ability of RDNs to provide timely, cost-effective, and evidence-based nutrition services to our patients. It also places additional responsibility and liability on RDNs resulting from their ability to order nutrition care for the patient. Box 10.2 compares the new wording (effective 2014) of section 482.28(b) of the CoP Food and Dietetic Services with the old wording (written in 2008); the relevant addition is "all patient diets, including therapeutic diets, must be ordered by a practitioner responsible for the care of the patient, *or by a qualified dietitian or other clinically qualified nutrition professional as authorized by the medical staff and in accordance with*

State law.[21,23] This new language eliminates the previous requirement that physicians or another licensed independent practitioner write all diet orders.

> **BOX 10.2** Comparison of the 2008 and 2014 Conditions of Participation from the Centers for Medicare & Medicaid Services for Therapeutic Diet Orders[21,23]

CMS CoP Food and Dietetic Services §482.28(b)(2) effective March 2008 to July 11, 2014[a,21]	CMS CoP Food and Dietetic Services §482.28(b)(2) effective July 11, 2014[23]
Regulation: Therapeutic diets must be prescribed by the practitioner or practitioners responsible for the care of the patient.	**Regulation:** All patient diets, including therapeutic diets, must be ordered by a practitioner responsible for the care of the patient, or by a qualified dietitian or other clinically qualified nutrition professional as authorized by the medical staff and in accordance with state law.
Interpretive Guidelines: Therapeutic diets *must* be: » prescribed in writing by *the practitioner responsible for the patient's care*; » documented in the patient's medical record (including documentation about the patient's tolerance to the therapeutic diet as ordered); and » evaluated for nutritional adequacy. *In accordance with state law and hospital policy, a dietitian may assess a patient's nutritional needs and provide recommendations or consultations for patients, but the patient's diet must be prescribed by the practitioner responsible for the patient's care.*	**Interpretive Guidelines:** The hospital's governing body may choose, when permitted under state law and upon recommendation of the medical staff, to grant qualified dietitians or qualified nutrition professionals diet-ordering privileges. In many cases, state law determines what criteria an individual must satisfy in order to be a *qualified dietitian*; state law may define the term to mean a *registered dietitian* registered with a private organization, such as the Commission on Dietetic Registration, or state law may impose different or additional requirements. Terms such as nutritionists, nutrition professionals, certified clinical nutritionists, and certified nutrition specialists are also used to refer to individuals who are not dietitians, but who may also be qualified under state law to order patient diets. It is the responsibility of the hospital to ensure individuals are qualified under state law before appointing them to the medical staff or granting them privileges to order diets. If the hospital chooses not to grant diet-ordering privileges to dietitians or other nutrition professionals, even when permitted under state law, the patient's diet must be prescribed by a practitioner responsible for the patient's care. In this situation, a dietitian or nutrition professional who does not have privileges to order diets may nevertheless assess a patient's nutritional needs and provide recommendations or consultations for patients to a practitioner responsible for the care of the patient.

[a] CMS CoP = Centers for Medicare & Medicaid Services Conditions of Participation

The definition of the term *therapeutic diet* is important in this setting. As published in the *Federal Register* on May 12, 2014, CMS considers "all patient diets to be therapeutic in nature, regardless of the modality used to support the nutritional needs of the patient."[23] CMS allows individual hospital governing boards to decide which orders may be written by RDNs in their facilities, including enteral and parenteral nutrition. The scope of these privileges must be delineated by each hospital's privileging policy and only applies to patients admitted to that hospital.

In addition to defining *therapeutic diets* in the *Federal Register* comments,[23] CMS outlined the privileging process for qualified dietitians in hospitals. The intent is to ensure oversight of RDNs and their ordering privileges by medical staff—either by appointing RDNs to the medical staff or by authorizing ordering privileges without appointment to the medical staff, all through the hospital's relevant rules, regulations, and bylaws.[23] Many hospitals have chosen one of the following two methods to authorize RDN nutrition order-writing privileges:

> Follow existing processes for granting privileges for other allied health practitioners, such as speech–language pathologists, physical therapists, or occupational therapists.

> Implement policies and procedures for the physician to delegate to the RDN the authority to write nutrition orders for individual patients admitted to that health care facility.

The ability to implement independent nutrition order-writing privileges is also dependent on each state's professional licensure regulations or the absence of restrictions to this privilege. State laws governing other health care professions must also be considered, such as state pharmacy laws that may affect pharmacies accepting RDN orders for parenteral nutrition support. The Academy of Nutrition and Dietetics professional website provides a state-by-state guide to laws and regulations that should be considered in addition to the CMS CoP (this online resource might not be exhaustive and may not be updated on the same schedule as changes in state laws; www.eatrightPRO.org/advocacy/licensure/licensure-map-and-statutes-by-state/statutes-by-state-list). It is the CNM's responsibility to verify all applicable rules, regulations, or laws that can affect privileges being requested. CNMs should consult their facility's legal counsel and quality director or compliance officer for support in this review. The Academy of Nutrition and Dietetics Quality Management Committee also publishes practice tips (www.eatrightPRO.org/advocacy/licensure/therapeutic-diet-orders/hospitals-and-critical-access-hospitals), two of which are particularly helpful for implementation of order-writing privileges for RDNs in hospitals: Practice Tips: Hospital Regulation—Ordering Privileges for the RDN[24] and Practice Tips: Implementation Steps—Ordering Privileges for the RDN.[25]

CNMs may also access helpful resources on this subject through the Clinical Nutrition Management Dietetic Practice Group website (www.cnmdpg.org), including articles published in the peer-reviewed publication *Future Dimensions in Clinical Nutrition Management* after the 2014 rule change. These include the following articles:

> "Are Your RDNs Competent to Write Orders? Assessing Practice Based Competency"[26]

> "Timeline of Events Leading to Allowance of RDN Order Writing Privileges by CMS"[27]

> "Implementation of Order Writing Privileges in Acute Care Hospitals"[28]

The *Journal of the Academy of Nutrition and Dietetics* and *Nutrition in Clinical Practice* also publish articles to guide implementation of RDN order-writing privileges.

Nutrition Order-Writing Privileges for Registered Dietitian Nutritionists in Long-Term Care Facilities

On September 28, 2016, CMS released the revised Requirements for Participation for Medicare and Medicaid-Certified Nursing Facilities.[29] This was the first time CMS had updated the regulations for long-term care (LTC) facilities in 27 years, and the document therefore contained a very comprehensive set of regulatory updates. One of the major items of interest to CNMs was a new provision effective November 28, 2016, for delegation of the task of writing dietary orders to a qualified dietitian[29]:

> *Section 483.30(e)(2): A resident's attending physician may delegate the task of writing dietary orders, consistent with §483.60, to a qualified dietitian or other clinically qualified nutrition professional who is acting within the scope of practice as defined by State law and is under the supervision of the physician.*

CMS provides additional guidance for this section in the SOM.[20] Note that the guidance following sections refer to delegation of tasks to *qualified therapists* because a second, related section authorizes the attending physician to delegate to qualified therapists the task of writing therapy orders.

Guidance Section 483.30(e)(2)-(3)

Physicians and non-physician practitioners (NPPs) may delegate the task of writing orders to qualified dietitians or clinically qualified nutrition professionals and qualified therapists if the State practice act allows the delegation of the task, and the State practice act for the qualified individual being delegated the task of writing orders permits such performance. Delegation of this task does not relieve the physician of the obligation to supervise the medical care of his/her residents. Physician responsibilities related to physician supervision of resident care are located in §483.30(a), F710, and physician obligations for conducting resident visits are located at §483.30(b), F711.

Dietary orders written by a qualified dietitian/clinically qualified nutritional professional, or therapy orders written by therapists, do not require physician cosignature, except as required by State law.

CNMs can help themselves and their staff prepare for surveyors' questions related to this provision by reviewing the probing questions in the CMS SOM for LTC facilities, as listed below from the SOM version last updated on November 22, 2017.[20]

Probes 483.30(e)(2)-(3)

- *If the dietitian/other clinically qualified nutrition professional is writing dietary orders, did the attending physician delegate this task?*

- *If State law allows dietitians or other clinically qualified nutrition professionals to write dietary orders, are they functioning within the scope of practice defined by State law?*

- *Do physicians cosign dietitian/other clinically qualified nutrition professional orders and/or therapists orders, if required by State law?*

- *Is there evidence of physician supervision of dietitians/other clinically qualified nutritional professionals and/or qualified therapists who write orders? Examples of supervision may include face-to-face encounters, clinical record reviews, telephone consults, e-mail, telehealth, and electronic health records.*

- *When facility policy and State law allows physicians to delegate the task of writing orders to qualified dietitians, other clinically qualified nutrition professionals, and qualified therapists, how does the facility ensure physician supervision of individuals performing these tasks?*

While the update improves the efficiency of nutrition care and the autonomy for RDNs working in these facilities, it is critical to note the substantial difference between the ability of RDNs to write nutrition orders in hospitals compared to LTC facilities. In LTC facilities, the attending physician must first delegate the task of writing nutrition orders to the RDN for that individual resident, ensuring oversight by the attending physician.[20]

The definition of a therapeutic diet in LTC facilities, as stated in the CMS SOM,[20] is as follows:

Therapeutic diet refers to a diet ordered by a physician or other delegated provider that is part of the treatment for a disease or clinical condition, to eliminate, decrease, or increase certain substances in the diet (eg, sodium or potassium), or to provide mechanically altered food when indicated.

The issue of enteral or parenteral nutrition is not addressed in the LTC setting as it was in the hospital SOM from CMS. Since it is not expressly prohibited, some LTC facilities are allowing RDNs to write enteral and parenteral nutrition orders when that authority is delegated by the attending physician for a resident receiving one or both of those therapies. Again, CNMs must review all applicable state laws in partnership with the facility's legal counsel before proceeding with order-writing privileges for RDNs. The guidance provided on the Academy of Nutrition and Dietetics professional website (www.eatrightPRO.org/dietorders) includes LTC facilities, and the Academy of Nutrition and Dietetics Quality Management Committee published a Practice Tip on this topic, as well (Reform Requirements for RDNs and NDTRs in Long Term Care Facilities[30]).

Compliance Guidelines and Suggestions

As the previous review of compliance issues demonstrates, the regulatory landscape is continually changing. Therefore, CNMs must be vigilant to maintain compliance within the facility where they are employed. How does a CNM ensure that all accreditation standards pertinent to clinical nutrition services or food services are appropriately and adequately adopted and incorporated and that procedures are in place to address and maintain compliance? The following steps are essential:

> Identify the applicable accreditation organization, such as the state agency or agencies, TJC, AOA/HFAP, DNV, or CIHQ.

> Read the accreditation standards in their entirety, not just those directly referencing food and nutrition services.

> Identify the standards that apply specifically to clinical nutrition services, such as screening, assessment, and reassessment. Consider application of those standards to the provision of care throughout the Nutrition Care Process, nutrition screening, nutrition counseling and education, and nutrition care coordination and discharge planning.

> Identify the standards that apply specifically to other related nutrition services, such as food services and emergency or disaster preparedness plans.

> Identify the standards that apply specifically to staff resources, such as requirements related to hiring, immunization, training, performance reviews, and competency documentation.

> Identify the standards that require service coordination with other departments, services, or disciplines, such as nursing, pharmacy, or social services. Many standards are interdepartmental and contain shared aspects of care or service delivery. The following steps should be used to address interdepartmental standards:

  • Meet one-on-one with the managers or supervisors of interdisciplinary areas and jointly develop, implement, test, analyze, and revise (as necessary) the pertinent coordinated policies and procedures, which should ensure all entities have components in place to achieve compliance.

  • Become a part of an interdisciplinary team or group of facility managers that meets on a regular basis to identify and address possible compliance concerns.

> Meet one-on-one with the facility's compliance manager (or other designated person). Do this at least twice a year, if possible, and more frequently, if necessary, to identify areas of strengths and concerns and to develop, coordinate, and assess action plans to maximize compliance.

> Attend facility meetings and briefings on standards compliance. Follow through on those items or areas of concern promptly and within a reasonable time frame, as dictated by the situation.

> Read facility communications related to regulations, compliance, documentation, and other need-to-know topics. Complete all required tasks promptly.

> Attend and participate in conferences, webinars, or other related opportunities, to learn the challenges CNMs in other organizations and facilities have encountered in addressing standards compliance. Reading blogs and listservs, such as the one provided by the Clinical Nutrition Management Dietetic Practice Group, can also help keep you informed and provide resources on best practices.

> Keep a resource file of information, examples, documents, and notes related to standards and compliance components affecting the applicable setting.

> Continuously view the "compliance world" from both the food and nutrition services perspective and a facility-wide perspective.

> Regularly communicate activities and compliance strategies from the food and nutrition department to key facility personnel, such as the quality director, chief nursing officer, and hospital administration. This ensures coordination of activities between departments and their ability to answer surveyors' questions on behalf of the CNM, if needed.

> Regularly communicate activities and compliance strategies to RDNs and NDTRs so they are aware of the regulatory standards and how to follow them in their daily practice.

A continually changing regulatory landscape can be challenging, but it also provides the unique opportunity for CNMs to advocate for new services to be provided by RDNs. Both the Academy of Nutrition and Dietetics and the American Society for Parenteral and Enteral Nutrition (ASPEN) have active public policy and legislative workplans that CNMs can both inform and influence.

Nutrition Services Compliance Requirements

Throughout this chapter, a great deal of information has been provided about various accrediting agencies, CMS CoPs and CfCs, and accreditation standards. What is most important is that CNMs focus on the standards relevant to the organizations in which they are employed or to which they provide contracted services.

Developing Facility and Department Checklists

Over the years, CNMs at many facilities have developed their own facility-specific checklists or guides to help them keep track of all standards specific to nutrition and food services as well as standards with more interdisciplinary and global content, such as patient education, infection control, and human resources. When developing a facility-specific checklist, start with any guides that the accreditation entity might provide, such as the annual Survey Activity Guide for Health Care Organizations developed by TJC and available on its website (www.jointcommission.org),[31] or DNV's Accreditation Requirements, Interpretive Guidelines and Surveyor Guidance.[32]

Since TJC is the most widely used accreditation agency, we will use their process to discuss survey readiness recommendations for CNMs. TJC's website provides guidance about the documents that site surveyors for the Hospital Accreditation Program will request, including the following[31]:

> performance improvement data from the past 12 months

> documentation of performance improvement projects being conducted and reported to a centralized facility-specific committee (eg, the quality committee), including the reasons for conducting the projects and the measurable progress achieved

> environment of care management plans and annual evaluations

> environment of care multidisciplinary team meeting minutes for the 12 months prior to the survey

> infection control surveillance data from the past 12 months

> an organization chart

> a list of departments, units, areas, programs, and services within the organization (if applicable)

> a list of approved or prohibited abbreviations

Other documents that may be requested include:

> a list of all contracted services,

> the complaint or grievance policy,

> medical staff bylaws and rules and regulations, or

> medical executive committee meeting minutes.

Although CNMs are not directly responsible for maintaining or providing all of the items and documents listed by TJC, they should nonetheless understand how facility-wide compliance and compliance specifically within the nutrition department are interwoven. For some individuals, it is helpful first to view "the big picture" and then gradually break that holistic view down into its specific components, such as personnel and departmental requirements, that are directly relevant to their compliance responsibilities. As applicable checklists are developed or adopted for areas of responsibility, consider the policies and procedures of the entire facility and how the CNM's areas of responsibility might overlap with those of other units or departments. Should checklists be crafted using examples from other facilities, peers, or publications, they should be carefully reviewed and altered, as necessary, to ensure they are consistent with facility-specific policies and procedures and any existing state requirements.

Personnel Documentation

The CNM is responsible for hiring competent individuals who meet the minimum credentials outlined in the job description to perform activities in a specified area of nutrition services and ensuring that these individuals continue to develop the knowledge, skills, and competencies required to provide safe and adequate care that meets accreditation standards. In small facilities, CNMs can perform a variety of jobs, such as overseeing aspects of foodservice management while also directing clinical nutrition services. In a larger facility, staffing allotments may include additional foodservice managers, allowing the CNM to provide focused attention to clinical nutrition service needs. In both circumstances, certain requirements apply and the facility is responsible for specifying and defining for each position both the job responsibilities (job description) and the qualifications specific to performance of the activities within the job description. For example, the job description and the specified qualifications for an RDN to provide clinical nutrition services or clinical nutrition services management would be distinct from the job description and specified qualifications for an NDTR, a nutrition services clerk, or a foodservice worker.

All job descriptions and their specified qualifications must be kept up to date and used consistently across all applicable individuals in performance appraisals and reviews to ensure every employee is performing activities consistent with the applicable job description. If the facility has both employed and contracted individuals providing services, employees and contractors who do the same work should have the same job description, meet the same job qualifications, and be evaluated using the same standards.

Review of employee files is part of the survey process and certain components of employee files must be available at all times. Depending on the facility's policies and procedures, the employee file in the human resources department and the employee file in the food and nutrition services department may require different documents. A checklist can help ensure that the required items are maintained in each employee file and updated as needed.

Files Kept by the Human Resources Department

Accreditation surveyors will expect to find the following items in employee files kept by the human resources department:

> initial employment application as completed by the applicant

> documentation of all applicable background checks

> new hire orientation (to the facility) documentation, including proof that the employee attended orientation, whether in person or virtually

> signed job description

> verification of any required license(s)—that is, a copy of each license printed from the primary verification source at the time of hire and during each renewal period

> verification of required certifications as stated in the job description, such as Basic Life Support (BLS), Advanced Cardiovascular Life Support (ACLS), or Certified Specialist in Renal Nutrition (CSR)

Files Kept by the Food and Nutrition Department

Within the food and nutrition services department or designated unit or area, each employee file should contain documentation of the following:

> orientation to the department, unit, or area in which the employee is *currently* working

> job description pertinent to the *current* assigned duties with evidence (employee's signature and date) that the job description was reviewed with the employee

> verification of all *current* certifications that are either specific to the job description or required or both (eg, BLS/ACLS, a food handler's card, or other certifications specified in the *current* job description, such as those available from CDR, the National Board of Nutrition Support Certification, or the Association of Diabetes Care and Education Specialists)

> *current* verification of *current* RDN or NDTR status from CDR, including date of verification

> verification of any required state licenses or certifications, printed from the primary verification source at time of hire and for each renewal period

> evidence of specified competency knowledge, skills, and abilities for *current* positions

> performance evaluations, signed by required parties (usually the employee and manager) and dated within the last 12 months, with documentation of specified competency knowledge, skills, and abilities for *current* positions

> verification of successful completion of required in-service education

Nutrition-Related Accreditation Standards

In coordination with staff from other pertinent departments or units, CNMs must ensure that facility activities, services, policies, and procedures comply with all accreditation standards and CoP with a nutrition component (eg, assessment and reassessment of patients; or planning, providing, and coordinating patient care, treatment, and services). The essential elements of the standards are fundamentally the same for all accrediting organizations, although the details vary. Several important nutrition-related, surveyable areas are discussed in the following sections.

Nutrition Screening, Assessment, and Reassessment

A facility's scope of service must have a written definition of the scale and content of nutrition screening, assessment, and reassessment that includes time frames in which these activities are to be performed.[33] For example, nutritional risk screening within 24 hours of hospital admission is currently a standard procedure in many facilities. If there are any concerns as to whether existing nutrition screening, assessment, and reassessment policies and procedures are in compliance with accreditation standards, the CNM should review, in detail, the accreditation organization's standards and discuss those concerns immediately with the appropriate person or department within the organization or facility. Participation in ongoing internal audits may be recommended.

Facility policies and procedures must define in writing the criteria that lead to a more detailed assessment of the patient[34]; the CNM is responsible for the department's formulation of nutrition care policies and procedures that identify conditions and concerns that may indicate a possible need for nutrition education or another nutrition intervention. These policies and procedures should be coordinated with other patient care departments, such as nursing, pharmacy, or social services. The content of the policies and procedures must be specific to the facility and tailored to patient types and units, such as the intensive care unit, within that facility.

Once the policies and procedures have been finalized, approved, and implemented, the CNM must ensure processes are adequately monitored and any faults or deficiencies are identified and corrected. Common methods of assessing compliance include monthly chart audit reviews, automated reports from the electronic health record, and attention during initial and annual competency evaluations. If corrective actions such as staff education or creation of improved follow-up procedures are taken, the CNM should document the actions to confirm compliance.

Discharge Planning

Transitions of care planning, also known as discharge planning, have recently gained focus. CMS's SOM for hospitals contains an entire CoP dedicated to discharge planning (section 482.43, Condition of Participation: Discharge Planning). Refer to the full SOM for more details.[8] Likewise, the accreditation agencies have developed standards related to discharge planning, with resources dedicated to improving a patient's transition from one care setting to another. CNMs should provide education to RDNs and NDTRs to incorporate nutrition discharge planning into every step of the Nutrition Care Process and assess for compliance through regular chart audit reviews.

Food Service and Therapeutic Diets

To maintain accreditation, facilities must have documented procedures to ensure the provision of safe food and nutrition products to patients (see Chapter 13 for information on quality control in food services).[34] In addition, facilities must have a documented plan in place to provide adequate and appropriate food and foodservice-related supplies to patients, staff, and visitors in a variety of emergency situations. The Emergency Operations Plan must include procedures to procure, store, prepare, deliver, and dispose of food and related single-use supplies.[33] For the CNM, the provision of adequate and appropriate food (and nutrition) often involves three components: therapeutic or specialized oral diets, oral nutritional supplements, and enteral nutrition support products. Therapeutic or specialized diets and nutritional supplements are available from the food and nutrition services department, but the availability of enteral nutrition products and selected nutrient modular components within the department will be based on an approved formulary and interdepartmental policies and procedures. Provision and delivery of parenteral nutrition support is the domain of the facility's pharmacy department; the nutritional monitoring of this intervention should be an interdepartmental undertaking between the food and nutrition services and pharmacy departments.

There are several CMS regulations related to therapeutic diets, nutrient adequacy, and a therapeutic diet manual, as presented in Box 10.3.[8] It is the CNM's responsibility to ensure the facility has a readily available therapeutic diet manual that can be accessed readily by staff in the food and nutrition services department as well as medical and nursing staff in all patient care areas. A hard copy must also be available in the event of computer or network downtime. At a minimum, the manual should contain therapeutic diet information pertinent to the facility's patient population.

BOX 10.3 Conditions of Participation From the Centers for Medicare & Medicaid Services for the Food and Nutrition Department[8]

Centers for Medicare & Medicaid Services Condition of Participation (CMS CoP)	Practical Implementation Tips
Section 482.28(b): Menus must meet the needs of patients. (1) Individual patient nutritional needs must be met in accordance with recognized dietary practices.	Nutrition adequacy of diets should be based on the Dietary Reference Intakes and analyzed and compared using nutrient analysis software. Menus should be established for at least 1-week cycles (or longer if dictated by the patient population type or the average length of stay), and the nutritional analysis should be available as part of the diet manual. Facility-specific diet sheets or a diet definitions list, or both, should be developed and distributed to each nursing unit. Nursing staff and physicians must know what foods are allowed or not allowed based on each diet that may be ordered in the facility.
Section 482.28(b)(3): A current therapeutic diet manual approved by the dietitian and medical staff must be readily available to all medical, nursing, and foodservice personnel. **Interpretive Guidelines for Section 482.28(b)(3):** The therapeutic diet manual must be approved by the dietitian and the medical staff. The publication or revision date of the approved therapeutic diet manual must not be more than 5 years old. The therapeutic diet manual (or copies of it) must be available to all medical, nursing, and foodservice personnel.	Clinical nutrition managers should purchase online access to the Academy of Nutrition and Dietetics Nutrition Care Manual or another nationally recognized, evidence-based diet manual.

Content in the manual should be reviewed annually or within the time frame specified by the accreditation entity. CMS requires that the content be reviewed at least every 5 years, but most facilities update this more frequently as new research is published.[8] The Academy of Nutrition and Dietetics publishes the Nutrition Care Manual, with rolling updates. The CNM and a representative from the facility's medical governing board should sign for approval of these updates each time they occur. Typically, at least one knowledgeable and skilled RDN in the food and nutrition services department will analyze the content. The CNM then reviews the analysis before it is presented to the appropriate medical staff entity for evaluation, approval, and signature. An approval signature page contained within each manual can be used to document proof of the annual review. If the facility uses an online-only electronic manual, the approval signature page can be printed, signed, and filed in the departmental policy manual for future reference.

All therapeutic diets ordered by the physician, RDN, or other licensed independent practitioner responsible for the individual's care in a facility should be consistent with the diet content and prescription as defined and delineated in the therapeutic diet manual or Nutrition Care Manual.[8] If a patient has a known or suspected food or food-related allergy or refuses food or oral nutrition supplementation, the CNM must ensure the availability of food substitutes of equal nutritional value and provide these substitutes within a reasonable time frame, such as at the scheduled meal time or nourishment time or at a time preferred by the patient. The facility should develop a standardized list of readily available and applicable food substitutes for a variety of therapeutic diets and food and beverage consistencies and have this list of substitutes ready when a patient requests an alternative to any foods or beverages usually provided. In addition, accreditation standards require that the facility recognize and accommodate a patient's cultural, religious, or ethnic food and beverage preferences within the therapeutic diet order.[33]

Some CNMs, particularly in smaller facilities, are responsible for ensuring that food is procured, delivered, stored, prepared, and served in a safe, timely, and sanitary manner, for scheduled meals and between-meal nourishments. In larger facilities, these activities and responsibilities are usually overseen by foodservice managers and directors.

Staff Education and Credentials

Accreditation standards place a high priority on ongoing training and education for facility staff and employees. As noted previously in this chapter, the facility must document that staff and employees are qualified and have the necessary training and credentialing to perform the duties and functions required of their assigned positions. The CNM should require documentation that RDNs and NDTRs have attained the continuing professional education units (CPEUs) that CDR requires to maintain their credential (75 CPEUs every 5 years for the RDN, and 50 CPEUs every 5 years for the NDTR). In addition, CNMs should closely monitor state-mandated continuing education requirements and verify that employees are meeting those requirements. Be aware that state regulations vary in their continuing education requirements, and the number of CPEUs required by a particular state in a given time frame may differ from CDR requirements.

To reduce the chance that credentials could lapse, procedures should be in place to remind credentialed or licensed employees of their continuing education obligations in a timely manner. Individuals who have let their RDN or NDTR credential, license, or certification lapse should not be employed in positions requiring proof of current registration, license, or certification until they have successfully reinstated their credential and have an action plan to prevent recurrence.

The work of employed individuals who have met the requirements for CDR credentialing but not yet taken the appropriate credentialing examination should be closely monitored. A qualified and credentialed staff person (an RDN) should cosign medical record documentation by these individuals to confirm that nutrition care is appropriate, safe, and in compliance with facility procedures and requirements.

In addition, the CNM should confirm that all employees attend required in-service education and training sessions. Timely and appropriate documentation of attendance should be included in each employee's personnel file.

Patient Education

To be accredited in compliance with CMS CoPs and CfCs, a facility must provide education to patients. The type of education provided depends on the individual patient's needs, the facility's patient care protocols, and the orders of the physician or other licensed independent practitioner.

All patient education should be provided in a manner that maximizes the patient's ability to comprehend the content. The CNM should ensure that patient nutrition education is provided for a variety of diseases, conditions, and disorders, with the necessary information delivered in a way that is understandable to the patient or to the patient's caregiver.

Nutrition education, with the RDN as a member of a multidisciplinary team, is often incorporated into facility protocols related to other types of patient education, such as education about medications, treatments, or specific diseases or conditions. Documentation of the education provided and of the patient's (or caregiver's) comprehension of and anticipated compliance with the information provided, is required. As relevant, the documentation should include evidence about the method of education used and what efforts were taken to facilitate patient comprehension.

The Survey Process

An on-site survey may be an intense, stressful time for all management and staff, including the CNM, even when the facility is prepared and ready for the survey. Accredited facilities should always be ready for a survey, but knowing a survey is impending can magnify the stress level regardless of how prepared you and your team are. However, a knowledgeable, skilled, responsible, and responsive CNM can reduce this stress and ensure the survey goes well. To that end, the following tips may help.

Checklists, Checklists, Checklists

As noted previously in this chapter, checklists are extremely helpful in preparation for surveys. Figures 10.2 and 10.3 are examples that may help you create checklists for your specific facility, department, or unit. You can also obtain checklists created

FIGURE 10.2 Sample checklist for registered dietitians' personnel files

Personnel File Checklist

Employee Name:	Date:

Instructions: For each item, check that appropriate documentation is on file for the employee. Supervisors should keep the department or unit file current at all times.

Human Resources (HR) file:

☐ Initial application for employment

☐ Completed background check

☐ Registration and license verification printed from primary source at time of hire (signed by hiring HR consultant or manager)

☐ Verification of other certification(s) at time of hire

Unit or department file:

☐ Orientation to *current* unit or department

☐ *Current* job description (signed and dated by employee)

☐ Subsequent verification of certification(s), if required

☐ Subsequent registration and license verification (printed from primary source or obtained from the licensing or accrediting agency website, signed by the supervisor or manager, and dated prior to expiration date)

☐ Initial competency skills check-off for *current* position

☐ Most recent performance evaluation (within the last 12 months), with evidence of annual competency skills check-off (signed and dated by employee and manager)

☐ Verification of in-service education

☐ Documentation of continuing education (CE), including topics relevant to the position (eg, if the dietitian works in the neonatal intensive care unit, CE in this area should be completed)

☐ Proof of attendance at orientation for new hires

FIGURE 10.3 Checklist for preparing staff for a survey

Be able to describe or explain the following:

☐ Registered dietitian nutritionists' and nutrition and dietetics technicians', registered (NDTR) involvement with National Patient Safety Goals

☐ nutrition screening and assessment policy (including time frames for assessment and reassessment)

☐ interdisciplinary interaction

☐ education of patients (how identified, where you document, what you take into consideration)

☐ how you know to see patients

☐ how you communicate nutrition discharge needs

☐ knowledge of emergency and disaster protocols specific to the food and nutrition department

☐ performance improvement activities

☐ how you are competent to take care of a patient population

☐ Wear your badge. It should be facing the right way, and visible.

☐ Work with the NDTR (if applicable) to review all medical records on nursing units to be sure every patient marked with a positive nutrition trigger has been assessed and all notes are timely.

☐ Ensure timely completion of all temperature and cleaning logs for the patient food refrigerator on nursing units.

☐ Keep pager, phone, or other communication devices with you and turned on at all times, in case the surveyor on the nursing unit needs to reach you.

☐ If spoken to by a surveyor, notify your manager as soon as possible after the interview regarding the questions you were asked and how you responded to them.

by others and modify them to your specific setting.

Effective checklists are specific, relevant, and easy for all users to understand. Use the following guidelines to create effective checklists in preparation for a survey:

> Every checklist should have a clear title and include fields for dates and signatures.

> The items to be checked should be specific and clearly defined. As appropriate, incorporate the exact wording of the applicable standard, create status boxes to note conclusions or outcomes, and include space for comments, such as required follow-up steps.

- To ensure consistent use of a checklist, explain how to mark the status of each item. For example, indicate that users can enter a checkmark (✓) or a "Y" for "Yes"; an "N" for "No"; and "NA" for "Not Applicable."

> When creating a "Reminder" or "Don't Forget" checklist for a particular process, be sure to include all items and actions related to the process that must be completed or checked.

Once a checklist has been created, set a standard protocol regarding when it is used and by whom. Also, review each checklist periodically. If a checklist becomes outdated, modify or delete it and remove all printed copies of the previous version to prevent its reuse. Retain each completed checklist for at least the survey cycle, and be prepared to provide it to a surveyor in a timely manner, if requested. For example, TJC surveys facilities for accreditation every 3 years—therefore, best practice includes retaining full competency documentation for each RDN and NDTR for at least 3 years (or longer if TJC is delayed in performing its triennial survey).

Performing Mock Surveys

To prepare your department or unit for an actual survey, conduct mock survey exercises on a regular basis. Provide a list of questions a surveyor might ask employees and contractors who work in a certain area and help them practice their responses. Sample questions might include the following:

> What do you do if the fire alarm sounds?

> What job do you perform? What training did you have to perform this job?

> What do you do if you see an unidentified container in the kitchen and a ticking sound is coming from it?

> What action do you take if a patient refuses a meal because the temperature isn't "right"?

> What do you do if a chemical or unknown solution splashes on your face?

> Do you do nutritional risk screening here? Tell me about it.

> What do you do if you see a patient fall?

> Do you document your actions in the medical record? If so, what do you do and how do you do it?

> Is there a protocol you use to determine which patients you see and when?

> Can you tell me what National Patient Safety Goals are? Can you identify something being done in this facility to meet these goals, and tell me about your role in this effort?

> What is the correct temperature for the dish machine in the "wash" mode?

> What are universal precautions? How are you impacted by them?

> As a CNM, foodservice manager, or director of food and nutrition services, how do you know that the employees you supervise are competent to perform their assigned duties and tasks? What steps do you take if there is a concern about their competency?

> How do you assess and document competence in the employees you supervise?

> How do members of the nursing staff know what foods their patients can have based on their ordered diet? How do physicians know what diet they should order for their patients?

> How do you know that your menu cycle is meeting nutritional needs?

Assess the outcome of each mock survey so you and your staff can build on strengths, identify weaknesses and their causes, and restructure processes and procedures to overcome weaknesses and reinforce strengths. Many accreditation agencies provide sample questions with desired answers on their websites; it is helpful to review this material with staff on a periodic (at least annual) basis.

Postsurvey Follow-Up

After a survey ends, begin preparing for the next one by taking the following steps:

> Meet with other managers and supervisors in your department as well as managerial and supervisory staff from other relevant areas of the facility. Share input and insights about facets of the survey that went well and facets that did not. For those parts of the survey that went well, solicit input about how to maintain or improve performance. If deficiencies were identified, discuss how they can be corrected.

> Attend the postsurvey exit interview or exit conference and take notes about concerns related to your department. Devise and implement a follow-up plan to respond to those concerns. Have the plan implemented within 2 weeks, if possible.

> Share information gathered at the exit interview with staff. At this time, thank employees and contractors for their involvement and efforts before and during the survey; emphasize the value of teamwork in the survey process; highlight positive aspects and findings of the survey; underscore the negative aspects and findings of the survey; and present initial ideas to improve performance.

> Above all, be open, be honest, and be a leader in setting the stage for staying "survey ready" at all times.

Hospital-Acquired Conditions

The following "never events," or hospital-acquired conditions (HACs), are defined by CMS as events that "could reasonably have been prevented through the application of evidence-based guidelines."[35] HACs include the following:

> pressure injuries (stages III and IV)

> falls and trauma

> vascular catheter-related infection

> manifestations of poor glycemic control (diabetic ketoacidosis, nonketotic hyperosmolar coma, hypoglycemic coma, secondary diabetes with ketoacidosis or hyperosmolarity)

> surgical site infections and mediastinitis following coronary artery bypass graft

Since these conditions or complications should never occur during a patient's hospitalization, CMS will not reimburse the hospital for the costs associated with treating them unless they are documented as *present on admission* (POA).

Malnutrition and weight loss have been shown to play a role in HACs.[36] Therefore, CNMs should educate clinical nutrition staff about HACs and partner with nurses, physicians, and other departments (eg, risk management and quality improvement) to optimize the delivery of nutrition interventions to patients at high risk for HACs.

For example, malnourished patients are at higher risk for infection; depending on the etiology, parenteral nutrition (PN) may be the treatment for the malnutrition. Patients receiving PN are at high risk for catheter-related infections.[37] If PN is being used inappropriately in patients who could tolerate enteral nutrition, the CNM should provide this information to the appropriate physician leaders so they can establish steps to reduce inappropriate PN use. In addition, the CNM should coach RDNs to question and advise against PN use when an evidence-based indication is not present. Peterson and colleagues found that incidence of inappropriate PN use was lowered when RDN order-writing privileges were established and RDNs had the authority to deny PN when an indication was not present.[38]

Summary

Regulations are an integral and indelible part of health care delivery that ensure the delivery of safe, quality care. Individuals charged with ensuring compliance are continually challenged as the rules become narrower in focus, more detailed in content, and perpetually more difficult to incorporate into daily operations. For CNMs, the need to be compliant, safe, and creative in the delivery of food and nutrition services is a given. The methods by which those ends are accomplished are as numerous as the challenges that precipitate them.

REFERENCES

1   About the Federal Register. GovInfo website. Accessed December 26, 2019. www.govinfo.gov /help/fr

2   National Archives, Office of the Federal Register. About the Code of Federal Regulations. National Archives website. Accessed December 26, 2019. www.archives.gov/federal-register/cfr /about.html

3   Centers for Medicare & Medicaid Services. The Medicare Learning Network. Accessed December 26, 2019. CMS website. www.cms.gov/Outreach-and-Education/Medicare-Learning -Network-MLN/MLNGenInfo/Index

4   Centers for Medicare & Medicaid Services. Conditions for coverage (CfCs) & conditions of participations (CoPs). CMS website. Accessed December 26, 2019. www.cms.gov/Regulations -and-Guidance/Legislation/CFCsAndCoPs/index

5   Department of Health and Human Services, Centers for Medicare & Medicaid Services. *CMS Manual System Pub 100-16 Medicare Managed Care.* January 20, 2006. Centers for Medicare & Medicaid Services. Accessed December 26, 2019. www.cms.gov/Regulations-and-Guidance /Guidance/Transmittals/Downloads/R78MCM.pdf

6   Centers for Medicare & Medicaid Services. CMS-Approved Accrediting Organizations. Centers for Medicare & Medicaid Services; July 22, 2022. Accessed December 26, 2019. www.cms.gov /Medicare/Provider-Enrollment-and-Certification/SurveyCertificationGenInfo/Downloads /Accrediting-Organization-Contacts-for-Prospective-Clients-.pdf

7   Centers for Medicare & Medicaid Services. State Operations Manual, appendix. Updated December 1, 2021. CMS website. Accessed May 11,2022. www.cms.gov/regulations-and -guidance/legislation/cfcsandcops

8   Centers for Medicare & Medicaid Services. *State Operations Manual, Appendix A—Survey Protocol, Regulations and Interpretive Guidelines For Hospitals.* Centers for Medicare & Medicaid Services; Updated October 12, 2018. Accessed December 27, 2019. www.cms.gov/Regulations -and-Guidance/Guidance/Manuals/downloads/som107ap_a_hospitals.pdf

9   Academy of Nutrition and Dietetics. Quality Management Committee and Scope of Practice Subcommittee. Academy definition of terms list. eatrightPRO website. Updated September 10, 2019. Accessed December 27, 2019. www.eatrightPRO.org/-/media/eatrightPRO-files/practice /scope-standards-of-practice/20190910-academy-definition-of-terms-list.pdf?la=en&hash =1DB6495E0B94CB5FA3E7443B1E8436A32E50B8B8

10 Academy of Nutrition and Dietetics Quality Management Committee. Academy of Nutrition and Dietetics: revised 2017 scope of practice for the Registered dietitian nutritionist. *J Acad Nutr Diet.* 2018;118(1):141–165. doi:10.1016/j.jand.2017.10.002

11 Academy of Nutrition and Dietetics Quality Management Committee. Academy of Nutrition and Dietetics: revised 2017 scope of practice for the nutrition and dietetics technician, registered. *J Acad Nutr Diet.* 2018;118(2):327-342. doi:10.1016/j.jand.2017.10.005

12 Academy of Nutrition and Dietetics Quality Management Committee. Academy of Nutrition and Dietetics: revised 2017 standards of practice in nutrition care and standards of professional performance for Registered dietitian nutritionists. *J Acad Nutr Diet.* 2018;118(1):132-140.e15. doi:10 .1016/j.jand.2017.10.003

13 Academy of Nutrition and Dietetics Quality Management Committee. Academy of Nutrition and Dietetics: revised 2017 standards of practice in nutrition care and standards of professional performance for Nutrition and Dietetics Technicians, Registered. *J Acad Nutr Diet.* 2018;118(2):317-326.e13. doi:10.1016/j.jand.2017.10.004

14 Focus area standards for RDNs collection. *Journal of the Academy of Nutrition and Dietetics* website. Accessed December 28, 2019. www.jandonline.org/content

15 Focus area standards for CDR specialist credentials. *Journal of the Academy of Nutrition and Dietetics* website. Accessed December 28, 2019. https://jandonline.org/content/credentialed

16 Doley J, Clark K, Roper S. Academy of Nutrition and Dietetics: revised 2019 standards of professional performance for registered dietitian nutritionists (competent, proficient, and expert) in clinical nutrition management. *J Acad Nutr Diet.* 2019;119(9):1545-1560.e32. doi:10.1016/j.jand.2019.05.013

17 Brantley SL, Russell MK, Mogensen KM, et al. American Society for Parenteral and Enteral Nutrition and Academy of Nutrition and Dietetics: revised 2014 standards of practice and standards of professional performance for registered dietitian nutritionists (competent, proficient, and expert) in nutrition support. *J Acad Nutr Diet.* 2014;114(12)2001-2008.e37. doi:10.1016/j.jand.2014.08.018

18 Davidson P, Ross T, Castor C. Academy of Nutrition and Dietetics: revised 2017 standards of practice and standards of professional performance for registered dietitian nutritionists (competent, proficient, and expert) in diabetes care. *J Acad Nutr Diet.* 2018;118(5):932-946.e48. doi:10.1016/j.jand.2018.03.007

19 Academy of Nutrition and Dietetics. Scope of practice decision algorithm. EatrightPRO website. Updated 2019. Accessed December 28, 2019. www.eatrightPRO.org/-/media/eatrightPRO-files/practice/scope-standards-of-practice/20190510-scope-of-practice-decision-tool-algorithm-final.pdf?la=en&hash=5987E388A61D43EAD2690776EAC2AA1278FA4070

20 Centers for Medicare & Medicaid Services. *State Operations Manual, Appendix PP—Guidance to Surveyors for Long Term Care Facilities.* Centers for Medicare & Medicaid Services; February 3, 2023. Accessed December 27, 2019. www.cms.gov/Regulations-and-Guidance/Guidance/Manuals/downloads/som107ap_pp_guidelines_ltcf.pdf

21 Centers for Medicare & Medicaid Services. *State Operations Manual, Appendix A—Survey Protocol, Regulations and Interpretive Guidelines for Hospitals.* Centers for Medicare & Medicaid Services; February 21, 2020. Accessed December 15, 2013. www.cms.gov/Regulations-and-Guidance/Guidance/Manuals/downloads /som107ap_a_hospitals.pdf

22 The White House, Office of the Press Secretary. Executive order 13563—improving regulation and regulatory review. Whitehouse.gov website. Updated January 18, 2011. Accessed December 27, 2019. www.whitehouse.gov/the-press-office/2011/01/18/improving-regulation-and-regulatory-review-executive-order

23 Medicare and Medicaid programs; regulatory provisions to promote program efficiency, transparency, and burden reduction; part II. Updated May 12, 2014. *Fed Regist.* 2014;79:27105-27157. Accessed December 27, 2019. www.federalregister.gov/articles/2014/05/12/2014-10687/medicare-and-medicaid-programs-regulatory-provisions-to-promote-program-efficiency-transparency-and#h-22

24 Academy of Nutrition and Dietetics. *Practice Tips: Hospital Regulation—Ordering Privileges for the RDN.* Academy of Nutrition and Dietetics; 2021. Accessed January 31, 2023. www.eatrightPRO.org/-/media/files/eatrightPRO/advocacy/practicetips-hospitalregulationorderingprivileges.pdf

25 Academy of Nutrition and Dietetics. *Practice Tips: Implementation Steps—Ordering Privileges for the RDN.* Academy of Nutrition and Dietetics; 2021. Accessed January 31, 2023. www.eatrightPRO.org/-/media/files/eatrightPRO/advocacy/practicetips-implementationsteps orderingprivileges.pdfF

26 Phillips W. Are your RDNs competent to write orders? Assessing practice based competency. *Future Dimensions.* 2017;36(4):11-15.

27 Phillips W. Timeline of events leading to allowance of RDN order writing privileges by CMS. *Future Dimensions.* 2016;35:10-12.

28 Phillips W, Wagner E, Reiner J, LeBlanc G. Implementation of order writing privileges in acute care hospitals. *Future Dimensions.* 2015;34:3-9.

29 Medicare and Medicaid programs. Reform of requirements for long term care facilities. *Fed Regist.* 2016;81:68688-68872. Published October 4, 2016. Accessed December 27, 2019. www.federalregister.gov/documents/2016/10/04/2016-23503/medicare-and-medicaid-programs-reformof-requirements-for-long-term-care-facilities

30 Academy of Nutrition and Dietetics. Practice tips: reform requirements for RDNs and NDTRs in long term care facilities. Updated September 2021. eatrightPRO website. Accessed March 15, 2022. www.eatrightPRO.org/-/media/eatrightPRO-files/practice/quality-management /quality-care-basics/practicetips-reformrequirementsltcfacilities.pdf?la=en&hash =EE376133A1F892FB89FF682D3BC49ADD80FDC3D0

31 The Joint Commission. Snapshot of survey day. Updated January 2019. Accessed December 27, 2019. Joint Commission website. www.jointcommission.org/accreditation-and-certification /health-care-settings/hospital/prepare/snapshot-of-survey-day

32 DNV GL Healthcare USA. *National Integrated Accreditation for Healthcare Organizations (NIAHO) Accreditation Requirements, Interpretive Guidelines and Surveyor Guidance— Revision 18-2*. DNV GL Healthcare USA, Inc.; September 21, 2020. Accessed December 28, 2019. https://brandcentral.dnvgl.com/original/gallery/10651/files/original /0d9513b108d847808df973607dd5b32e.pdf

33 The Joint Commission. Emergency management EM.02.02.03 EP 3. In: *Comprehensive Accreditation Manual for Hospitals (CAMH): The Official Handbook.* Joint Commission Resources; January 1, 2020.

34 The Joint Commission. Provision of care, treatment, and services PC.04.01.01. In: *Comprehensive Accreditation Manual for Hospitals (CAMH): The Official Handbook.* Joint Commission Resources; December 23, 2019.

35 Centers for Medicare & Medicaid Services. Hospital-acquired conditions reduction program. CMS website. Updated July 16, 2019. Accessed December 27, 2019. www.cms.gov/Medicare /Medicare-Fee-for-Service-Payment/AcuteInpatientPPS/HAC-Reduction-Program

36 Fry DE, Pine M, Jones BL, Meimban RJ. Patient characteristics and the occurrence of never events. *Arch Surg.* 2010;145(2):148-151. doi:10.1001/archsurg.2009.277

37 Matsushima K, Cook A, Tyner T, et al. Parenteral nutrition: a clear and present danger unabated by tight glucose control. *Am J Surg.* 2010;200(3):386-390. doi:10.1016/j.amjsurg.2009.10.023

38 Peterson SJ, Chen Y, Sullivan CA, et al. Assessing the influence of registered dietitian order-writing privileges on parenteral nutrition use. *J Am Diet Assoc.* 2010;110(11):1703-1711. doi:10.1016/j .jada.2010.08.003

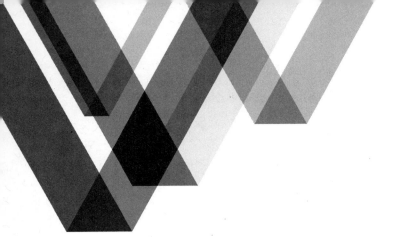

CHAPTER 11

Human Resources 101

Julie Grim, MPH, RDN, LD

Introduction

In nutrition and dietetics, as in many service businesses, people are the most valuable resource. Registered dietitian nutritionists (RDNs) are often promoted to management positions due to qualities such as strong technical skills, work ethic, and personal desire for advancement. However, the skills that lead to a clinician's promotion might not be the skills necessary to be an effective manager. Clinical nutrition manager (CNM) or foodservice manager positions are often an RDN's first exposure to management and the human resources (HR) functions of hiring, counseling, scheduling, budgeting, and so on. Navigating labor laws and the hiring process in general can be a challenge, and mistakes can have legal, financial, and emotional costs. It is important to understand the basic HR functions as well as the laws that govern them.

Becoming a manager does not automatically mean you know how to interview, coach, train, evaluate, or otherwise effectively manage employees. However, all of these skills can be learned, and there are many people available to help you do so. Many HR and management skills are best learned from interactions with people, but it is worthwhile to start with a basic understanding of important processes and concepts. In this chapter, we discuss the hiring process, employee management, and how best to partner with your HR team to maximize your effectiveness.

The Hiring Process

Research shows that sound hiring choices are directly linked to a company's financial returns.[1] As a manager, you may be responsible for hiring RDNs; nutrition and dietetics technicians, registered (NDTRs); kitchen supervisors; diet office staff; and cooks and foodservice workers. This chapter reviews five key components of the hiring process: recruiting, applicant screening, interviewing, checking references, and making the job offer.

Recruiting

Recruitment, typically the first step in the hiring process, refers to the attraction, screening, and selection of qualified people to interview for a position within your organization. However, an open position presents an opportunity to assess the appropriateness of the current staffing in your department. This is the time to consider whether the position is still necessary and whether there have been any changes in the credentials or skill sets you require of the individual filling the position.

Working With Human Resources

The role of HR in the recruitment process varies from institution to institution. In some cases, the HR department closely manages the process, from sourcing candidates and completing the screening interview to determining the appropriate salary level and extending the job offer. In other organizations, HR plays a smaller role in this process, and you may be responsible for some or all of these steps. It is important to meet with your HR staff before you begin recruiting so you have a clear understanding of their role in the process and yours. The following are important questions to answer:

> What methods will be used for recruitment? What resources are available to you and how are costs allocated?

> Who is responsible for verification of a candidate's licensure and registration status, or other required credentials?

> What kind of paperwork is involved in opening a position for recruitment and selecting a candidate? For example, your organization may have specific forms, requisitions, or worksheets that you must complete to create the job description, set its pay grade, and get approval for new hires.

> How soon can someone start work after an offer is made? The amount of time typically depends on how long the background check, preemployment physical, and employment verification processes take.

Establishing a Recruitment Strategy

When determining your recruitment strategy, it is essential to know your environment and competition and ensure the job description posted by HR makes sense and is current. For example, if you are recruiting for clerical or foodservice workers, consider who your local competition is for such employees and how your organization's pay scale compares to that of the competition for similar jobs. Candidates for these types of positions may also want to know whether your organization is accessible via public transportation and what types of advancement and educational opportunities your organization offers employees in the role. It is good to include this information in the job posting so potential applicants know what to expect ahead of time.

If you need to hire RDNs or NDTRs, potential recruitment resources include the following:

> dietetic internship directors, NDTR program directors, and university faculty, who typically keep in touch with their students and may be able to provide specific recommendations (Program directors often belong to online professional groups through which they could publicize your job description to a larger audience.)

> local sales representatives for pharmaceutical companies, who often travel to multiple institutions and know many of the clinical dietitians in their service area

> local professional dietetics associations that offer online job posting opportunities as well as free networking opportunities at meetings; also, many dietetic practice groups offer the opportunity to share information about open positions at no cost

> online job sites, such as Indeed, Glassdoor, Monster, or others

> social or professional networking sites (Find out whether your organization hosts various social media outlets or has a Facebook page and, if so, whether you can advertise there. Can you use one of the professional networking sites, such as LinkedIn or Yahoo?)

You can accelerate your recruitment learning curve by asking other managers within your organization what strategies they have found successful for hiring frontline staff. For example, if the laboratory manager has been consistently successful posting open positions on community college bulletin boards or websites such as Craigslist, you might consider a similar strategy. If your organization hosts or participates in job fairs, find out how you can be included. If there are dietetics or culinary programs in your local area, you might consider recruiting undergraduate or graduate students looking for nutrition or food preparation experience; these students may become valuable employees with a passion to learn.

Ask your staff how they found out about their jobs at your organization. Current employees can also be a great source of referrals. In fact, many institutions pay bonuses for employee referrals. If your organization has such a bonus program, find out if your positions are, or can be, included—and tell your staff.

Writing the Job Posting

All effective job postings include key information in a succinct format that grabs the attention of your desired audience. Figures 11.1 and 11.2 (on page 218) provide two different examples of complete job postings. The following key elements should be included in all job postings:

> job title

> company (brief description and why it is a good place to work)

> overview of responsibilities

> reason for job opening, if applicable (eg, department growth or new project)

> requirements or qualifications, distinguishing between what is desirable (eg, nutrition support order-writing experience) and what is mandatory (eg, RDN credential or licensure, a specified level of education or degree, or a minimum number of years of experience)

> any required "soft skills" (eg, communications skills or leadership ability)

FIGURE 11.1 Sample job posting for a clinical dietitian

Location:	Regency Medical Center, Dallas, Texas
Posting date:	September 1, 2019
Open position number:	01678
Job title	Clinical Dietitian
Work type:	Full-time
Work schedule:	Monday through Friday, 8:00 AM to 4:30 PM
Hiring manager:	Alice Smith, MBA, RDN, LD

Job Summary:
» Provides medical nutrition therapy using evidence-based practice to optimize patient care. Provides consultation to the health care team to ensure efficient and effective nutrition care of patients. Monitors and evaluates patient care and nutrition outcomes on an ongoing basis. Educates patients, health care team members, dietetic interns, and members of the community. Participates in ongoing process improvement activities within the Department of Nutrition Services and the institution.
» Maintains a customer-service, patient-centered approach at all times when fulfilling job duties. Meets the qualifications to provide care for patients in the specific age range of assigned clinical area. Works under the direction of the Clinical Nutrition Manager in the Department of Nutrition Services.

Competencies and Skills:
» Demonstrates competence in written, oral, and electronic communication skills.
» Demonstrates ability to function effectively in an interdisciplinary environment.

Education and Experience:
» Bachelor's or advanced degree in dietetics or nutrition required.
» Registration with the Commission on Dietetic Registration, or eligibility for registration when hired, required. If eligible for registration, must obtain registration and licensure within 6 months of hire date.
» At least 2 years of clinical experience preferred.

Working Conditions and Physical Demands:
» Work is typically performed in both inpatient and ambulatory care settings.

Regency Health System:

Regency Health System serves nearly 2 million people in North Texas and has been nationally recognized for innovative practices and quality care. Regency is a not-for-profit health system and a premier teaching institute. Regency was named to the Becker's Hospital Review "150 Best Places to Work in Health Care" list for 2018.

Regency offers a competitive compensation package beginning on the date of hire, including comprehensive medical and retirement program benefits and more.

We are an Affirmative Action, Equal Opportunity Employer.

TO APPLY: www.regencyhealth.com/employment

FIGURE 11.2 Sample job posting for a foodservice manager

Location:	Lakeland School District, Lakeland, Florida
Posting date:	March 1, 2022
Job title	Foodservice Manager
Work schedule:	Day Shift, Monday through Friday
Work type:	Full-time
Salary range:	$45,000–$60,000 per year
Hiring manager:	Frank Mendez, RDN, Foodservice Director

Primary Purpose:

» Supervise, train, and manage campus foodservice operation. Ensure that appropriate quantities of food are prepared and served. Meet time constraints set by menu and other requirements established by central office administration and regulatory agencies. Process and update student meal applications. Meet health codes. Carry out other duties as assigned by Foodservice Director.

Qualifications:

» High School Diploma/GED

Required Knowledge or Skills:

» Knowledge of methods, materials, equipment, and appliances used in food preparation
» Ability to manage personnel
» Effective planning and organizational skills
» Ability to use personal computer and software to develop spreadsheets, perform word processing, and use software designed for foodservice programs
» Knowledge of Child Nutrition Program policies and other relevant regulations

Experience:

» 3 years' experience in institutional foodservice operations
» Supervisory experience in foodservice operations (preferred)

Major Responsibilities and Duties:

» Produce and maintain work schedules and production records.
» Direct daily activities in kitchen and cafeteria.
» Maintain all serving schedules and serve all food items according to menu specifications defined by departmental policies and procedures.
» Work cooperatively with campus principal to accommodate temporary schedule changes, and special serving requirements and to resolve personnel problems.
» Supervise and train employees at campus level, promoting efficiency, morale, and teamwork.
» Ensure food is produced safely and is of high quality according to policies, procedures, and department requirements.
» Maintain accurate reports of daily and monthly financial, production, and activity records.
» Ensure food items are stored in a safe and hazard-free environment.
» Establish and enforce standards of cleanliness, health, and safety following health and safety codes and regulations.
» Maintain a safe work environment.
» Ensure appropriate quantities of food and supplies are available through daily orders and periodic inventories.
» Maintain maintenance logs for all equipment within the campus foodservice department.
» Perform preventive maintenance to equipment and report necessary repairs.
» Recommend replacement of existing equipment to meet department needs.
» Conduct periodic physical inventory of equipment and supplies.
» Promote teamwork and interaction with fellow staff members.
» Help screen, select, and train cafeteria workers and make sound recommendations about the assignment, discipline, and retention of cafeteria personnel.

Job Contact Information:
Name: Frank Mendez, Foodservice Director
Phone: 555-555-5555
Email: fmendez@emailaddress.org
TO APPLY: www.lakelandschool.com/employment

Applicant Screening

The second step in the hiring process is applicant screening. An effective screening process should provide you with initial insight into which applicants are likely to be the best matches for the position, allow you to narrow your list of which applicants you will interview more thoroughly, and save you substantial time and frustration in the hiring process. To help ensure you screen applicants effectively and efficiently, take the following steps:

1. Provide your HR department with an accurate position description. The description should include licensure or registration requirements, shift or schedule requirements (such as the need to alternate early or late shifts, work weekends, or attend early morning rounds), and soft-skill requirements, such as collaborative teamwork skills or strong verbal communication skills.

2. Review resumes and cover letters. Cover letters should be well written and error free and should include succinct summaries of an applicant's qualifications and why they are interested in the position. Resumes should also be well formatted and error free and should reflect the skills and experience listed in the job posting. Look for keywords that match the qualities you are seeking and identify anything you may want to know more about (eg, long gaps in employment or multiple positions over a short period of time).

3. Review job applications closely. For hourly positions that do not require a resume, look for job applications that are complete and error free. Carefully evaluate how well a candidate's skills, education, and experience match the position you have posted, and note anything you want to clarify should you meet the candidate for an interview.

4. Conduct a brief phone interview with each promising candidate. Speaking with candidates will help you evaluate their verbal communication skills, explore their qualifications in greater detail, and identify whether their salary expectations align with what the position pays, if this is a concern. (In some organizations, this function may be performed by the HR department.)

Preparing for the Interviews

The third, and perhaps most challenging, step in the hiring process is conducting interviews. Interviewing candidates is an art, but it also requires certain skills. You have to be a good listener, know how to redirect a conversation, distinguish between applicants who simply want the job and those who can get the job done, and ensure you are abiding by employment laws and the requirements of your institution.

Understanding Legal Requirements

To master the interview process, begin by learning the laws that govern this process. Although sometimes confusing and complex, employment regulations are designed to eliminate bias, discrimination, prejudice, and unfair hiring practices and to ensure that all candidates are judged solely on the basis of their ability to do the job. There are a number of federal Equal Employment Opportunity Commission (EEOC) laws you need to understand. Most employers with at least 15 employees are covered by EEOC regulations, so the following laws are almost certainly applicable at your organization[2]:

> **Title VII of the Civil Rights Act of 1964**: This law, which applies to employers of 15 or more individuals, prohibits employers from discrimination based on race, color, gender, national origin, or religion.

> **Equal Employment Opportunity (EEO) laws**: EEO rules prohibit specific types of employment discrimination, including discrimination on the basis of race, color, religion, sex, age (older than 40), national origin, or status either as an individual with a disability or as a protected veteran.

> **Americans with Disabilities Act (ADA) of 1990**: The ADA bars employers of more than 15 employees from discrimination based on physical or mental disability and requires reasonable accommodation of individuals with disabilities during hiring and employment.

> **Age Discrimination in Employment Act (ADEA) of 1967**: The ADEA, which applies to employers of 20 or more individuals, prohibits discrimination against employees age 40 years or older (in favor of younger employees). There is no upper age limit specified; therefore, mandatory retirement is illegal in most cases.

The US Department of Labor (DOL) administers and enforces most labor laws and is a reliable resource for information about any of these statutes. To avoid potential violations of antidiscrimination statutes during the hiring process, it is essential that you understand whether interview questions are legal or illegal. Box 11.1 provides some examples of legal and illegal questions; *this list is not exhaustive*.[3] If you are in doubt about whether you can legally ask a specific question, a good rule of

BOX 11.1 Examples of Illegal and Legal Interview Questions[3]

	Illegal questions	Legal questions
Age	How old are you? When is your birthday? In what year were you born? In what year did you graduate from college or high school?	Are you over the age of 18? Can you, after employment, provide proof of age?
Marital and family status	Are you married? With whom do you live? Do you have children? How many children do you have? Are you pregnant? Do you expect to have a family? What are your childcare arrangements? How is your family's health?	This job requires 25% travel. Do you have any restrictions on your ability to travel? Do you have responsibilities or commitments that will prevent you from meeting specified work schedules? Do you anticipate any absences from work on a regular basis? If so, please explain the circumstances.
Religion	What religion do you follow?	Are you able to work Saturdays or Sundays? **Note:** Tread carefully here. If the respondents say that they have religious obligations that limit availability, you should indicate that your company makes reasonable efforts to accommodate religious beliefs or practices. However, you are not required to make an accommodation if doing so would create an undue hardship to the business.
Ethnic origin	Do you speak Spanish?	What languages do you speak?

thumb is to ask yourself whether it relates to the specific functions of the job. If it doesn't, don't ask the question.

In addition to employment law, you must also know your state's professional licensure laws and your facility's policies related to registration and licensure. Can you hire a candidate who is RDN-eligible but does not yet have the credential? Is a license required to practice in your state? In many states, a dietitian must be licensed to practice.[4] If you reside in one of those states, is there an option for provisional licensure and, if there is, how long does it take to obtain a provisional license?

Doing Your Homework

Far too often, busy managers find themselves rushing to prepare for interviews at the last minute, and, as a result, they fail to get the key information during the interview that they need to make an informed decision. Be sure to prepare ahead of time and write out your questions so you remember to ask them in the interview to obtain the information you need about the applicant. According to Davila and Kursmark,[1] managers most often make hiring errors because they do not gather enough information and make improper assumptions. In fact, research reveals that more than 70% of managers spend less than 5 minutes preparing for interviews.[1] The following Stories From the Field box describes a hiring error of this nature.

> ## STORIES FROM THE FIELD: A Hiring Error
>
> A newly promoted clinical nutrition manager's first task was to hire a dietitian replacement for the open staff position. The manager's personal friend (also an experienced dietitian) recommended a friend of theirs for the position. The candidate interviewed well, but the new manager did not fully investigate the candidate's job history and did not interview any other applicants. Soon after hiring the new employee, the manager noticed several red flags: the employee was openly critical of previous bosses, abused their salaried status, and became sloppy with their work. After the new employee did not show up for a weekend shift, the manager took action and began formal performance coaching. The manager found this very challenging, given the personal connection to the employee. However, once the employee realized the manager was serious and that their job was in jeopardy, performance improved. Simply because someone is a personal friend does not mean they are the best candidate for the job. In addition, being a manager means it's not always possible to be everyone's friend.

The following points may be helpful in organizing your interviews before they begin:

> **Determine the skills and competencies needed for the position.** Make a list of what you are looking for. For example, if you are interviewing for an outpatient RDN, requirements might include experience with motivational interviewing, proven coaching skills, program marketing and development experience, and demonstrable public speaking skills. When interviewing candidates for a diet office supervisor position, you would want to find out about their management skills, employee counseling experience, attention to detail, problem-solving skills, customer service abilities, and knowledge of your particular computerized diet office system, such as CBORD or Computrition. Also determine what soft skills (or "people skills") the candidate needs to have; these may be even more important than technical skills because they involve how people relate

to each other. Examples include skills in communicating, listening, giving feed-back, showing initiative, negotiating, collaborating and cooperating as a team member, solving problems, and resolving conflicts.

> **Write out appropriate interview questions.** Your interview questions should reveal your candidate's technical skills, knowledge, behaviors, likes, dislikes, and key motivators.[1] Start with the job description if you are unfamiliar with the job's requirements. Determine what questions will elicit answers that let you know whether or not a candidate has the skills and traits needed for the position. A scripted list of job-related questions will prevent you from straying into a quicksand of illegal questions. Also, preparing questions in advance helps ensure consistency among interviews for the same position. When you gather the same information from all candidates, you can more objectively compare their suitability for the job.

> **Review each candidate's application materials (eg, resume, cover letter, completed application form) prior to the interview.** You create a poor impression of your managerial skills if you review application materials in front of interviewees. They may conclude that you are disorganized and do not prepare in advance. It is important to remember that interviewing is a two-way process and you want to create the best impression possible on every interviewee.

> **Conduct the interview in a private space where you are not easily distracted.** The diet office and the cafeteria are not good places to conduct an interview. If you do not have a private office, schedule a room or borrow an office for the interview.

> **Plan several "ice-breaker" questions.** A few casual questions unrelated to work at the start of the interview can enable you to establish rapport and put the applicant at ease. Questions about weather and traffic are usually safe.

> **Learn from experienced interviewers.** If your interviewing experience is limited, you may want to ask your HR team if you can observe them (or another skilled manager within your institution) interviewing job candidates. Another option would be to have someone from HR sit in with you during your first few interviews and provide coaching and feedback as appropriate. In the absence of these shadowing opportunities, or in addition to them, ask your HR team to suggest recordings of mock interviews or similar online resources you could benefit from watching.

> **Plan to interview multiple promising candidates and ask others to help you evaluate them.** Other people can and should help evaluate your pool of candidates. Feedback from others can help you avoid making choices based on the natural bias to choose someone similar to yourself.[5] You may find input from people who will be colleagues or collaborators with the new hire to be especially helpful. This also helps the potential new hire to determine if the work setting and new colleagues are a good match for them, facilitating their decision-making process.

Conducting the Interview

At the start of the interview, set a collegial tone. Let your candidates know that you are glad to meet them and express your appreciation for the time they have taken to interview with you. Use your prepared ice-breaker questions to get the conversation started. Remember, you may be nervous, but your candidates are likely even more anxious. It is important to build rapport and set them at ease, so you can get a clear picture of what they might bring to your team.

Occasionally, a candidate will volunteer personal information. Take care to avoid pursuing these topics in ways that might run afoul of labor laws or your institution's hiring policies. For example, if your job applicant shares that they are arriving to the interview late because their child missed the school bus, avoid asking questions about the child, other children, a spouse, and so on, as doing so could make you vulnerable to potential charges of discrimination based on marital or family status. Instead, guide the interview back to your structured questions.

After breaking the ice, explain how the interview will proceed and try to follow that format as closely as possible. State that you will be taking notes to help you remember so that candidates do not get concerned when they see you writing things down.

The notes you take should be clear and factual. Avoid writing your opinions or interpretations of what you think a candidate said. Focus on the degree to which the candidate meets the competencies. Careful note-taking is especially important if you are interviewing many people for the same position, as doing so enables you to remember and distinguish one candidate from another. In addition, these notes serve as your documentation of how you reached your hiring decision. Be aware that your HR department may require you to keep interview notes for a designated period of time in case questions about hiring practices arise.

Be sure to manage your time. If you've set aside an hour for an interview, do your best to stick with that schedule. However, it is good to be prepared to cut the meeting short and jump to the "wrap up" questions if the interview does not require the full amount of time. Do not waste your time or the candidate's by stretching the meeting out.

As you talk with the candidate, share relevant information about the job. Be sure job requirements and performance expectations are clear. For example, explain whether employees are expected to work on weekends or take calls outside of their scheduled working hours. Managers often make hiring errors because they do not gather enough information or confirm that the candidate fully understands what the job involves. If you are hiring for a clinical position that requires working every fourth weekend, teaching a class one evening each week, or attending early morning bedside rounds, share that information during the interview and get agreement from the candidate that they can accept these responsibilities.

During interviews, focus on hiring the right candidate. Do not rush the interviewing phase just to fill the position, even if you are under pressure to do so. You will potentially be living with the decision for a long time. If the individual you hired turns out not to be a good fit for the team or the organization, there can be any number of consequences, including the potential for poor team morale, team member resignations, and decreases in productivity. In addition, the number of steps required to document poor performance can be time consuming, stressful, and cumbersome.

If the candidate seems like they may be a good fit for the position and the team, provide a brief tour of the work area, if possible. This helps the candidate make a more informed decision about whether to accept the job if an offer is made and provides informal interaction time that may help you decide whether to make the job offer.

Types and Methods of Interviewing

Two common interviewing methods are used in health care: (a) standard/psychological/job-related and (b) behavioral/situational. In this section, we will also discuss peer interviews and various common ways to conduct an interview.

Standard Interviewing

Standard/psychological/job-related interviewing involves general questions related to job qualifications, education, experience, and accomplishments of applicants (sample questions of this type are listed in Box 11.2). If an applicant meets requirements and responds appropriately to the interview questions, they are judged qualified for the position. Traditional interviewing has been criticized because candidates who are skilled at interviewing can anticipate what the interviewer will want to hear and prepare answers ahead of time.

BOX 11.2 Standard Interviewing Questions

» Tell me about your experience working on teams.

» What has been your greatest work accomplishment, and why?

» Why have you changed jobs so frequently?

» What are your strengths and weaknesses?

» What did you enjoy most about your last or present job?

» What is the greatest value you bring to your organization?

» What have you done to improve your professional skills this year?

» What are you looking for in a new opportunity?

Behavioral Interviewing

Unlike standard interviewing questions, behavioral interviewing uses preselected questions correlated to key competencies and requires that candidates answer by giving specific examples of past behavior. Box 11.3 provides some samples of this type of questioning. This method presumes that the best predictor of future performance is past performance. Many consider behavioral interviewing to be the most accurate interviewing method for identifying performance effectiveness.[1] The advantages of behavioral interviewing include the following[1,3,6]:

> Behavioral interviewing is inherently nondiscriminatory and focuses on abilities, not disabilities.

> Interviewers avoid asking careless questions and sharply reduce the risk of straying into potentially biased areas of questioning.

> Candidates must give detailed examples illustrating how they have performed a specific skill or demonstrated a specific competency.

> Interviewers can make hiring decisions based on the proven capabilities of applicants as detailed or demonstrated in the interview process.

Peer Interviewing

Peer interviewing is an interviewing process that uses a panel of people within the organization to gain a more complete idea of a candidate's appropriateness for a position. For peer interviewing to be effective, several factors must be in place. First, prepare a decision matrix that identifies for the panel interviewers the key attributes an employee should have for that particular position (see Figures 11.3 and 11.4 on page 226). This matrix ensures interviews are consistent and helps provide objective, accurate data about the various candidates. Second, select high-performing employees to participate in the peer interviewing process and make sure these employees are trained on use of the matrix, the selection process, performance standards for the position to be filled, improper and illegal questions, and how to ask behavioral questions.[7] Your facility may offer training in peer or team interviewing or may require specific training to be completed before allowing employees to take part in peer or team interviews. If training is available, take advantage of this resource. Third, only present peer teams with candidates after you have interviewed them and determined that they seem qualified for the job. Finally, participating candidates should be sufficiently briefed and informed so that they can prepare for what might be a new interview experience for them.[8]

FIGURE 11.3 Sample decision matrix for hiring a diet office supervisor

Diet Office Supervisor: Hiring Worksheet

Desired Competency	Behavioral Question/Qualification	Scoring Guidelines (1 = poor; 3 = fair; 5 = excellent)
Problem solving	Give me an example of a time you solved a tough problem.	
Prioritizing	Think of a day when you had plenty of things to do. Describe how you scheduled your time.	
Initiative	Give me an example of a time you went beyond the normal job expectations for your role in order to get the job done.	
Diligence	Tell me about a time when you had to do a job that was particularly uninteresting. How did you deal with it?	
Technical skills and experience	Minimum of 2 years supervisory experience. Experience in diet office	
Communication effectiveness	Written and verbal communication prior to, during, and after the interview	
Professionalism	Poise, professional attire, language, thank-you note sent, etc	
	Total:	

FIGURE 11.4 Sample decision matrix for hiring an outpatient dietitian

Outpatient Dietitian: Hiring Worksheet

Competency	Behavioral Question/Qualification	Scoring Guidelines (1 = poor; 3 = fair; 5 = excellent)
Creativity	What have you done that was innovative?	
Initiative	Give me an example of a time when you went beyond the normal job expectations for your role in order to get the job done.	
Interpersonal savvy	Describe a situation in which you tried but were unable to build rapport with someone. Why didn't your efforts work?	
Action oriented	Can you tell me about a time that you seized an opportunity and "took the ball and ran with it?"	
Experience	Registered dietitian nutritionist (RDN) with state licensure; minimum 2 years of experience as outpatient RDN. Motivational interviewing, program development, and media skills/experience	
Professionalism	Poise, professional attire, language, thank-you note sent, etc	
Communication effectiveness	Written and verbal communication prior to, during, and after the interview	
	Total:	

There are several reasons to conduct peer interviews, including the following[7,9]:

> Peer interviews can help develop a sense of cohesiveness among interviewers.

> Participation in peer interviewing allows employees to have ownership in the selection process. They are truly invested in the success of the new hire.

> When the new hire starts, employees who were involved in the interviews already believe they can get along with the new team member.

> Research indicates that peer interviewing enhances employee retention.

> Peer interviewing is fairly easy to learn how to do.

> This type of interview gives the candidate (who is also evaluating the company) a chance to interact with your best and brightest.

Although peer interviewing has proven to be very advantageous, there are several disadvantages to the peer interview process that, while not outweighing the advantages, should also be considered. These include the following[7,9]:

> The time spent preparing for and conducting peer interviews can become too much for employees when they have other responsibilities.

> Peer interviewing does not work if the team is not high performing and capable of collaboration. You have to make sure you have the right employees doing the interviews. For example, some employees may be determined to reject talented applicants they see as potential competition for promotions.

> Candidates are more likely to feel intimidated facing a panel of several people.

> Employees may misunderstand their role in the hiring process and become upset if you do not follow their recommendations. You must make sure to explain to your employees what impact their input will have on the final decision. Consider how your employees will handle it if you do not select their favorite candidate.

> Candidates may ask the panel sensitive questions about management or salary. Train your employees to expect these questions and advise them on how to defer those issues to the hiring manager.

> Employees with little experience in interviewing may not be objective in their evaluations. Even experienced interviewers can struggle with this challenge.

As noted earlier, a decision matrix can make the peer interviewing process more objective. Before the interviews begin, review the matrix with all panel members and run through questions that can be used to collect relevant information about the candidates. Shortly after an interview, the interviewers should use the matrix to rate the interviewee based on how well the interviewee answered the questions. After multiple candidates are interviewed, they then can be ranked on the basis of these scores (as discussed later in this chapter). The matrix is important because it makes evaluation of all candidates more objective and consistent, ensures the interview team selects the right questions for the attributes identified, and facilitates decision making and prevents emotional decisions.

Telephone, Online, and Other Remote Interview Methods

Telephone interviews are often used as an expedient, cost-effective interviewing method. Telephone interviews can be very helpful in screening, especially if a candidate is not local; however, they tend to be unpopular with both candidates and managers. If you use telephone interviewing in your recruiting process, be aware that you probably will not learn as much about the candidate as you would from an in-person interview. To obtain the best information possible, telephone interviews should be just as structured as face-to-face interviews are.

Video conferencing, Skype, FaceTime, and Zoom are all remote alternatives to in-person interviewing. These options may be worth investigating at your institution, especially if face-to-face contact is restricted or candidates are not local. When using a remote interviewing technique, it is especially important to ensure that all candidates are interviewed consistently and equitably. Some candidates may have limited access to technology or be unfamiliar with its use. Background and lighting may not be ideal, which can limit your ability to read body language. Also, be aware that less-than-ideal eye contact is common in video interviews because individuals instinctively look at the faces on the screen instead of the camera.

Ranking and Selection

Once the interviews are complete, you will need to review the completed decision matrix and rank your candidates. It is best to complete the decision matrix on each candidate as soon as the interview is complete, while your notes make sense and the interview is still fresh in your mind. Ideally, all interviewers rate the candidates separately and then get together to discuss their findings, compare their ratings, and tally the scores if a numerical rating system has been used. Ranking competencies in order of importance can help identify the strongest candidate for the position if two or more promising applicants have similar overall scores. No candidate is a perfect match. In addition to interview rankings, when making your decision you should also consider background and reference checks, salary requirements, information obtained from other sources, and credentials.

Reference Checks

The fourth component in the hiring process is the reference check. Before you make a job offer, you or your HR department should check the candidate's references. Some, but not all, HR departments do this as their standard operating procedure. Due to liability concerns, many references will not provide much information about previous employees other than verification of their entry and exit dates and possibly the reason for exit and eligibility for rehire. Keep in mind that the same discrimination laws that apply to interviewing also apply to reference checking. Do not ask about marital status, age, disabilities, religion, ethnicity, or other issues related to any EEOC protected class.

Do not let your excitement or relief in finding the "perfect" candidate or your impatience to fill the position lead you to make the critical error of skipping reference checks. Even when a candidate's resume and interview responses seem highly credible, you need to conduct due diligence. If you are serious about specific candidates, make sure their work history is accurate, and check at least a reference or two. It is also critical to verify a candidate's licensure and registration status before making a job offer. At a minimum, the reference check should include the following[10]:

> verification of employment dates

> verification of position or title held

> eligibility status for rehire

> reason for separation

> recommendation for another position/role

The following Stories From the Field box provides a cautionary tale of what could happen if these steps are not followed.

STORIES FROM THE FIELD: Checking References

A clinical nutrition manager had an employee with a bachelor's degree in nutrition who worked in the diet office. The employee was an excellent worker and well loved by everyone. The employee had applied to the local dietetic internship several times and was repeatedly rejected. The manager wrote a letter on the employee's behalf, and the employee was accepted into the program. After the employee completed clinical rotations, the manager hired them back into a per diem dietitian position. After several months, the director of the dietetic internship program told the manager that the employee had not completed *any* classroom assignments for the internship. The internship director gave the employee a few months to complete the assignments, but the employee did not do so. The manager was forced to terminate the employee, as they did not meet the standards for a registration-eligible dietitian. It's always important to check credentials and references, and not work on trust alone, even with someone who may seem familiar.

Making the Job Offer

The fifth and final step in the hiring process is making the job offer. Be sure to work with your HR team to understand your facility's salary guidelines and determine whether your salary range is competitive in the marketplace. For example, your employer might have data showing what your company and multiple direct competitors pay employees with jobs similar to the one you are filling. The Academy of Nutrition and Dietetics also conducts biannual compensation and benefits surveys for the dietetics profession, which can be a source of regional and position-specific salary trends.[11]

Work with HR to learn how salary negotiations should take place, who is responsible for making the offer, and what type of flexibility you have. If you as the hiring manager are responsible for the making the offer, ask an HR team member for assistance if you feel unsure. The availability of online sources of compensation information (eg, salary.com or payscale.com) has leveled the playing field between employer and prospective employee when it comes to negotiations and job offers. This makes it more important than ever to be proactive so you can hire top-quality candidates. If you have the option, be prepared to counteroffer when a candidate asks for more money. However, the reality is that most RDN positions are set within the facility or company's budget, and nutrition managers have little flexibility in salary negotiations. If you cannot negotiate on salary, your facility's benefits package may be a selling point to candidates. Be sure you can articulate its advantages to prospective employees. For example, if your organization offers a 401(k) retirement plan and matches up to 5% of employee contributions, let candidates know that this offering is above average and translates to dollars beyond the salary alone. Are you able to offer a sign-on bonus in lieu of a higher initial salary? Do you use a career ladder program that offers the potential for additional compensation? Does your facility pay higher salaries to RDNs with advanced degrees or advanced certification, such as Certified Diabetes Care and Education Specialist (CDCES) or Certified Nutrition Support Clinician (CNSC)? Does your organization pay registration and licensure fees or Academy of Nutrition and Dietetics membership dues? Is there an allowance for professional development or conferences and continuing education events?

Other benefits, such as free parking, subsidized bus or train transportation, reduced rates for health insurance, free or reduced-rate health club memberships, subsidized day care, summer vacations, and flexible scheduling or no weekend work, may all give you the edge over your competition. Tuition reimbursement is an important but often overlooked benefit that might be very enticing to your prospective employee.

Finally, as you prepare to make an offer, make sure you think about its implications for salary equity within your department. Work with your HR team to ensure the offer aligns with what other staff members earn.

If you are having difficulty attracting and hiring quality candidates, do your homework. Where are these desirable candidates accepting jobs, and why? If candidates are choosing sales positions over your offerings, keep in mind that very few hospital positions can compete with the salary and benefits of sales positions. If candidates are electing to work at other hospitals, you may have more leverage. Find out when and how salary budgets are set at your institution. Ensure that the data used to determine salary budgets are up to date, especially if your facility hasn't hired someone new in a particular position in several years. With the constantly changing role of the RDN, try making a case for increased salary based on the current value your team brings. Do you have any data about outcomes to demonstrate your department's value? What skills do your RDNs have, and what are their responsibilities? How long has it been since you last updated job descriptions for your staff? If your RDNs are performing tasks typically associated with advanced practice, such as enteral and parenteral nutrition order writing, research, and feeding tube placement, you may be able to get job descriptions revised and regraded. To gain ideas, look at other advanced practice clinician job descriptions, such as those for advanced practice nurses, and talk to other professionals at your institution who have successfully raised salaries.

New Employee Orientation

New employee orientation is one of the most important but most neglected functions in the workplace. Research has shown that organizations with strong onboarding processes improve new hire retention by 82% and productivity by more than 70%.[12] To succeed in their jobs, new employees need to be drawn into the team and the organizational family. Recruitment Solutions found that 47% of employee turnover occurs in the first 90 days.[3] An employee handbook and reams of policies and procedures do not comprise a sufficient orientation program. Employees often complain that orientation is boring or overwhelming or that they are left to "sink or swim" after they are hired. As a result, new employees are not productive and may leave the organization within the year.

Orientation programs for new employees in health care settings typically include the following goals:

> Reduce start-up costs associated with new hires.

> Reduce new employees' anxiety.

> Reduce employee turnover.

> Prepare new employees to have realistic job expectations.

> Ensure that new employees understand and can meet regulatory agency requirements.

> Reduce ongoing training and retraining needs.

Following are some effective methods for engaging new employees:

> Assign your best performers to "buddy" or mentor new employees.

> Make sure the new employee's workspace is clean, ready, and comfortable before their first day of work.

> Ensure that key coworkers know the employee is starting and that introductions are made. For example, arrange a group breakfast or lunch on the employee's first day.

> Develop an effective orientation program that starts with the basics and does not cram everything into a 1-day session.

> Make the orientation process fun and interesting.

> As a manager, remain involved. Meet regularly during the first 30 to 90 days to evaluate the new employee's progress, clear up any confusion about job responsibilities, and develop your relationship.

Effective orientation programs in health care include the following key information and elements:

> Training on all relevant regulatory requirements, such as Health Information Portability and Accountability Act (HIPAA) compliance, fire safety, and patient rights and responsibilities, all of which are common components of your hospital's orientation program and typically must be completed within 30 days of hire

> Important department policies

> Key job responsibilities

> Skill competency verification, documentation of which is typically required within 30 to 90 days of hire (check with your institution to ensure your process meets its standards)

> Introductions to teammates and other staff the new employee needs to know

> Regularly scheduled meetings between the new employee and their direct supervisor

The goal of regularly scheduled meetings is to build the relationship between the employee and the manager and evaluate the employee's initial progress. In *Hardwiring Excellence*, Studor recommends that managers ask every new hire the following four questions after 30 days of employment[7]:

> **How do we compare with who we said we were?** In responding, employees might bring up issues such as real or perceived discrepancies between actual schedules and what hours they are expected to work. This provides an opportunity to clear up any confusion.

> **What are we doing well?**

> **What are some things you saw at your previous facility that you think could make us better?** This question invites the employee to help maximize the department's opportunities for process improvement.[7]

> **Is there anything that you are uncomfortable with that might cause you to leave?**

Common Management Challenges

First-time leaders often encounter HR situations that are completely new to them. This section covers several issues that many leaders identify as having been particularly problematic for them as new managers.

Managing in a Union Environment

In addition to the HR issues typical in any food or nutrition department, managing in a union environment poses distinctive challenges. The union contract, otherwise known as the collective bargaining agreement, sets specific parameters for a variety of employment-related issues, such as compensation and benefits, working conditions, job security, disciplinary procedures, employees' rights, management's rights, and contract length. If you are new to the union environment or new to a particular institution with a union contract, you must take it upon yourself to learn about several aspects of the union environment right away, including the following:

> Learn about the historical and current relationship between the union (or unions) and management, including past and present grievances, negotiating points during the last contract renewal, and key players involved on both sides.

> Be knowledgeable of the tenets of the collective bargaining agreement that could affect how you address performance management challenges. Learn the meaning of every paragraph that relates to items such as performance management evaluations, scheduling, job tasks, and so on. For example, what options do you have if the cashier staff needs to be trained on a new cash register system? Can you ask them to come in early or work extra hours? When staff or management take issue with a policy or action, people will likely refer to the contract repeatedly to "prove" a point. You will be surprised at the variation in each person's interpretation of the contract, so make sure you know its true meaning.

> Learn to work closely with union representatives as well as management experts in the staff relations or HR department. These people can serve as resources who

can help you decide how best to respond to myriad situations that may arise. Ask your HR team to identify a department leader who can mentor you in navigating the union environment.

Documentation and communication take on even more importance in the union environment. Be sure that you communicate pertinent information regarding any changes, new initiatives, and other relevant matters to union leaders before you share it with the rest of the team. This way, the union can be prepared for any questions or concerns from its members. The steps in the performance management process are similar in union and nonunion environments. In either setting, you usually begin by coaching an employee whose performance is unsatisfactory. Then, if performance does not improve sufficiently, issue a verbal warning, followed by a written warning. If these steps do not work, disciplinary action, such as suspension or termination, is an option. However, there are some important differences to note when you work with unionized employees rather than nonunion employees. One important example is that a unionized employee typically has the right to have a union representative present during any disciplinary meeting that includes a written warning or suspension. This right to union representation is usually restricted to disciplinary meetings.

By keeping the union informed and involved in the performance management process, you may avoid defensive actions and disputes regarding disciplinary decisions. However, you should not expect that involving and informing the union will mean it will necessarily accept your decision to discipline an employee. The union's role is to represent the employee appropriately, and it may act if the employee's contractual rights appear to have been violated. In addition, it is often recommended that you have another manager present to take notes and serve as a witness of the interaction and ensure its fairness. Be sure to keep complete, factual, detailed, and timely documentation of performance situations and actions. You will need this documentation to justify any performance management decisions if the union initiates proceedings that challenge these decisions, such as grievance hearings or arbitration.

Managing Various Generations

Managers and supervisors in most organizations today are faced with the prospect of managing employees from four generations: Baby Boomers (those born between 1946 and 1964), Generation X (born between 1965 and 1980), Millennials (born between 1981 and 1996), and Generation Z (born between 1997 and 2012). Each generation comes to the workforce with its own priorities, preferences, and work styles, as summarized in Box 11.4 on page 234.[13-20]

To maximize your managerial effectiveness, you should understand the key motivators of each generation, how they learn best, and how they prefer to receive information. For example, with members of Generation X and Millennials being the predominant groups in the workplace today, the traditional management model of "top-down, boss-is-always-right" may not be effective. Therefore, a new manager should expect that it may take time for their employees to trust them. You can build your relationship with your employees by taking the opportunity to hear their individual needs and concerns through one-on-one meetings scheduled at least monthly. Many food and nutrition managers talk about the increased demands of their younger employees for flexible work schedules, frequent feedback, and input on policies such as the dress code. The issues described in the following Stories From the Field box are common for many food and nutrition managers today.

> **BOX 11.4** Generational Snapshots[13-20]

Baby Boomers[19,20]

» Born between 1946 and 1964

» Traditional upbringing, followed by youthful rebellion

» Have entered or are nearing retirement

Values and characteristics

» Optimism

» Involvement with and loyalty to the organization

» Strong work ethic

» Limited work-family balance

» Question authority

» Desire quality

» Continuous learners

Generation X[19,20]

» Born between 1965 and 1980

» Shaped by the AIDS epidemic, the fall of the Berlin Wall, and the personal computer boom

» Comfortable with technology

Values and characteristics

» Skeptical of institutions

» Reluctant

» Respect efficiency and performance over tenure

Millennials[13-15,19,20]

» Born between 1981 and 1996

» Also referred to as the Echo Boomer Generation because many are the offspring of Baby Boomers and their demographic "echo"

» The largest generation in the workforce

» Extremely comfortable with technology

Values and characteristics

» Realism

» Parental involvement and structured upbringing

» Social, confident, and inclusive

» Merged families

» Multitaskers, entrepreneurial

» Work-life balance

» Demanding and questioning

Generation Z[14,16-19]

» Born between 1997 and 2012

» The most ethnically and racially diverse generation

» Currently entering the workplace in large numbers

» Shaped by nearly a decade of war and economic uncertainty due to Great Recession and wars in Iraq

» Characterized by total and continuous connectivity and communication

Values and characteristics

» Anxiety at work

» Even though identify as digital, request more face-to-face interaction at work

» Company culture, stance on social issues, and retention practices are critical

» Likely to take a nonbinary view of gender

Perhaps the biggest challenge for many nutrition leaders is effectively managing Millennials and Generation Z employees. Research suggests that Millennials and Generation Z employees learn best from a "coaching" style of leadership and are looking for a mentoring relationship with their supervisors or their team.[15-17] Business leaders suggest that Millennial employees can benefit from mentors who can help them understand corporate culture and how decisions are made in the business world. In return, ask these employees to mentor other workers on new trends, such as advances in technology, social media best practices for product and service marketing, and word-of-mouth marketing.[14,15]

Following are other recommendations for working with Millennials[14,15]:

> Let them set their goals.

> Praise sincerely, but often.

> Listen to them.

> Don't assume they share your goals.

> Address performance issues quickly. Provide direct, prompt feedback.

> Explain the "why" behind the decisions you make.

The following Stories From the Field box provides a CNM success story with Millennial employees.

Although Generation Z is not the largest percentage of today's workforce, that will soon change. Things to consider for employees in Generation Z include being able to articulate your organization's social mission during the interview, ensuring frequent face-to-face contact, having strong initiatives to address retention, and having robust recruitment and succession planning processes in place.[15,16]

Of course, in addition to generational differences, individual employees are shaped by other social and personal factors including gender, race or ethnicity, personality, and thinking style. Many organizations employing RDNs and NDTRs need to provide excellent and efficient service every day of the year, and in this demanding environment, managers cannot possibly cater to every desire of their employees regarding working conditions. However, your team will benefit greatly if you aim to accommodate individual differences and provide options when possible in the following areas:

> **Supervision:** Can you individualize the method and amount of supervision for each employee?

> **Feedback:** What types of constructive criticism and acknowledgment are best for different employees?

> **Technology and equipment:** Can you make tools available that reduce tedious processes and increase the time your employees can spend providing patient care?

> **Scheduling:** Is there room for scheduling flexibility that prioritizes factors other than seniority? For example, can you set up a rotating schedule for covering less-desirable shifts or have teams self-schedule within defined parameters?

> **Work assignments:** How can assignments and tasks be delegated to provide the right balance of opportunity for specific individuals and team growth?

> **Professional development:** Can training and opportunities for skill building be offered in different formats to suit different learning styles? For example, could a training program blend traditional, instructor-led classes (which might appeal more to Baby Boomers) and web-based self-study classes (such as those that might appeal more to Generation X, Millennials, or Generation Z)?

> **Communication:** Can your staff communicate effectively across multiple channels, such as print, email, internet and intranet, phone and voicemail, and face-to-face encounters? What communication methods work best for the individuals being addressed? If you think intergenerational communication styles may be a source of friction or conflict for your team, consider group discussions with your team about generational differences. During your meetings, ask your team members which generational profile best seems to describe them. You may find that some identify with a group older or younger than the generation into which they were born. Ask team members which of the characteristics attributed to their generation are most important to them.

> **Opportunities for innovation:** Are you prepared to capitalize on the entrepreneurial strengths of employees by outsourcing challenging problems to special teams? For example, can your staff help develop a marketing plan, choose a new productivity system, or sketch the format to be used for nutrition documentation in the electronic health record system? Consider assigning special projects to small teams deliberately composed of people from several generations, to gain the synergy of their complementary strengths.

Diversity, Inclusion, and Cultural Humility

Diversity, inclusion, and cultural humility are important components of effective HR management in the 21st century, as we explored in Chapter 3. Cultural competence and humility are key components in the ongoing work of reducing disparities in access to and quality of health and nutrition care. A culturally competent staff is prepared to tailor the delivery of health and nutrition services to meet patients' and clients' social, cultural, and linguistic needs. The practice of cultural humility is a lifelong learning endeavor involving self-reflection and self-critique to not only learn about another's culture but also to examine one's own beliefs and cultural identities.[21]

As a nutrition leader, you should strive to be culturally competent and model the practice of cultural humility for your team members and ensure they are adequately trained on these key concepts. Your team needs cultural competence and humility to work with each other and other teams' members and, even more importantly, to provide culturally appropriate care to patients with diverse values, beliefs, and behaviors.

Many organizations provide training resources on cultural humility and inclusion through their HR departments or offices of diversity. Examples of additional training resources include the Network of the National Library of Medicine, The Joint Commission, and the Academy of Nutrition and Dietetics professional website (www.eatrightPRO.org).[21-23]

It is important to consider diversity as a key factor in the hiring process and be intentional about maximizing the diversity of your team. Developing a diverse team can enhance workforce effectiveness and team problem-solving skills.[24,25] When thinking about diversity, consider gender, age, race, ethnicity, and cultural heritage. To hire, onboard, manage, and develop your diverse team effectively, it is critical to practice inclusive leadership.[24]

Inclusive leadership is defined as leadership practices that ensure all team members feel they are treated respectfully and fairly and are valued for who they are. Leaders need to be mindful of their own biases and strive to ensure that all team members have a sense of belongingness and empowerment.[24-26] Inclusive leadership practices will help you ensure your diverse team is positioned to perform at its maximum potential. For a deeper discussion of these topics, see Chapter 3.

Partnering With Human Resources to Maximize Your Effectiveness

Unfortunately, many nutrition leaders do not receive training on problematic situations relating to HR. The following sections cover several issues you may encounter in health care and foodservice management and offer suggestions and resources to help you address each of them.

Harassment

Harassment may or may not be sexual in nature. Sexual harassment is a form of sex discrimination that violates Title VII of the Civil Rights Act of 1964. Sexual harassment can occur in a variety of circumstances, as the following points explain[27]:

> All gender identities can be victims of sexual harassment, and all genders can be instigators. The victim and harasser do not have to be of different sexes.

> The harasser can be the victim's supervisor, an agent of the employer, a supervisor in another area, a coworker, or a nonemployee.

> Victims do not have to be the person harassed. They can be anyone affected by the offensive conduct.

> Sexual harassment in the workplace does not necessarily involve economic injury to or discharge of the victim.

> The harasser's conduct must be unwelcome.

Harassment at work unreasonably interferes with or alters the employee's work performance or creates a hostile, abusive, or offensive work environment.[24] Examples of hostile behavior could include bullying, gossiping about someone, or excluding one or more coworkers from team activities. To determine whether a workplace environment qualifies as being hostile, the following factors are typically examined:

> whether the conduct was verbal, physical, or both

> how often the conduct was repeated

> whether the conduct was hostile or patently offensive

> whether the alleged harasser was a coworker or a supervisor

> whether others joined in perpetrating or perpetuating the harassment

Examples of inappropriate conduct of a sexual nature include sexually oriented jokes; sexually explicit emails, screen savers, posters, cartoons, or graffiti; and unwanted verbal or physical contact. The standard used by civil rights agencies and courts in determining whether a hostile work environment exists is whether a reasonable person, in the same or similar circumstances, would find the conduct offensive.[27] A single incident may be sufficient to establish a *quid pro quo* harassment claim, but typically a pattern of conduct is required to establish a hostile work environment.

As a manager, you need to take any and all steps necessary to prevent harassment from occurring in your department.[27,28] It is critical that you clearly communicate to employees that harassment will not be tolerated. You must set the example by being alert to others' behavior, by not participating in anything that might be construed as harassment (no matter how subtle), and by stopping inappropriate behavior immediately if you observe it. Carol Merchasin, lawyer and noted training consultant in harassment prevention, states that a manager must use caution in the "danger zones, such as comments on personal appearance, jokes, cartoons, and nicknames that demean others on the basis of their race, gender, ethnic origin, religion, age, disability, and sexual orientation."[28]

You must also take immediate and appropriate action when an employee alleges harassment. Know your facility's complaint or grievance process and ensure your employees also understand the process. Even if no one complains, you need to be alert to conduct that is inappropriate and immediately put an end to it. The first step is to contact your HR representative for assistance.

Patient Privacy

Health care leaders need to be knowledgeable of the component of HIPAA that addresses the privacy of protected health information (PHI), understand the policies and procedures that the institution has put in place to comply, and be proactive in educating their staff on how HIPAA pertains to the teams' tasks and responsibilities.[29] For example, PHI can be electronic or printed. What does your organization's policy state about students accessing computerized medical records? Also, what patient information is allowed on tray tickets, and what is your procedure for verifying two patient identifiers?

Make sure you and your staff comprehend the requirements for reporting suspected violations of patients' privacy rights. Become familiar with your facility's policy to better understand which suspected violations need to be reported, and to whom. Also be aware that health care organizations routinely audit patient electronic health records to ensure only appropriate individuals are accessing PHI. The following Stories From the Field box below describes a situation in which HIPAA was violated.

STORIES FROM THE FIELD: Protecting Patient Privacy

A clinical nutrition manager was approached by the facility's information technology department after they noticed a suspicious pattern of unauthorized electronic medical record access from one of the dietitians. After an investigation, they found that the dietitian was reviewing medical records of other patients to learn about treatment options for a specific disease because their mother had recently been diagnosed with the condition. Even though the dietitian had been through HIPAA training, they did not realize their actions were in violation. Fortunately, administration took into account the dietitian's otherwise excellent work record, and the manager was able to keep the dietitian employed. It is easy to assume that the members of the clinical team know these rules, but it's not always wise to make that assumption.

Fair Labor Standards Act Compliance

The federal Fair Labor Standards Act (FLSA, 1938) established the minimum wage; rules for overtime pay; record keeping, which includes certain identifying information about the employee, such as name and Social Security number, as well as data about the hours worked and the wages earned; and standards for youth employment. FLSA policies are enforced by the DOL.[27] In recent years, the DOL has expanded enforcement of the FLSA, and multiple health care institutions have been found noncompliant. For example, DOL investigators found that nurses at multiple facilities in a large health care system were owed money because the health care system's timekeeping system automatically deducted time for meal periods whether or not the employees were fully relieved of their duties and also found that employees at multiple nursing care facilities were owed money for overtime and minimum wage violations.[30,31]

Even if appropriate compensation policies and procedures are in place, violations can arise from failures in policy administration and the day-to-day practices of managers and noncompliant employees.[30] The DOL may audit an employer at any time. Many investigations are initiated by employee complaints. Employers should be aware that an investigation can expand beyond the initial complaint to a review of all wage and hour practices. Following are a few examples of violations[31]:

> Computerized time systems automatically deduct meal periods, even when employees work during meal breaks.

> Employees work before and after their shifts without being paid properly.

> Employees are not paid for attending training sessions.

As a nutrition leader, you must understand the ramifications of the FLSA for both your exempt and nonexempt employees. It is important to properly distinguish exempt positions from nonexempt positions. A job title or job description does not necessarily grant exempt status; what matters is the actual work performed. Many people believe that all exempt workers are salaried and all nonexempt workers are paid an hourly wage. That is not the case. How employees are paid does not have anything to do with how they are classified. For example, a nonexempt worker may be paid a salary, but you still have to pay attention to minimum wage and overtime requirements for this employee. The FLSA website has many tools to assist leaders in increasing their understanding of and developing compliance strategies for this law.[30]

Family Medical Leave Act Compliance

The Family and Medical Leave Act (FMLA) was enacted in 1993 to provide workers the ability to better balance the needs of work, family, and personal health. Eligible employees may take up to 12 unpaid workweeks of leave in a 12-month period. Examples of qualifying events include the birth or adoption of a child and to bond with the newborn child within 1 year of birth; to care for the employee's spouse, child, or parent who has a serious health condition, including incapacity due to pregnancy; and for prenatal medical care. A complete list is available on the DOL's website (www.dol.gov) .[32] There is also a provision in the FMLA stating that eligible employees may take up to 26 workweeks of leave in a single 12-month period to care for a covered military service member with a serious injury or illness if the employee is the service member's spouse, child, parent, or next of kin. In addition, the FMLA requires that employers maintain employees' health benefits during leave and restore employees to their same or an equivalent job after the leave ends.[27] When serving in a leadership role, it is important to be aware of the provisions of this statute and be proactive in anticipating needed staffing adjustments to manage during an employee's absence. The FMLA includes multiple requirements for compliance. Nutrition leaders should familiarize themselves with the tenets of the law and work closely with their HR teams to ensure they are in compliance with it.

Summary

The skills required to manage various HR processes are often new to nutrition leaders and may be outside their comfort zone. Therefore, it is vital that you partner with your HR department to understand your role and theirs, including how they can best support you. Your people are your most important resource. Understanding and gaining competence in the hiring, orientation, and ongoing management and development of your staff is vital to creating and maintaining a highly functioning team that provides safe, timely, effective, and efficient care and service.

REFERENCES

1   Davila L, Kursmark L. *How to Choose the Right Person for the Right Job Every Time*. McGraw Hill; 2005.

2   US Equal Employment Opportunity Commission. Laws & guidance. EEOC website. Accessed March 8, 2021. www.eeoc.gov/laws-guidance

3   Armstrong S, Mitchell B. *The Essential HR Handbook: A Quick and Handy Resource for Any Manager or HR Professional*. Career Press; 2008.

4   Academy of Nutrition and Dietetics. Licensure and professional regulation of dietitians. eatrightPRO.org website. Accessed March 20, 2021. www.eatrightPRO.org/advocacy/licensure /professional-regulation-of-dietitians

5   Cottrell D. *Monday Morning Leadership: 8 Mentoring Sessions You Can't Afford to Miss*. Cornerstone Leadership Institute; 2002.

6   Yeung R. *Successful Interviewing and Recruitment*. Kogan Page; 2008.

7   Studor Q. *Hardwiring Excellence*. Fire Starter Publishing; 2003.

8   Hayton E. The complete guide to peer interviewing. Harver website. 2019. Accessed March 25, 2021. https://harver.com/blog/peer-interviewing

9   Pentilla C. Peering in. *Entrepreneur*. 2005;33(1):70-72.

10 Podmoroff D. *How to Hire, Train, and Keep the Best Employees for Your Small Business*. Atlanta Publishing Group; 2005.

11 Griswold K, Rogers D. Compensation and benefits survey 2019. *J Acad Nutr Diet*. 2020;120(3):448-464. doi:10.1016/j.jand.2019.12.015

12 Laurano, M. *The True Cost of a Bad Hire*. Brandon Hall Group; 2015. Accessed March 16, 2021. https://b2b-assets.glassdoor.com/the-true-cost-of-a-bad-hire.pdf

13 Banta C, Grim JA. Successful management across the millennium. Presented at: Clinical Nutrition Management Annual Symposium; April 1, 2008; San Antonio, TX.

14 Delcampo RG, Haggerty LA, Haney MJ, Knippel LA. *Managing the Multi-Generational Workforce: From the GI Generation to the Millennials*. Routledge; 2016.

15 Erickson T. Gen Y in the workforce. *Harvard Business Review*. Accessed January 9, 2020. https://hbr.org/2009/02/gen-y-in-the-workforce-2

16 Tulgan B; RainmakerThinking, Inc. Meet generation Z: the second generation within the giant Millennial cohort. The Art of Service website. 2013. Accessed October 28, 2019. https://theartofservice.com/meet-generation-z-the-second-generation-within-the-giant -millennial-cohort.html

17 Singh AP, Dangmei J. Understanding the Generation Z: the future workforce. *South Asia J Multidiscip*. 2016;3:1-5.

18 Generations: demographic trends in population and workforce (quick take). Catalyst website. 2021. Accessed March 17, 2021. www.catalyst.org/research/generations-demographic-trends -in-population-and-workforce

19 Generational differences in the workplace. Purdue University Global. Accessed March 25, 2022. www.purdueglobal.edu/education-partnerships/generational-workforce-differences -infographic

20 Smith, A. General mindsets affect the workplace. SHRM website. September 10, 2021. Accessed March 25, 2022. www.shrm.org/resourcesandtools/hr-topics/global-hr/pages/generational -mindsets-affect-workforce.aspx

21 Martin C. Clinical Conversations Training Program. Network of the National Library of Medicine website. July 14, 2020. Accessed March 25, 2022. www.nnlm.gov/guides/clinical-conversations -training-program

22 The Joint Commission. Health equity. Joint Commission website. Accessed March 29, 2021. www.jointcommission.org/resources/patient-safety-topics/health-equity/#t=_Tab _StandardsFAQs&sort=relevancy

23 Academy of Nutrition and Dietetics. Inclusion, diversity, equity and access hub. eatrightPRO website. Accessed March 20, 2021. www.eatrightPRO.org/idea/inclusion-diversity-equity-and-access

24 Bourke J, Titus A. Why inclusive leaders are good for organizations, and how to become one. *Harvard Business Review.* 2019. Accessed March 25, 2021. https://hbr.org/2019/03/why-inclusive-leaders-are-good-for-organizations-and-how-to-become-one

25 Hunt V, Layton D, Price S. Why diversity matters. McKinsey website. 2015. Accessed March 20, 2021. www.mckinsey.com/business-functions/organization/our-insights/why-diversity-matters#

26 Ceambur A. The challenge of managing a diverse team. Alle Ceambur website. 2016. Accessed March 20, 2021. https://alexandraceambur.com/2016/10/24/the-challenge-of-managing-diverse-teams

27 US Equal Employment Opportunity Commission. Facts about sexual harassment. EEOC.gov website. Accessed July 1, 2011. www.eeoc.gov/facts/fs-sex.html

28 Merchasin CM, Chapman MH, Polisky J. *Case Dismissed! Taking Your Harassment Prevention Training to Trial.* 2nd ed. American Bar Association; 2005.

29 US Department of Health and Human Services. HIPAA for professionals. HHS website. Accessed November 27, 2019. www.hhs.gov/hipaa/for-professionals/index.html

30 US Department of Labor. Wages and the Fair Labor Standards Act. US Department of Labor website. Accessed November 27, 2019. www.dol.gov/agencies/whd/flsa

31 Pear R. Pay practices in health care are investigated. *New York Times.* August 8, 2010. Accessed January 9, 2020. www.nytimes.com/2010/08/10/health/policy/10health.html

32 Nursing care facilities pay $261,418 in back wages, penalties, and damages after US Department of Labor investigation. US Department of Labor website. September 5, 2019. Accessed January 9, 2020. www.dol.gov/newsroom/releases/whd/whd20190905

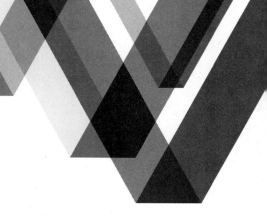

CHAPTER 12
Getting Involved in Research

Susan Renee Roberts, DCN, RDN, LDN, CNSC, FAND

Introduction

Does the thought of conducting research excite you and your staff, or does research seem like a daunting endeavor? It is a common misconception among registered dietitian nutritionists (RDNs) that research can only be conducted by those with a doctorate degree or in academic settings. However, there are many types of research, and RDNs can incorporate research activities into their practice, no matter where they work. Essential elements for research success are an inquisitive nature and personal desire to solve a problem or answer a question.[1] The intent of this chapter is to help you and your staff increase your understanding of and comfort level with research. Research can initially seem like an overwhelming task but can foster the desire to conduct more research to answer the inevitable, subsequent unanswered questions.

Why Research Is Important and Why Registered Dietitian Nutritionists Should Conduct It

Research is important and necessary for a number of reasons. Think about all the amazing advances in science, technology, medicine, and nutrition that have been possible only because someone was willing to commit to researching a new method or different treatment. By collecting data and analyzing evidence, researchers allow us to confidently and successfully implement processes and interventions that improve patient outcomes and achieve other important objectives. Data demonstrating improved patient outcomes or cost savings can also influence public policy at the state and national levels. The Academy of Nutrition and Dietetics states, "research forms the backbone of dietetics practice and the basis for the Academy of Nutrition and Dietetics work in education and policy,"[2] and for that reason, it promotes RDN participation in research activities. The importance of research is also emphasized in the standards of professional practice (SOPP) for registered dietitian nutritionists, Standard 4: Application of Research,[3] which states the RDN "applies, participates in, and/or generates research to enhance practice." Evidence-based practice (EBP) incorporates the best available research, evidence, and information in the delivery of nutrition and dietetics services. The rationale for including research activities in the SOPP is to "promote improved safety and quality of nutrition and dietetics practice and services," which is an essential, practical, and relevant goal for those of us practicing in the field of food and nutrition. Within Standard 4, the following five indicators describe ways that the RDN can demonstrate the standard in practice[3]:

> **4.1**: Reviews best available research, evidence, and information for application to practice

> **4.1A**: Understands basic research design and methodology

> **4.2**: Uses best available research, evidence, and information as the foundation for evidence-based practice

> **4.3**: Integrates best available research, evidence, and information with best practices, clinical and managerial expertise, and customer values

> **4.4**: Contributes to the development of new knowledge and research in nutrition and dietetics

> **4.5**: Promotes application of research through alliances and collaboration with food and nutrition and other professionals and organizations

The first three indicators direct practitioners to stay current on research and use the best evidence in their practice environment. Without ongoing research, RDNs cannot carry out these foundational indicators. The last two indicators advance the RDN's role as an active participant in research activities, which is the primary focus of this chapter.

Research is essential to the advancement of the nutrition and dietetics profession. In addition, research includes specific professional and personal benefits you and your staff may gain by engaging in research activities. These benefits include professional development, interdisciplinary collaboration, enhanced respect for yourself and your staff, justification of the need for additional staffing, expanded career opportunities, and greater job satisfaction. RDNs who have participated in research provided their perspective on how it has enriched their career and benefited their practice; as reflected in the responses featured in the Stories From the Field box on the next page, many RDNs find that research gives them a great sense of accomplishment, helps them keep abreast of developments in the science of nutrition, elevates their critical thinking skills, and improves patient care.[4]

Barriers to Participation in Research (and How to Overcome Them)

Despite the benefits and value of research to our patients and profession, participation in and publication of research are not routine activities for most RDNs.[5] Sustained RDN involvement in clinical nutrition research has been associated with exposure to the research process, research mentors, administrative support and personal drive to be involved with research.[1] You will find that the benefits of research, such as increased recognition and opportunities to present and publish, can help motivate your staff to participate, but you must also help them identify and overcome barriers to participation. In one study using focus groups of clinical dietitians, researchers found that the most frequently identified barriers to research involvement were insufficient support from administration, lack of time, inadequate understanding of research methodology, knowledge deficits regarding statistical analysis, and access to statistical software.[6] These barriers may be challenging, but they are not insurmountable.

STORIES FROM THE FIELD: Registered Dietitian Nutritionists Who Participate in Research in Various Settings

"I get great joy and satisfaction from compiling the results and discussing them with colleagues. It's a tremendous feeling of accomplishment and completion when you finish a project that seems so huge when you first start out. Continuously having to read the literature in the area of study is also a great educational benefit to research."

    —Faculty member, large state university[a]

"The research process has helped me become a critical thinker and given me the confidence to defend my synthesis of the literature, thereby allowing me to provide the best clinical consultations I can as a dietitian. It has also enhanced my acceptance by academic medicine professionals and provided me with opportunities for networking with other health care professionals in my field."

    —Clinical nutrition manager, large pediatric hospital[a]

"Research can be very difficult, but it is so rewarding to see a project come to fruition, especially if you can design an experiment that answers a question that has not been answered before. [Research] will make you a greater asset to the medical team and sharpen your critical thinking skills. In the end, you will be a better clinician."

    —Intestinal rehabilitation program director, large tertiary care academic hospital[a]

"Research has benefited my career most by broadening my scope of practice, and my job satisfaction has been improved because I am more familiar with why I practice the way I do. I see the evidence behind [my practice], and I am able to better represent our career to a multidisciplinary staff by being informed by current research. Also, I enjoy seeing the outcomes of research; it is rewarding to see something that you have worked so hard on for so long end up being an example for other RDs all around the country."

    —Clinical dietitian specializing in trauma, large tertiary care academic hospital[b]

"I have enjoyed doing research, especially when it has led to sharing the results at the national level. It's been great to share what we've done with others to help enhance their practices, too. Specific to the nutrition protocol pilot study, this is a great project to be involved in because it directly affects our scope of practice and allows more independence in the care of our patients. We can show the doctors and other disciplines that we are capable of managing our patients safely and effectively."

    —Clinical dietitian specializing in hematopoietic stem cell transplant, large tertiary care academic hospital[b]

"After completing a research project for my dietetic internship, I found I enjoyed being able to work with data, numbers, statistics, and see the outcomes of my work. It's harder to see those outcomes in the inpatient setting due to quick discharges and the time it takes to make lifestyle changes. Research allows our profession to validate the current procedures as well as lead changes for future procedures. Ultimately it shows the importance and value of our profession, including our salary."

    —Clinical dietitian in first year of practice at a large tertiary care academic hospital[b]

"Completing my research project was one of the most rewarding parts of the internship. The excitement I experienced when I reviewed our results and the pride I felt when presenting our project made all the work we poured into the project worth it. Being a part of the entire process from beginning to end allowed me to better understand why evidenced-based practice truly is the gold standard. The hard work that goes into research is a vital part of the care we provide to our patients."

    —Clinical dietitian who recently graduated from a dietetic internship program[b]

[a] Robien K. Making research happen: the real world of clinical nutrition research. *Support Line.* 2003;25:3–6.
[b] Personal communications with the author (email, 2015)

Lack of Support From Administrators

If you lack adequate financial support from your facility's administration to conduct a large study, consider starting with a small pilot project. If a pilot project suggests your research could lead to cost savings, an improvement in the quality of care, or increased patient safety, you may increase your odds of getting funding from the administration for additional staffing or monetary incentives for the researchers. Another tactic to enhance the administration's interest in your research is to ask a nurse or physician leader to join you in championing and presenting the research project.

Lack of Time

If you and your staff RDNs perceive lack of time to be the main obstacle to research, consider whether any of the following strategies would work for you:

> Start with a small project that combines clinical care and data collection (eg, collect data in the intensive care unit [ICU] on the day nutrition support is initiated, to determine whether early feeding is consistently being done).

> Break the research project into manageable pieces with specific and realistic timelines.

> Spread the research workload among a team of RDNs.

> Involve students or interns in the project to assist with the literature review, data collection, preliminary analysis, and draft report.

> Determine whether any of the researchers' clinical or administrative activities could temporarily or permanently be delegated to other individuals.

> If you have a large staff, establish a rotating project day on which one RDN conducts research while other RDNs cover patient care responsibilities, thereby allowing the researchers to commit a block of time to their project without the department incurring the additional cost of supplemental staff.

Lack of Knowledge or Expertise

If the RDNs on your staff avoid research because they are not knowledgeable about research methodology, direct them to investigate and learn through books[7,8] and online resources about the topic, such as the Academy of Nutrition and Dietetics Research Toolkit.[9] Research courses, either through a university or a Massive Open Online Course (MOOC), are also options. In addition, a physician or other clinician with research experience may be willing to serve as a mentor. RDNs who are Academy of Nutrition and Dietetics members can also learn about and get more involved in the research process by participating in the Academy of Nutrition and Dietetics Nutrition Research Network (NRN), which "conducts, supports, promotes and advocates for practice-based research that answers questions important to dietetics practice."[10] A number of studies based on research conducted by the NRN (formerly known as the Dietetics Practice-Based Research Network) are in process or have been published, including projects related to nutrition diagnosis, critical thinking skills in professional practice, pediatric obesity, adult weight management, validation of malnutrition clinical characteristics, and clinical staffing models.[11-15]

RDNs can participate in the NRN in a variety of ways, such as sharing ideas for research, participating on the advisory committee that determines which research projects to conduct, collecting data, and disseminating results. Since participants are not required to have research experience, NRN membership is a good way for RDNs who are interested but not confident about research participation to get exposure and gain experience.[10]

Research has shown that RDNs with a graduate degree and those with more knowledge of and affinity for EBP are more likely to be involved in research.[1,16] As of January 1, 2024, all RDNs will be required to have a master's degree to practice, which should translate into more RDNs with an interest in and skills to participate in research. However, in the meantime, as a nutrition leader or manager, you can increase the probability of research activities occurring in your organization by including research opportunities or expectations in job descriptions and development plans for nutrition managers and staff.

You can also foster your staff's knowledge of EBP in a number of ways, such as the following:

> Encourage exploration of articles about EBP, research methodology, and critical evaluation of published research as well as research presented at conferences or in webinars.[17-19]

> Host regular journal club sessions led by staff members where your team discusses required readings on relevant topics and explores why EBP is important in nutrition.[20]

> Encourage your staff to use the Academy of Nutrition and Dietetics Evidence Analysis Library (www.andeal.org), which is a member benefit.

> Refer RDNs to other online EBP resources, such as clinical guidelines from organizations in their area of practice.[21]

Finally, you and your staff may be reluctant to conduct research because you do not feel prepared to handle the statistical analysis requirements. While many RDNs have taken a course in statistics as an undergraduate or graduate student, most of us are not experts in statistics. To overcome this barrier, keep in mind that we cannot be experts in all areas. Lack of advanced knowledge and expertise in statistics should not deter you from participating in research. Instead, look for ways to collaborate with others who have these skills, and take the initiative to learn a bit about the statistics relevant to your particular research study (see Box 12.1 on page 248 for online resources). For example, Parrott[22] suggests the following ways to become more comfortable with and competent in statistical analysis:

> Learn the basics by talking with colleagues about what resources or statistical software they would recommend, obtaining a book about statistics designed for nonstatisticians, taking a course in statistics, and exploring different software programs and their accompanying instruction manuals.

> Become familiar with the types of statistical tests generally used in the type of research you plan to conduct (from the research you reviewed in your literature review phase).

> Don't go it alone; get involved with others who are skilled researchers.

You can overcome the barrier of insufficient statistical knowledge by involving a statistician early in the research process. Many health care facilities or health systems affiliated with universities have statisticians on staff who will provide help for free or at a nominal cost. If this is not an option, consider a consultant (usually costly) or requesting an RDN with a doctorate degree on the faculty at a nearby university to provide mentorship. Individuals with expertise in statistics can help determine the necessary sample size and type of analysis, which in turn can affect the research question and study design.

The Research Process

The research process involves choosing a question to answer, designing and implementing the study, analyzing the data, and disseminating the results. The following sections touch briefly on these issues, but the research process is certainly more complex than what can be described in this chapter. Other references should be explored for more information on this topic.[7,8]

Choosing the Research Question and Designing the Study

The research process begins with the identification of a concern or question that is both relevant and important. A research question often originates from problems encountered in everyday clinical practice or management. To define your research question, you must begin by being knowledgeable about the published literature in the area of interest. That understanding enables you to focus your research efforts on an issue that is lacking evidence or requires further confirmation. A good research question can be described using the acronym FINER, which stands for feasible, interesting, novel, ethical, and relevant[8] (see Box 12.2). The research question you develop is critical because it drives the rest of the research process; it is the key to conducting good research. If written well, the research question dictates the type of study design as well as the type of statistical analysis. Variables in the research question should be operationally defined so that a better assessment of how to analyze the data can be made. Research questions can be descriptive (eg, What is the prevalence of malnutrition in a facility?), relationship or association oriented (eg, What is the association between type of feeding and 30-day mortality in critical illness?), or causal (eg, What is the difference in glycemic control in patients who receive enteral vs parenteral nutrition support?). Creating a specific and measurable question will also help you use time and resources more effectively and assist with determining what research design is most appropriate. See Box 12.3 on page 250 for examples of ways to narrow down the research question.

BOX 12.2 Using FINER to Help Define a Research Question

F = Feasible
If you want to compare resting energy expenditure (REE) of patients who are critically ill as measured with indirect calorimetry to REE calculated using a predictive equation, you need a metabolic cart and someone to operate it correctly to make this study feasible. Another important consideration is your required sample size (the minimum number of subjects required to produce statistically relevant or meaningful results) and the length of time required to obtain it. If you have funding for 1 year but need 5 years to accrue the required sample, the study is not feasible as designed; you must either restructure it or find additional funding. Even if funding is not limiting the length of the study, you need to consider the time involved in terms of feasibility. Consider collaborating with others who have expertise in the area to make your study more feasible and your subject pool more diverse.

I = Interesting
The research topic should be of interest to you but also to the dietetics profession and other stakeholders, such as administrators, potential funding groups, physician or nurse leaders, and your staff. Their interest in your topic can assist in making the project more successful, and interesting research is more likely to be selected for presentation or publication.

N = Novel
Research should lead to new evidence that answers a question. However, it is not always necessary (or possible) to ask a completely original question. In the area of nutrition, there is also opportunity for additional research to determine whether findings from previous research can be confirmed or validated. If you review evidence-based guidelines, such as those in the Academy of Nutrition and Dietetics Evidence Analysis Library, you will notice that many of the recommendations do not have a "strong" rating because more evidence is needed. Therefore, replicating a study that has already been carried out can add to the evidence in a particular area, as evidence-based practice is established through results from multiple studies.

continued on next page

continued from previous page

E = Ethical

Research practices must always be ethical. To present and publish research outside of your organization, approval of the research protocol from an authorized institutional review board (IRB) is required prior to any data collection. The role of the IRB is to protect human and animal research study participants from potential harm and unethical research practices. For example, an IRB would not approve a study comparing the potential benefits of feeding patients vs starving them. In this context, keep in mind the burdens (eg, time, discomfort, invasion of privacy, and risks) on participants as you are planning your research study.

R = Relevant

A research question must be relevant. Always consider the potential significance of your research. For example, if you propose to research whether feeding a specific type of formula to oncology patients results in higher albumin levels, you may be selecting an end point that is not relevant enough to justify the effort. An outcome that involves quality of life, financial costs, or medical complications may be more relevant and more applicable to clinical practice. In addition, you must be able to use a valid instrument (eg, a scale for weight changes or a validated instrument for surveying quality of life) to measure what you are studying.

BOX 12.3 Focusing a Research Question

Broad topic	Narrowed topic	Focused topic	Research question (Narrowly focused and measurable)
Females	Females and breast cancer	Postmenopausal females and breast cancer	Do postmenopausal females with a breast cancer diagnosis alter their dietary intake of fat from baseline (precancer diagnosis)?
Critically ill patients	Critically ill patients and enteral nutrition (EN)	Critically ill patients with obesity who are receiving EN	As compared to eucaloric EN, does hypocaloric EN administered to critically ill patients with obesity result in improved glycemic control after 5 intensive care unit days?
Outpatients	Outpatients with hyperlipidemia	Outpatients with overweight and hyperlipidemia who are not taking statins	Does intensive nutrition counseling of outpatients with overweight and hyperlipidemia help them attain and maintain healthful fasting serum lipid levels, thereby avoiding treatment with statins?

Once you have identified your research question, you must design a study that will answer it. Steps include choosing the type of study design, identifying primary and secondary outcomes, determining the specific population to be studied, selecting a sample size, establishing research methods, planning what data will be collected, and pretesting and revising the study protocol.

Different types of study designs produce different types of evidence, with varying levels of quality and reliability (see Figure 12.1 and Box 12.4 on page 252).[23,24] Randomized controlled trials (RCTs) and systematic reviews provide the highest level of evidence for intervention questions, but these types of research are not always feasible due to factors, such as a lack of resources (including time), insufficient expertise, or ethical concerns. Although observational studies (eg, cohort studies, case-control studies, case series, and reports) produce a lower level of evidence than RCTs for intervention questions, they are often a good way for clinicians to become involved in and more comfortable with the research process, especially if time and expertise are limited. Furthermore, evidence from descriptive and correlational studies can answer other practice-relevant questions and be useful in determining whether an RCT is warranted.

As you design the study, you will need to set expectations regarding its logistics and publication. For example, the responsibilities of all study personnel should be clearly outlined from the start. Before any data collection begins, it is essential to establish who does what, how they will receive credit (eg, author order in publications), and how they will be compensated if compensation is an option (eg, days off, time off, or monetary rewards).

FIGURE 12.1 Levels of evidence for various research study designs[23]

Study designs with more rigor are associated with a higher quality of evidence as well as less chance for bias and confounding factors.

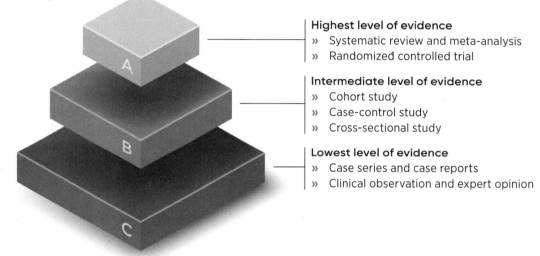

Highest level of evidence
» Systematic review and meta-analysis
» Randomized controlled trial

Intermediate level of evidence
» Cohort study
» Case-control study
» Cross-sectional study

Lowest level of evidence
» Case series and case reports
» Clinical observation and expert opinion

Prospective vs Retrospective Study Designs

As you think about the appropriate research design for your research question, consider whether data should be collected prospectively or retrospectively. Each approach has benefits and limitations. Examples of prospective research include RCTs and cohort studies, although cohort studies can also be carried out retrospectively. A cohort study involves two or more groups, one or more of which has a risk factor, prognostic feature, or specific intervention that one group does not. Cohort studies differ from RCTs in that the subjects are not assigned an intervention by the researcher. Instead, the intervention they receive is determined by a clinician or subject. The groups are then followed prospectively (or retrospectively) and observed for specific predetermined outcomes. With cohort studies, confounding variables can be controlled or accounted for using logistic or linear regression analysis. These statistical tests can provide greater confidence that the outcomes are related to the intervention. Confounding variables are variables that also affect the outcome of interest and, if not accounted for, make it difficult to determine whether the intervention and outcome

> **BOX 12.4** Selected Types of Research Studies[23,24]

Descriptive Study Design

Research that examines and describes a group of patients, a situation, or an area of interest in a systematic manner; usually as a precursor to a quantitative study (which includes an intervention or randomization).

Types of descriptive research include qualitative studies, case studies, and survey research.

Examples:

» The nutritional status of patients who are critically ill (malnourished vs at risk for malnutrition) upon admission (descriptive)

» Use of a focus group of individuals with celiac disease to understand their perceptions about the etiology of their gastrointestinal complaints and how they manage them (qualitative)

» Nursing staff's beliefs about the value of measuring gastric residual volumes in patients who are enterally fed (survey)

Correlational Study Design

Research that predicts the association or correlation between two or more variables. Note that correlation and causation are very different, and a correlational study *cannot* imply a causal relationship.

Types of correlational research include case-control and cohort studies:

» *In case-control studies,* researchers compare two groups of patients; one group has an outcome condition or disease and the other group does not. The researchers retrospectively study the effect of a predictor or exposure to a risk factor on the development of the disease. Cases with the disease are matched to controls who do not have the disease.

  Example of a case-control study: Comparison of the influence of a high-fiber diet (predictor) on the development of colon cancer (outcome). Two groups, one with colon cancer and one without colon cancer, are compared (development).

» *In cohort studies*, which can be prospective or retrospective, researchers follow patients either over time or back in time to assess the association between identified risk factors and an outcome.

  Example of a retrospective cohort study: Comparison of the complication and readmission rates of patients with head and neck cancer who receive nutrition support with a percutaneous endoscopic gastrostomy tube vs rates for those who do not receive nutrition support via a feeding tube.

Experimental or Analytic Study Design

Research involving application of an intervention to establish a cause and effect.

Types of experimental or analytic research include randomized controlled trials (RCTs), and randomized crossover trials. In RCTs, study participants are randomly assigned to one or more groups exposed to a treatment or intervention or to a control group that is not exposed to the treatment or intervention. Randomized crossover trials are another type of experimental or analytical study. In this study design, the subjects are assigned one treatment or another (or a placebo), then undergo a washout period before they receive the alternate treatment (eg, the treatment they did not receive during the first phase of the study). Subjects in randomized crossover trials serve as their own controls.

Examples:

» Differences in hospitalization rates for exacerbation of congestive heart failure (CHF) for individuals with CHF who are randomly assigned to receive nutrition counseling from a registered dietitian nutritionist or receive an educational handout only (RCT)

» Incidence of diarrhea as measured by frequency and stool consistency in patients who are enterally fed a standard isotonic formula and randomly assigned to receive a probiotic, fiber supplement, or placebo (RCT)

» In individuals with irritable bowel syndrome, two types of fiber are evaluated for their effect on abdominal pain, constipation, and diarrhea. Half of the participants are randomly assigned to an insoluble fiber supplement for 1 month and the other half are assigned to take a soluble fiber supplement over the same time period. After a 1-month washout period, the two groups receive the other type of fiber for an additional month. (randomized crossover design) are related. For example, if glucose control in patients receiving enteral vs parenteral nutrition is the outcome of interest, confounding variables such as diabetes, intravenous dextrose, acuity, and BMI may also influence glucose control and should be collected and accounted for using regression analysis. If the baseline characteristics of the groups are similar or individuals with confounding variables are excluded, the researcher can also be more confident that the factor or intervention is truly related to the outcome.[23] RCTs are less affected by confounding factors because these trials are designed to use the principles of control, randomization, and replication. When key confounders are mitigated in an RCT through the use of rigorous eligibility criteria, the researcher can conclude from statistically significant results that there is a causal relationship between the intervention and outcomes. The limitations of these types of prospective studies are that they are typically expensive to conduct, may require a relatively large sample size, and can take longer to complete.

New researchers should consider beginning their research experience with case studies, case series (both of which are typically retrospective), or a cross-sectional study. Because electronic medical records are utilized in most clinical settings, retrieval of lists of patients with a particular International Classification of Diseases (ICD-10) code or procedural code is more feasible. Nutrition managers and RDNs should collaborate with their information technology departments for assistance identifying patients of interest for the research. These studies are usually faster to complete and less expensive than RCTs or cohort studies, and they can be an effective way to gather the data about a population or group of patients needed to design a prospective trial. However, retrospective data collection can be hampered by selection bias, missing information from a database or medical record, or poor recall by study subjects.

Box 12.5 on page 254 details a series of related study designs for research about enteral nutrition delivery among patients who are critically ill.

Outcomes Research

Outcomes research focuses on maximizing the quality of care and is conducted at a practice site or in a real-world setting.[25-27] Because outcomes research is not as controlled as RCTs, outcomes research has lower internal validity (eg, cause-and-effect relationship between the independent and dependent variables) and higher external validity (eg, generalizability of the results to persons, settings, and times other than those used in the study) in comparison to RCTs. The outcomes studied can be clinical (eg, ventilator-free days, infectious complications, or mortality), functional (eg, quality of life or patient satisfaction measures), or economic (eg, cost of services). The aim of an outcomes study is to determine "the impact of an intervention on one segment of the sample (intervention group) compared with the impact on a segment of the sample not receiving the intervention (comparison or control group)."[25] Because many variables in the practice setting can influence outcomes, the "selected intervention should be one that can be tested realistically within the dietetics professional's span of control and expected to show measurable difference if implemented."[19] Box 12.6 on page 254 guides you through the steps of an outcomes project. The PICO (patient group, intervention, control or comparison group, outcome) format, which can also be used in RCTs, is recommended to organize your research question for an outcomes project.[25]

BOX 12.5 Study Design Examples for Enteral Nutrition Delivery in Critical Illness

Study design	Aim of study
Descriptive	Survey of registered dietitian nutritionists (RDNs) to determine their experience regarding percentage of enteral nutrition (EN) delivered compared to prescribed and what the most prevalent causes are for under delivery. The survey results indicate that RDNs perceived that most patients who are critically ill receive 50% to 70% of their prescribed EN, and the most prevalent causes of cessation of feedings were having to hold feeds for procedures and gastrointestinal intolerance.
Correlational (retrospective cohort)	Based on the survey results, a retrospective review of medical records of patients in the intensive care unit for at least 1 week and receiving EN for at least 3 days was conducted. Patients were divided into two groups: those who received 80% or higher of prescribed EN and those who received less than 80%. The reasons (predictor or risk factor) for not attaining at least 80% of EN prescription (outcome) were identified and compared between the groups. The study results found an association between cessation of feedings for procedures or surgeries and percentage of EN prescription delivered.
Correlational (prospective cohort)	Based on the retrospective cohort study, the researchers implemented a volume-based feeding (VBF) protocol to overcome the EN missed while feedings were held for procedures or surgeries. Patients were observed prospectively over 3 months to determine whether there was an association between VBF vs traditional rate-based feeding (RBF) and EN delivery. The study results found an association between the type of feeding protocol and the percentage of prescribed EN delivered. Percentage of prescribed EN delivered was 85% in the VBF group compared to 65% in the RBF group.
Randomized controlled trial (RCT)	Subsequently, an RCT was conducted to compare the effect of VBF vs RBF on percentage of prescribed EN delivered. Glycemic control was a secondary outcome. The patients' baseline characteristics, including history of diabetes, BMI, acuity, and age, were similar. VBF compared to RBF resulted in 83% vs 68% of prescribed EN delivery, respectively. The difference in EN delivery was statistically significant ($P<.05$) although there was no statistical difference in glycemic control. The researchers concluded that VBF vs RBF leads to improved EN delivery without adversely affecting glycemic control.

BOX 12.6 Steps in an Outcomes Research Project

Step 1: Develop the practice question.
Typically, a desirable question is one that is not answered by existing evidence or for which the available evidence is not very strong or is conflicting.

The question should be stated in PICO format, where P = patient group, I = intervention, C = control or comparison group, and O = outcome(s). For example:

» Do inpatients receiving tube feedings (P) who are monitored daily by the registered dietitian nutritionist (RDN) (I) compared to inpatients receiving tube feedings who are monitored twice a week by the RDN (C) receive more of their nutrition prescription and have a shorter hospital length of stay (O)?

» Do inpatients with congestive heart failure (P) who receive nutrition education provided by an RDN (I) compared to members of the same patient population who receive nutrition education provided by a nurse (C) have better dietary compliance and fewer hospital readmissions (O)?

Step 2: Conduct an exhaustive literature review.
What studies have already been completed and published in the area you are researching?

Are there gaps in the evidence?

What methodologies and research techniques are used and accepted in studying this question?

continued on next page

continued from previous page

Step 3: Determine the study design.

Define the comparison in your study by identifying which intervention will be tested and what type of care the comparison group will receive.

Establish the necessary sample size (discuss with a statistician), a description of the participants, and inclusion and exclusion criteria.

Plan appropriate data collection methods. Data should include patient characteristics, information about the intervention (eg, did it happen consistently, and was it carried out by one individual or multiple individuals?), outcome indicators, how the outcomes are being measured, and any covariates or confounders that could also influence the outcomes. Establish the frequency of data collection and confirm that any individuals collecting data will follow the same procedure. Fidelity within a research study is key to a quality study and confidence that the outcomes are related to the intervention. Fidelity within the context of research means the treatment or intervention is delivered as intended per the predefined protocol.

Step 4: Institute study methods.

If the study design is prospective, prepare to enroll participants. Enrollment includes recruitment, screening for eligibility (be prepared to keep records of how many participants were screened but not enrolled), informed consent procedure, and assignment of participants to the intervention or control group. If the study design is retrospective, screen potential participants for eligibility: based on the inclusion and exclusion criteria, examine the electronic medical records to determine whether the patient can be included.

Standardize procedures by using a study manual and data collection forms and tools. Take care to identify potential sources of bias and, if possible, remove them.

Obtain commitment to the study from all participating sites. Although novice researchers are unlikely to conduct a multisite study, it may be feasible if the researchers are part of a health care system with multiple hospitals interested in the same research question.

Secure institutional review board (IRB) approval from the primary site, followed by approval from other sites (if any). If the other sites are within one health care system, the submission for approval from the IRB would include all participating sites and further approval at each site would usually not be required.

Provide appropriate training for staff involved in the study.

If appropriate, conduct a pilot study before launching a larger study.

Plan a method to check the accuracy of data collection during the study.

Step 5: Analyze and report data.

Create a database for data entry. Various free software programs exist for use in spreadsheets. If you are using multiple research sites, a central, blinded data collection site is preferred.

Identify a coding method. Statistical analysis usually requires the data to be entered as a number, so a number must be assigned to data collected in words (eg, if you are collecting information on diagnoses, the various diagnosis categories need to be assigned their own numbers for entry into the database, and you need to keep a record of what each code means).

Engage the help of a statistician, if needed, to conduct the statistical analysis.

Prepare results for presentation and publication. Dissemination of the evidence is essential to promote the dietetics profession and enhance knowledge. The results should be used to demonstrate to department and organization leaders the value of nutrition interventions, of the RDN, as well as to change practice to improve patient care.

Adapted with permission from Biesemeier C. Outcomes research in nutrition support. *Support Line.* 2003;25:7-13.[25]

Outcomes research that evaluates and documents the benefits of interventions provided by the RDN can help you and your staff improve performance, gain respect, and increase funding and revenues, and it can advance the dietetics profession more generally. When conducting outcomes research, focus on measuring outcomes that can demonstrate the value of our profession to patients, payers, and administrators. Ideally, the evidence or data you collect should be used to ensure quality of care, patient safety, and/or cost savings.

Outcomes research using an existing database, such as the electronic health record (EHR), is a good way for a clinical dietitian or clinical nutrition manager (CNM) to begin participating in research activity. The EHR can help you learn about specific practice patterns (eg, initiation of enteral feedings in the ICU, or nutrition interventions used for patients with pressure ulcers or injuries). Ask your facility's information technology personnel whether they can assist in building reports that capture the desired data. The Academy of Nutrition and Dietetics Health Informatics Infrastructure (ANDHII) is another option for RDNs interested in participating in outcomes research. More information about ANDHII and how to participate is available on the ANDHII website (www.ANDHII.org).[28] This type of research, like any involving human subjects or their records, requires approval from the institutional review board (IRB).

Institutional Review Board Process

Before you initiate any research study, you should understand its legal and ethical dimensions, including those related to the IRB process. In the United States, health care and medical research is regulated by the federal government through the Department of Health and Human Services and the US Food and Drug Administration. US regulations have established the IRB as one way to ensure the protection of the rights and welfare of human beings who participate in research.[29-31] The principles of the IRB's work can be traced to the Nuremberg Code, developed in reaction to the coerced human experiments conducted by the Nazi party in World War II, and the Belmont Report, released in the 1970s, which declared that acceptable and ethical human research must embrace "respect for persons, beneficence, and justice."[29] To demonstrate respect for persons, researchers are obligated to ensure all study participants involved in research have voluntarily consented to participate and understand the risks and benefits associated with the study. Researchers must also protect participants' privacy and confidentiality and offer greater protections for vulnerable populations, such as children or those with disabilities. The application of beneficence requires that any possible benefits of research be maximized and that risks be minimized. Justice involves the equitable selection of subjects.

As a CNM, you will need to understand whether it is mandatory for your proposed research study to undergo the process of IRB approval. You will also need to ensure that any staff involved with the research study complete training on how to conduct research appropriately. The IRB will not grant study approval until all study personnel have completed the training.

To achieve IRB approval of your study, seek out and collaborate with the IRB staff at your organization. They can advise you about the IRB process and provide specific instructions and templates, which are often dictated by regulations, to assist you through the process. The IRB will typically have specific dates on which they meet to review and approve research studies. Take care to learn what the timeline is, ask whether prereview of a study is possible, pay close attention to all directions and deadlines, and call the IRB staff if you have questions or have not heard back about your study when you anticipated. Box 12.7 lists documents that the IRB potentially requires to review and approve a research study.[29]

BOX 12.7 Potential Documentation Required for Institutional Review Board Approval

» Research proposal and protocol, including how you plan to obtain informed consent

» Grant application, if applicable

» Institutional review board application (will differ among organizations)

» Documents related to informed consent (eg, sample consent form or consent cover letter) or an appeal for a waiver of consent

» Advertisements for recruitment of subjects, and plans and tools for recruitment

» Printed information you plan to provide to subjects

» Background information on study-related use of drugs, devices, or procedures

» Qualifications of research staff

» Specific information about the study site, to demonstrate it is an appropriate setting for the study

» Financial incentives for either researchers or subjects, if any

» Survey instruments, if applicable, with validity and reliability statistics

» Data collection tools

Adapted with permission from Cothran EH. Institutional review board review: a collaborative process. *Support Line.* 2010;32:22–27.[29]

Not all organizations have their own IRB. If your facility does not have one, additional options include starting an IRB at your institution; utilizing an external, commercial IRB; or partnering with another institution that has an IRB and is willing to serve as the IRB of record for the study.

The necessity for IRB approval will depend on the nature of the project. If the project's aim is quality or performance improvement and the findings will not be published or presented outside your organization, IRB approval may not be needed. However, you should still obtain project approval from upper management or the organization's administration. For example, suppose you wish to study whether your ICU patients on mechanical ventilation are positioned with the head of the bed inclined 30 degrees, and then use the data to determine the need for an intervention (eg, nursing in-services) to ensure beds at your hospital are positioned correctly. Your study probably does not need IRB approval as long as you do not plan to share the results outside of your hospital. However, if you designed a study to randomly assign ICU patients on mechanical ventilation to be positioned in beds with the heads inclined 30 degrees or left in a supine position in order to compare the incidence of ventilator-acquired pneumonia, your study would need IRB approval, even if the intent was to keep the results internal, because the research poses a risk to the patient and cannot be classified as merely a performance improvement project.

In general, any time you plan to present or publish research outside of your organization, you will need to obtain IRB approval for the study or project. Some studies are classified as exempt, meaning they involve minimal risk and do not have to undergo the IRB committee's review. Surveys, interviews, taste and food quality evaluation, or studies of existing records, as long as data is deidentified, are examples of exempt research. Typically, the IRB chairperson or vice-chair and one other IRB committee member review and approve studies for exempt status. Exempt studies may be eligible for waiver of informed consent. However, the criteria to meet waiver of informed consent are strictly defined by federal regulations. All of the following criteria must be met to get approval from the IRB for a waiver of consent[29]:

> The research involves no more than minimal risk to the subjects.

> The study will not adversely affect the rights and welfare of the subjects.

> The research could not practicably be carried out without the waiver or alteration.

> Whenever appropriate, the subjects will be provided with additional pertinent information after participation.

Prior to submitting a request for a waiver of consent, contact the IRB staff to discuss whether your study design meets the criteria listed here and ensure that you can provide the appropriate documentation to obtain the waiver.

The review process and associated obligations extend beyond the initial study approval. Annually, at a minimum, a report on the status of the study is required. If subjects enrolled in the study experience any adverse events, these must be reported to the IRB within a certain time frame, even if the adverse event is not related to the study intervention. Other types of information that must be reported include protocol deviations, patient complaints, and loss of data. The standards for submission of this type of information vary. Familiarize yourself with your organization's specific rules and reporting procedures.[29]

Communicating and Publishing Results

Once you have completed a study and analyzed the results, the next step is to communicate the information to others, both internally as well as externally to groups that will benefit from learning about your research. Even if your research results were not positive and don't support your hypothesis, the process of communicating and publishing should still occur. Negative findings or those that don't support what was hypothesized or what is accepted in practice should still be shared. After all your hard work conducting the research, the process of communicating your results brings a great sense of accomplishment and adds to the body of knowledge related to clinical nutrition—so don't skip this step!

Communicating Results Within Your Organization

First, determine what groups within your organization should hear about your research because their goals or practice are related and the information could make a substantial impact. In other words, if you share your study results with them, can you influence their actions or gain support for an initiative or change in practice to improve patient care? Think about including committees involved with quality improvement, patient safety, or a specific service line (eg, intensive care, surgical, or cardiovascular units). Also consider the value of reporting your findings to the pharmacy and therapeutics committee or nursing leadership committee. These committees often have physician and nursing champions who can drive change related to their discipline. Be sure you know the composition of the group (eg, identify potential supporters and opponents of your ideas), how long you have to present the information, and if a specific presentation format is required. Depending on the type of research study, you may want to share the results in an internal newsletter or publication to disseminate the information to a wider audience at your organization.

Abstracts

Submitting an abstract for an oral or poster presentation at your own institution as well as at local, state, or national meetings is a good initial way to share your study results. Frequently, the organization hosting the meeting will identify specific topics of interest for their meeting. Prior to submitting an abstract, you should review these topics and ensure you follow the submission guidelines. Each author is typically required to declare their role in the conduct of the research (eg, design, data collection, writing) and complete a conflict of interest statement as part of the abstract submission. Ask a colleague experienced in abstract submission to review your abstract and provide suggestions for improvement prior to submission. Once the abstract is accepted, be sure you understand and follow all instructions related to the presentation, whether it is a poster or an oral session.

Publishing Results

Publishing your research results is also important but will take more time and effort than the communication strategies previously described. When attempting to publish your findings, the first thing to determine is which journal or publication is most appropriate not only for your research focus but also for the type of research design you used.[32] For example, consider the journals that published the research you used in your literature review; some of these journals likely reach audiences who will be interested in your research. The publications of the various dietetic practice groups of the Academy of Nutrition and Dietetics are a good place to showcase pilot research, especially if the study is your initial effort or the study is lower on the hierarchy of study designs.

Once you have selected your target journal or publication, obtain a copy of its author and submission guidelines and follow these carefully. You may also want to read other articles published in the journal or publication to get ideas about how to format your manuscript.[33]

Regardless of where you decide to publish, be aware that publishers require a review and editing process for all manuscripts that they find worthy of consideration for publication. Do not be discouraged by the reviewers' comments and suggestions. Instead, if you feel overwhelmed by the requested changes, take a deep breath and put the manuscript aside for a day or two to gain perspective. The reviewers' comments and your subsequent revisions will only make the manuscript stronger. You do not have to incorporate all of the comments and suggestions into your manuscript. However, you will want to address each of the reviewer comments, and if you opt not to make a suggested change, explain why. At this time, you may want to contact a mentor who has published before and who may be able to help you discern which changes are most important to ensure that your manuscript is accepted for publication.

In addition, if your manuscript is rejected by a publisher, do not give up on publication. Perhaps the first journal you tried was not the right fit for your manuscript. Reevaluate your article, discuss your options with a mentor, and then submit your manuscript to a different, more appropriate journal. Keep in mind that the author and submission guidelines of the new journal will likely be different from those of the first journal, so some reformatting and rewriting may be necessary.

Embracing the Research Process

Now that we have progressed through the steps of the research process, from formulating the question to publishing the results, let's briefly consider an example of how your staff might progress from preliminary research to a complex trial. For each of the types of study examples, IRB approval is required. Imagine your staff becomes worried about diarrhea in patients who are tube fed, and they want to identify interventions that will decrease the incidence of this complication. You decide to conduct a cross-sectional observational study to identify how many patients on enteral feedings have diarrhea. The study shows that the incidence is high, so you decide to perform a correlational study to determine whether the incidence of diarrhea is associated with certain formulas, fiber supplements, or probiotics or whether it correlates with certain medications or conditions, such as infectious complications in the gastrointestinal tract. That study finds a negative association between the incidence of diarrhea and the use of a probiotic (ie, the incidence of diarrhea is lower in patients who are receiving a probiotic). This finding alone is of interest, may lead to a change in practice within your organization, and could be presented internally to your organization as well as outside your organization.

Based on this evidence and a review of published research, you explore the idea of conducting an RCT in which patients who are enterally fed are randomly selected to receive a probiotic or a placebo. Ideally, the study would be double-blind, meaning neither the patient nor the study investigators would be aware of which patients were receiving the actual treatment vs the placebo. Before launching a large RCT, your team of researchers carries out a pilot study. This small-scale study helps the team refine the research design and determine that the larger trial is logistically and financially feasible. Building on the pilot study, your team designs the RCT, gets it approved by the IRB, and conducts the trial. Upon completion, you communicate the results to key decision makers in your facility and publish the results in a leading nutrition journal.

At this point, you find yourself asking new questions or looking for more evidence—and the research cycle begins again.

Summary

Research is an exciting part of nutrition regardless of the research's specific focus area. If you have not yet gotten involved in the research process, you are heartily encouraged to do so for several reasons. First, RDNs need to be proactive in demonstrating how our interventions can improve outcomes. If we do not accomplish this task, we may find at some point that our roles are not valued or supported. Second, you and your staff will gain additional knowledge, professional skills (eg, writing, presentation, and leadership), recognition from others, including physicians and administrators, as well as job satisfaction. So take action! You can undoubtedly identify several problems or questions that need addressing in your organization, and a research study—even if simple and small in scope—can be the solution.

ADDITIONAL RESOURCES

Because there is a great deal more to research than can be covered in a single chapter, selected additional resources are listed here.

Academy of Nutrition and Dietetics: www.eatrightPRO.org
Offers many resources related to research, including many that are available to Academy of Nutrition and Dietetics members only.

Getting Started in Quality Improvement and Research for the RDN/DTR: www.eatrightSTORE .org/cpe-on-demand/cpe-on-demand/getting-started-in-quality-improvement-and-research-for-the-rdndtr
On-demand module explaining the importance of involvement in quality improvement and research projects.

Academy of Nutrition and Dietetics Evidence Analysis Library: www.andeal.org
The Academy of Nutrition and Dietetics site for evidence-based practice guidelines, evidence analysis projects, and related publications and tools (member benefit).

American Society for Parenteral and Enteral Nutrition (ASPEN): www.nutritioncare.org
Resources include a research toolkit (member benefit).

Cochrane Library: www.thecochranelibrary.com
Cochrane Reviews and other evidence-based health care resources.

Critical Care Nutrition: www.criticalcarenutrition.com
Site includes information about participating in the International Nutrition Survey project and other research led by this Canadian group

Cumulative Index to Nursing and Allied Health Literature (CINAHL): www.cinahl.com
Requires subscription to access (web address will vary by subscriber); an index of English-language and selected other-language journal articles about nursing, allied health, biomedicine, and health care.

***Journal of the Academy of Nutrition and Dietetics* collection on research methodology:** https://jandonline.org/content/researchDesign

PubMed: www.ncbi.nlm.nih.gov/pubmed
Essential database for conducting literature reviews.

***Research: Successful Approaches in Nutrition and Dietetics.* 4th ed.** Van Horn L, Beto J, eds. Academy of Nutrition and Dietetics; 2019.
Addresses designing, executing, analyzing, and communicating modern nutrition research that is essential for evidence-based practice.

REFERENCES

1   Boyd M, Gall SB, Rothpletz-Puglia P, et al. Characteristics and drivers of the registered dietitian nutritionist's sustained involvement in clinical research activities: a mixed methods study. *J Acad Nutr Diet.* 2019;119(12):2099-2108. doi:10.1016/j.jand.2019.03.018

2   Academy of Nutrition and Dietetics. Research. eatrightPRO website. Accessed July 19, 2020. www.eatrightPRO.org/research

3   Academy of Nutrition and Dietetics Quality Management Committee. Academy of Nutrition and Dietetics: revised 2017 standards of practice in nutrition care and standards of professional performance for registered dietitian nutritionists. *J Acad Nutr Diet.* 2018;118:132-140. doi:10.1016/j .jand.2017.10.003

4   Robien K. Making research happen: the real world of clinical nutrition research. *Support Line.* 2003;25:3-6.

5   Dougherty CM, Burrowes JD, Hand RK. Why registered dietitian nutritionists are not doing research—perceptions, barriers, and participation in research from the Academy's Dietetics Practice-Based Research Network needs assessment survey. *J Acad Nutr Diet.* 2015;115(6):1001-1007. doi:10.1016/j.jand.2015.01.012

6   Slawson DL, Clemens LH, Bol L. Research and the clinical dietitian: perceptions of the research process and preferred routes to obtaining research skills. *J Am Diet Assoc.* 2000;100(10):1144-1148. doi:10.1016/S0002-8223(00)00336-9

7   Van Horn L, Beto J, eds. *Research: Successful Approaches in Nutrition and Dietetics.* 4th ed. Academy of Nutrition and Dietetics; 2019.

8   Hulley SB, Cummings SR, Browner WS, Grady DG, Newman TB. *Designing Clinical Research.* 3rd ed. Lippincott Williams & Wilkins; 2007.

9   Academy of Nutrition and Dietetics. Academy research toolkit 2011. eatrightPRO website. Accessed August 23, 2020. www.eatrightPRO.org/research/projects-tools-and-initiatives /nutrition-research-network/academy-research-toolkit-2011

10 Academy of Nutrition and Dietetics. Nutrition Research Network. eatrightPRO website. Accessed August 23, 2020. www.eatrightPRO.org/research/projects-tools-and-initiatives/nutrition -research-network

11 Enrione EB. Content validation of nutrition diagnoses. *Topics Clin Nutr.* 2008;23(4):306-319.

12 Trostler N, Myers EF. Review of critical thinking in professional practice: application in making decisions to either measure or estimate resting metabolic rate. *Topics Clin Nutr.* 2008;23(4):278-291.

13 Resnicow K. McMaster F, Woolford S, et al. Study design and baseline description of the BMI2 trial: reducing paediatric obesity in primary care practices. *Pediatr Obes.* 2012;7(1):3-15. doi:10.1111 /j.2047-6310.2011.00001.x

14 Snetselaar L, Smith KL, Hollinger D, Myers E, Murphy G, Qualls L. Registered dietitian wellness insurance benefit makes a difference in adult weight management: a pre-post study. *Food Nutr Sci.* 2011;2(10):1043-1047.

15 Academy of Nutrition and Dietetics. Nutrition Research Network projects. eatrightPRO website. Accessed August 29, 2020. www.eatrightPRO.org/research/projects-tools-and-initiatives /nutrition-research-network/nutrition-research-network-projects

16 Byham-Gray LD, Gilbride JA, Dixon LB, Stage FK. Predictors for research involvement among registered dietitians. *J Am Diet Assoc.* 2006;106(12):2008-2015. doi:10.1016/j.jada.2006.09.017

17 Koretz RL. Assessing the evidence in evidence-based medicine. *Nutr Clin Pract.* 2019;34(1):60-72.

18 Koretz RL. Introduction to critical reading. *JPEN J Parenter Enteral Nutr.* 2014;3(1)8:122-123. doi:10 .1177/0148607113497761

19 Krenitsky J. Mastering critical appraisal of nutrition research for the busy clinician. *Support Line.* 2019;41:3-8.

20 Bowles PFD, Marenah K, Ricketts DM, Rogers BA. How to prepare for and present at a journal club. *Br J Hosp Med (Lond).* 2013;74:C150-C152.

21 McClave SA, Patel JJ. Evidence-based medicine and derivation of clinical guidelines. In: Mueller CM, ed. *The ASPEN Adult Nutrition Support Core Curriculum.* 3rd ed. American Society for Parenteral and Enteral Nutrition; 2017:819-828.

22 Parrott JS. Why dietitians can be great researchers. *Support Line.* 2010;32:17-21.

23 Hoppe DJ, Schemitsch EH, Morshed S, Tornetta P, Bhandari M. Hierarchy of evidence: where observational studies fit in and why we need them. *J Bone Joint Surg Am.* 2009;91(suppl 3):2-9. doi:10.2106/JBJS.H.01571

24 Boushey C, Harris J, Bruemmer B, Archer SL, Van Horn L. Publishing nutrition research: a review of study design, statistical analyses, and other key elements of manuscript preparation, Part 1. *J Am Diet Assoc.* 2006;106(1):89-96. doi:10.1016/j.jada.2005.11.007

25 Biesemeier C. Outcomes research in nutrition support. *Support Line.* 2003;25:7-13.

26 Carson SS. Outcomes research: methods and implications. *Semin Respir Crit Care Med.* 2010;31(1):3-12. doi:10.1055/s-0029-1246281

27 In H, Rosen JE. Primer on outcomes research. *J Surg Onc.* 2014;110(5):489-493. doi:10.1002/jso.23710

28 Academy of Nutrition and Dietetics. ANDHII. eatrightPRO website. Accessed September 5, 2021. www.eatrightPRO.org/research/projects-tools-and-initiatives/andhii

29 Cothran EH. Institutional review board review: a collaborative process. *Support Line.* 2010;32:22-27.

30 Pech C, Cob N, Cejka JT. Understanding institutional review boards: practical guidance to the IRB review process. *Nutr Clin Pract.* 2007;22(6):618-628. doi:10.1177/0115426507022006618

31 National Institutes of Health. Human subjects research–home page. NIH Central Resource for Grants and Funding Information website. Accessed August 30, 2020. http://grants.nih.gov/grants/policy/hs/ethical_guidelines.htm

32 Bliss DZ, Guenter PA, Heitkemper MM. From proposal to publication: are you writing research right? *Nutr Clin Pract.* 2000;15(6):299-305.

33 Gifford H, Ireton-Jones C. Taking your message to the street: presentation and publication. *Support Line.* 2010;32:16-19.

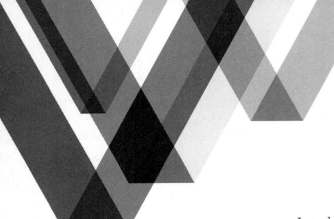

CHAPTER 13

Quality Management & Improvement

Janel Welch, MS, MPA, RDN, CDN, FAND, CPHQ, QCP, OHCC

Introduction

The importance of quality assurance in health care has never been as important as it is today. This chapter provides nutrition leaders with an overview of quality management as it relates to health care as well as the tools and resources commonly used to improve quality outcomes. Let's start with defining *quality*. Quality is an attribute of a product or service and is a subjective measure of how well that product or service meets or exceeds its perceived value from the perspective of the customer, consumer, client, and so on. It is measured against a standard of excellence. *Quality improvement* is the process of improving the quality, safety, efficiency and effectiveness of a product or service.

The National Academy of Medicine (formerly Institute of Medicine, or IOM) provides science-based advice on matters of medicine and health and defines *health care quality* as the "degree to which health services for individuals and populations increases the likelihood of desired health outcomes and are consistent with current professional knowledge."[1]

In 2001, the IOM Committee on Quality Health Care in America further clarified the concept of health care quality in its report, *Crossing the Quality Chasm: A New Health System for the 21st Century,* noting six dimensions of health care quality[1]:

> **Safe:** The patient's safety comes first.

> **Effective:** Care should be based on scientific knowledge and provided to patients who can benefit.

> **Patient centered:** Care should be respectful of and responsive to individual preferences, needs, and values, and patient values should guide all clinical decisions.

> **Timely:** Care should be provided promptly when the patient needs it.

> **Efficient:** Waste, including equipment, supplies, ideas, and energy, should be avoided.

> **Equitable:** The best possible care should be provided to everyone, regardless of age, sex, race, financial status, or any other demographic variable.

The National Quality Strategy was first published in 2011 under the guidance of the Agency for Healthcare Research and Quality (AHRQ) on behalf of the US Department of Health and Human Services (HHS).[2] The strategy's objective was to improve health care quality at the local, state, and national levels by providing a framework for improving patient care, health, and cost. The National Quality Strategy was developed in a collaborative research process that involved gathering input from more than 300 groups representing stakeholders from across the health care industry as well as the general public. This framework built on an earlier one known as the IHI (Institute for Healthcare Improvement) Triple Aim Framework, which had three aims for guiding and improving health care: providing better care, making care more affordable, and helping create better community and individual health.[3] The National Quality Strategy built on these three aims by adding the following six priorities[2]:

> **Patient safety,** with the goal of reducing harm caused in the delivery of care.

> **Person- and family-centered care,** with the goal of engaging the person and family as partners in their delivery of care.

> **Communication and coordination,** with the goal of improving the effectiveness of communication and care coordination.

> **Preventive care,** with the goal of promoting disease prevention with the most effective methods of treatment.

> **Community health,** with the goal of promoting community-wide best practices to enable healthy living.

> **Care affordability,** with the goal of developing care models that provide affordable health care.

Quality Improvement in Health Care

Quality management and improvement in health care ensures regulatory compliance and drives participation factors, reimbursement rates, performance ratings, and customer loyalty. As a nutrition leader, your contributions to driving quality outcomes are essential. Initiatives such as malnutrition coding, reducing hospital readmissions, reducing the risk of hospital-acquired infections, and reducing length of stay can all be influenced with the expertise of the registered dietitian nutritionist (RDN). Each organization has standards for which they are held accountable that correlate with clinical and financial outcomes.

As quality improvement methods and analysis becomes more rigorous and sophisticated, there can be a tendency to confuse it with research and label it as such. However, quality improvement differs from clinical research in a number of important ways. The first is that quality improvement does not control for extraneous variables (also known as external influences). As detailed in Chapter 12, clinical research utilizes standard protocols, tightly controls extraneous variables, generally requires prior institutional review board approval, and so on. Quality improvement projects, on the other hand, utilize data to evaluate processes and improve clinical outcomes, patient satisfaction, efficiency, and revenue generation. Quality improvement attempts to implement existing solutions that are likely to work, whereas research attempts to find new solutions. Quality improvement is often focused on institutional change, whereas research is focused on individual interventions. As an RDN, your work lies at the intersection of patients, procedures, and policies. Your work to improve the quality of care has a direct impact not only on your organization's bottom line but on the quality of care patients receive every day. Consistently working to evaluate, improve, and ensure quality care benefits you, your department, the organization, and patients alike.

Change Management

Health care is a complex system that changes quickly; it is not a question of whether change is needed but one of how much and how often change will take place. An important component in leading quality improvement efforts is the ability to guide the change management process. Change management helps ensure we listen to others, understand their concerns, and work with them wherever they are in the process of making a transition.[4] It addresses the human side of change, which helps the process go faster and improves the likelihood that change will be maintained.

Change entails moving from a current state to a future state via transitional stages, and change management increases the efficiency and effectiveness of this process by acknowledging and addressing some of the common and predictable responses people have when they are asked to change. The larger and more complex a project is, the greater the need for change management.

Organizations do not change just because new systems are put into place; they change when the people implementing the process also change. We need to be sure that individuals have input and buy into the changes being made. Box 13.1 highlights the four stages of change. Although the stages are nearly universal, the rate at which individuals move through them varies.

> **BOX 13.1** Four Stages of Making a Change
> 1. Denial or uncertainty
> 2. Anger or skepticism
> 3. Exploration or curiosity
> 4. Acceptance or commitment

Each stage of change requires slightly different strategies and approaches from you as a leader managing the process. Let's take a closer look at the stages in sequence to explore how people might react and how you can keep the process moving toward the desired outcome.

Stage 1: Denial or Uncertainty

This is the stage when change is announced. Stage 1 typically involves shock and often denial as people being asked to change realize that the familiar reality is shifting. If the change is not too challenging, getting through this first stage can happen quickly. If the change is larger, more complex, or creates a level of uncertainty, people will need time to adjust, absorb the information, and consider how they will be affected. As a leader, it is important to keep the lines of communication open; provide ample information, updates, and details; show care and concern; and listen attentively and respectfully as people process the change and their initial reaction to it.

Stage 2: Anger or Skepticism

Stage 2 is when people begin to react more directly to the change. They may start to feel concern, anger, resentment, or fear. They may resist the change actively or passively. They may feel the need to vent their anger. As a leader, you will need to talk to your staff about feelings they can expect at this stage, strengthen connections within the team, and encourage employees to think of new ways to do things. Start to train people on any new skills they will need during or after the change occurs and continue to explain the purpose and objectives of the change plan.

Stage 3: Exploration or Curiosity

Stage 3 is the turning point for individuals and for the organization. Individuals in this stage begin exploring and testing the implications of the change. They may also decide at this point whether they are going to accept the change or go in a different direction such as transferring to another department or leaving the organization. As the leader, continue to communicate the vision, clearly articulate timelines, encourage involvement, and be as transparent and patient as possible. In addition, if you anticipate staff turnover, develop a transition plan. People cannot be rushed through this stage, so do your best to support them.

Stage 4: Acceptance or Commitment

In stage 4, the changes start to become habitual, and people embrace the improvements to the way they work. The team or organization starts to become more productive and efficient, and the positive effects of change become apparent. Staff have a feeling of certainty similar to what they experienced prior to the change. This is the time to celebrate the success of the change transformation.

As a leader, always keep in mind that individuals tend to respond to change in similar ways (moving through these four stages), but at different paces. This can cause stress within a team if some of the team members have accepted the changes when others have not. It is important to focus on communication and work with each team member to determine what their needs are at any of the four stages.

As quality and process improvement are discussed in this chapter, remember the need to manage change throughout those processes. Change management is often overlooked when organizations attempt to fix problems too quickly or make drastic changes within the organization that affect staff. As a nutrition manager, you can remind leadership of the need to incorporate change management into any process improvement initiative.[5]

Quality Assurance Process Improvement

Quality assurance and quality improvement are two important but different concepts. It is vital to ensure that quality standards are a high priority in any organization, but especially in health care. *Quality assurance* is a method used to monitor a particular procedure or process to ensure that expected levels of quality are upheld. *Quality improvement* is a systematic approach to analyzing the organization's current performance to define and take any actions necessary to improve the quality of a process or procedure. Quality improvement can be considered an ongoing effort to improve the current performance of the organization, increasing its productivity by eliminating the waste and activities that do not add value.[6,7]

Quality assurance process improvement (QAPI) is a common term used in this work. QAPI projects are often initiated but not always completed. There are numerous reasons for this, including the following[8,9]:

> poor team selection

> inadequate training

> inadequate mentoring

> mismanagement of resources

> project scope being too small or too large

> no data or bad data

> unsuccessful implementation

> lack of synergy with organizational strategic plans

> lack of stakeholder buy-in

> lack of leadership support

Keep these potential barriers in mind as we discuss how to successfully complete a QAPI project.

Gather Your Team

The most important aspect of a project's success is leadership support. Find a leader (also called a champion) who will support your project from its beginning to its successful completion. Your project's champion should be someone influential who can help provide validity to the process you intend to create or improve. A champion also has the ability to support the necessary synergy between your project and organizational strategic plans.

Next, begin to pull together a team to evaluate and improve the area of need. Including the right people on a process improvement team is critical to a successful improvement effort. In health care, working with other departments and disciplines is very valuable because a change in one department could necessitate a change in another department. For example, if you were working on a project to change an old process such as paper menus to an electronic process, it would be important to consider having not only staff from the food and nutrition department on the team but representation from other areas as well, such as nursing, information technology, and education. Process improvement teams will vary in size and composition, with a frequent size recommendation from 8 to 10 members; this size team is not so large as to be unwieldy, but large enough to include members with varying perspectives.[1] Finally, when thinking about recruiting team members, try to get people involved who may be new to the process; in many organizations, the same people tend to sign up for virtually every project. Their expertise is valuable, but your project will also benefit from including different people with different perspectives.

Once a team is identified, hold an initial kickoff meeting to gain momentum. This is the time to get buy-in from the team. Introduce the problem, let the team know what will be expected of them, and ask whether this is an initiative they think they could support and commit to. Determine, with team input, whether you have identified all the right team members. Is there someone you overlooked who should be included? Box 13.2 delineates common roles for a member of this type of team.

Process Improvement

Once you are confident in your team's makeup, it is helpful to share the key drivers of a successful process improvement initiative with the team. Successful initiatives share the following qualities[1,8]:

> They align projects to business strategy.

> They drive both business results and performance outcomes.

> They focus on changes related to customers' top concerns or those having the greatest impact on revenue or expenses.

> They utilize a standard set of tools and methods.

> They are supported by the health system's infrastructure.

> They are supported by engaged leadership within the organization.

There are several methodologies you can follow when implementing a process improvement project that will be discussed later in the chapter. No matter which methodology or specific tool you use, you will need to follow a sequence of five steps, as highlighted in Box 13.3 and discussed in detail in the following sections.[10]

Process Improvement Step 1: Identify and Define the Problem

A quality improvement project often begins because there is a problem or perceived problem identified in an existing process. For example, there may be a concern about patients at your facility losing too much weight, or you are getting reports from the nursing team that they have found an abundance of unconsumed nutrition supplements in patient rooms. The first step in solving any problem is to clearly identify the problem. For example, you need to know the number of patients losing weight or the average number of unconsumed supplements found in patient rooms to define the scale or scope of the suspected problem. After gathering baseline data of this type, you may discover that there is no actual problem. More often, you find there is indeed a problem, and you need to evaluate the extent of the problem and state the goal you hope to achieve with the project.

A fundamental step in any process improvement project is determining the scope of the problem. Tools and techniques can help identify the problem, create buy-in among stakeholders, and promote consistent implementation of a new process. Key tools and techniques are discussed in the following paragraphs.

Benchmarking

Benchmarking is the process of comparing yourself to other organizations or to reference standards. Benchmarking enables you to set a target or goal for the process you are trying to improve and provides helpful guidance when determining the effectiveness of your improvement strategies. Benchmarking involves asking effective questions, such as the ones in Box 13.4.[11]

BOX 13.4 Effective Benchmarking Questions[11]

» What are we doing now?

» How well are we doing?

» What measurements determine how well we are doing?

» Why do we want to improve? What is our motivation?

» Are we using evidence-based practices?

» What are other organizations doing?

» How do we compare to other, similar organizations?

Benchmarking can be done at the national, state, or regional level; because benchmarking data are not always available, you may need to be flexible in sourcing them at a different level. Occasionally you may not have specific data elements available, in which case you need to rely on best practices. Research what exemplary organizations are doing and consider their processes as models. Utilize evidence-based research whenever it is available. Using our previous example of a trend of weight loss among patients at your facility, benchmarking could include a comparison of the average amount of weight lost in your patient population to the average amount of weight lost among patients in similar facilities, as recorded in state or national databases.

If you are unable to find benchmarks for comparison, consider the results that may be obtained through a successful intervention. Be realistic and set a goal that can be achieved if your intervention works, but not one so modest as to be inconsequential to patients. For example, if 65% of patients in your facility are experiencing weight loss, a reasonable goal might be to develop interventions so that only 40% of patients experience weight loss.

Stakeholder Analysis

A stakeholder is any person, group, team, or internal or external customers affected by your product or service. Internal customers include those with whom you work, colleagues in different departments, and departments that support your work. External customers include patients, families, visitors, suppliers, health care regulators, and auditors. Stakeholders can provide valuable input when identifying and defining the problem. When starting a project, always assess the needs of your stakeholders; never assume you already know what their needs are.[10]

A stakeholder analysis compares how much vested interest a stakeholder might have in a situation and enables you to plan the type and amount of communication they will require throughout the initiative. The first step in identifying stakeholders is to list all people touched or influenced by your project or process. This list should include names and titles of specific individuals. You will use this information when you start analyzing performance and then again when you begin to develop your communication plan.

Gathering Customer Voices

Once you have identified your customers in the stakeholder analysis, it is important to consider what your customers expect from your product, service, or process. Gathering voices of your customers captures their requirements and confirms their expectations.[12] This feedback helps you determine what is critical to quality: things that customers see as nonnegotiable and believe they cannot do without. One simple way to discover this information is to gather feedback from your internal and external customers through online or printed surveys, focus groups, comment cards, or one-on-one meetings in which you ask for feedback directly (eg, "In your opinion, how could we improve?"). In our example of patients losing weight, ask your nursing staff whether they are concerned and what they believe they need to help prevent this unwanted weight loss. Similarly, ask the medical team what they think might be contributing to this trend. Ask your food suppliers and other vendors for their input, as appropriate; perhaps they have valuable insight into trends they are seeing across the industry.

Process Improvement Step 2: Measure Current Performance

A successful process improvement project starts with measuring current process performance by collecting as much baseline data as possible. Current performance is measured to identify improvement opportunities and, once improvements have been implemented, to evaluate whether these changes have in fact improved the process. Health care organizations measure quality, productivity, efficacy, customer satisfaction, and cost-effectiveness. Performance quality and efficiency can be measured using standards called metrics. Common metrics used in health care include (but are not limited to) the following[9]:

> patient satisfaction data

> defect or error rates

> timeliness

> cycle time (time from the beginning to the end of a process)

> cost per unit

> waste

> environmental effects

> efficiency

> labor hours

> success rates

> safety risk

> volume

For each metric listed, there are different types of data you can collect. Historical data are data that were already collected in some capacity. Historical data can be collated and used as premeasures. Historical data are not always available, but when they are, they can be very valuable, saving you substantial time and providing insights on past trends. If it is not already available in a report, you may need to work with the information technology (IT) department to generate one. IT departments are generally busy places, so build realistic expectations into your projected timeline.

If historical data are not available, you will need to collect data manually and prospectively to serve as baseline data. The advantage to this is that you can collect the data you need and utilize a format you prefer. This can be time-consuming, but it is important to understand your current performance before you attempt to make improvements. One of the biggest mistakes seen in process improvement is stating that there is a problem without having data to support that claim. For example, you may perceive that there is an increase in the number of patients with weight loss in your organization, but once you actually gather and analyze the data, you may discover that the facts do not support your perception.

When gathering baseline data to determine if a problem exists, a sample size must be determined. Sampling in quality improvement work differs from research settings due to the variable nature of the population and the dynamic nature of the typical health care environment where many factors are uncontrolled. Since data collection involves staff time and resources, Perla and colleagues[13] recommend considering the following factors when determining the sample size for quality improvement work:

> the team's degree of belief that the change will result in improvement

> the costs associated with a failed test

> the readiness of those who have to make the change

Ways to Display Current Performance Data

After collecting and organizing data, the next step is to display them in a manner that makes them easy to read—highlighting similarities, disparities, trends, and other relationships (or the lack thereof) in the data set. These visual representations of data can then be used to compare metrics from before and after the implementation phase to determine whether an improvement was made. Some of the most common ways of displaying data are discussed in the following paragraphs.

Bar Graphs

A bar graph can be used to display and compare data in a manner that is easy to read and understand. In a bar graph, data categories are represented by bars of different colors or patterns. Bar graphs are used for nominal data. Nominal data is used for naming or labeling variables without any quantitative value; these variables are categorical in nature (eg, days of the week). A sample bar graph is provided in Figure 13.1.

FIGURE 13.1 Sample bar graph

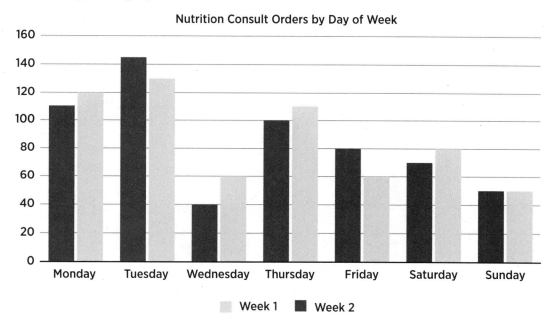

Histograms

Histograms provide a graphic representation that organizes a group of data points into specified ranges. Histograms are similar in appearance to bar graphs, but they condense a data series into an easily interpreted visual by taking many data points and grouping them together into ranges. On a histogram, the x-axis represents the range or group, and the y-axis represents the number count or percentage of occurrences for each group. A histogram displays a frequency distribution of the variable in question. Figure 13.2 shows a sample histogram of the age distribution of patient admissions into the emergency department of a hospital on a specific date; the age group is on the x-axis, and the number of patients in each group is found on the y-axis.

FIGURE 13.2 Sample histogram

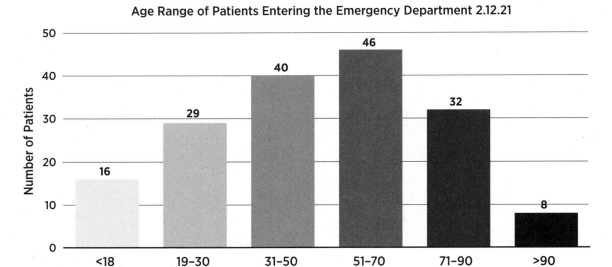

Age Range of Patients Entering the Emergency Department 2.12.21

Trend Charts

A trend chart, also called a run chart, shows data over time. This is a linear graph that allows you to track improvements by displaying data in a time sequence, usually over months. Time is generally displayed on the horizontal x-axis and the measure you are tracking is displayed on the vertical y-axis. A trend chart is a good way to evaluate at what point in time a process changed. Knowing this point in time subsequently enables you to determine whether improvement is actually taking place.[14] Figure 13.3 shows a sample trend chart tracking nursing home resident weight loss.

FIGURE 13.3 Sample trend chart

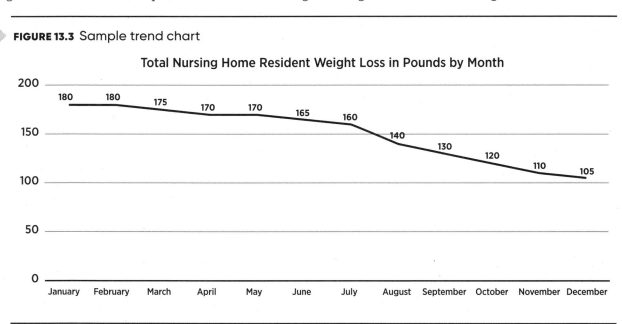

Total Nursing Home Resident Weight Loss in Pounds by Month

Pareto Charts

Pareto charts are used to help focus improvement efforts. They display the 80/20 rule (also known as the Pareto principle, which states that 80% of consequences result from 20% of causes).[15] Examples of the 80/20 rule are that 20% of criminals commit 80% of crimes, 20% of employees are responsible for 80% of the results, and 20% of the workplace hazards result in 80% of workplace injuries. To create a Pareto chart, data are organized into categories or classifications. Categories are ordered along the horizontal x-axis from those most frequently occurring to those least frequently occurring. Pareto charts are most useful when charting 50 or more data points, and they provide clues on where to direct your energy (namely, on the most important 20%). A Pareto chart is helpful when the process you are investigating produces data that are broken down into categories and you can count the number of times a measured event occurs in each category.[15] For example, if you are concerned about the overall quality of the food served in your facility, you survey your customers and find that 75% of those surveyed say that the food temperature is poor, and 20% state that there is not enough variety on the menu. Where would you start your improvements? By addressing the problem of food temperature first, you will address a variable that 75% of your customers think is a problem—as opposed to the 20% of customers who would like a greater variety of foods on the menu. Figure 13.4 shows a Pareto chart comparing diagnoses responsible for hospital readmissions.

FIGURE 13.4 Sample Pareto chart

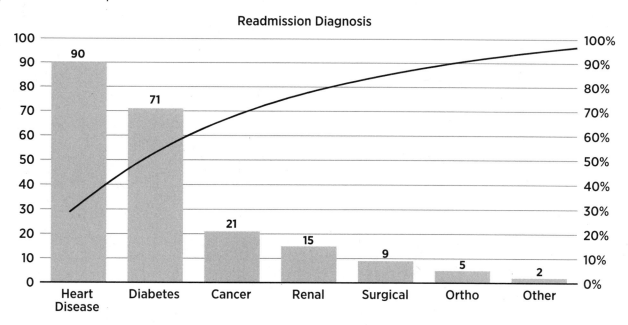

Pie Charts

Pie charts, also referred to as circle charts or circle graphs, represent data in a circular form resembling a pie. The graph is divided into labeled sections to visualize both absolute amounts or occurrences and relative proportions of the amount or frequency of data in each of the graph's sections. The sections of a pie chart are not only labeled (with numbers or percentages) but also color coded, which adds to their ease of use for readers. Pie charts are helpful when you need to compare groups of data quickly, as readers can easily compare the data to see how large each "slice" of data is and how these slices compare to the others in the chart. Familiar uses of pie charts include illustrating the distribution mix in an investment portfolio, results of public-opinion surveys, and a wide variety of demographic statistics. Figure 13.5 provides a sample pie chart illustrating the number and types of nutritional supplements ordered for patients in an intensive care unit during a 1-month period.

FIGURE 13.5 Sample pie chart

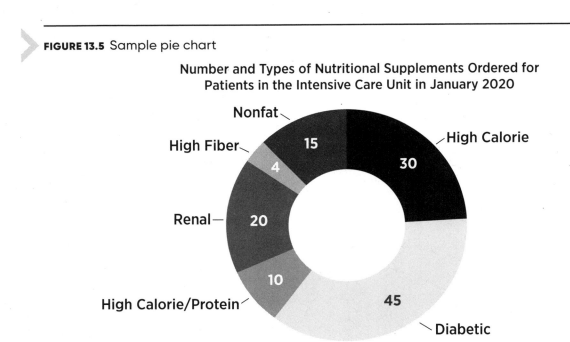

Number and Types of Nutritional Supplements Ordered for Patients in the Intensive Care Unit in January 2020

Process Improvement Step 3: Assess and Determine How Best to Improve the Process

Once a potential problem is identified, a systematic approach to analyzing data helps the team understand the reasons for process variation and poor performance and identify the root cause or causes of the issues and the systems involved. It is essential that the root causes identified are substantiated by the data collected in step 2. Some of the common tools used in this process are discussed in this section. No matter which tool is utilized, it is helpful to gather input from the members of the team in a process called brainstorming.

Brainstorming

Brainstorming is a valuable technique for generating ideas about potential causes of or solutions to a problem. It fosters creative thinking, incites enthusiasm, and allows transparency among team members through the open sharing of ideas. Brainstorming can be structured, unstructured, or even silent. The most commonly used of these is structured brainstorming, in which a problem is proposed to a group and each participant takes a turn identifying one thing that could be contributing to the problem. This gives everyone on the team a chance to share their ideas. A team member can skip their turn, but the facilitator continues the process until no further ideas are generated. All ideas are posted for the group to see, and then each idea is considered.[16,17]

In unstructured brainstorming, group members call out ideas as they think of them. This affords people the freedom to state what they would like to say without having to wait their turn. This approach to brainstorming allows people to share their frank opinions about what might be causing a problem, but it can also deter more introverted members of the team or those who prefer to take more time to consider their ideas before sharing them—especially in an animated group setting. If you use unstructured brainstorming, let the team know at the outset that you value everyone's ideas, whether they are shared during the brainstorming session or shortly after it.

In silent brainstorming, the facilitator asks each participant to take a few minutes to write down as many issues they can and then pass their lists to the facilitator. This allows participants to anonymously voice their opinions without the risk of being criticized by others.

It is important for the facilitator of a brainstorming session to promote open-mindedness and make it clear to participants that there are no wrong answers.

Regardless of which brainstorming technique you use, the more input you receive, the more valuable the brainstorming session is.

Tools for Process Assessment and Mapping

Value Stream Map or Flow Chart

Value stream mapping (VSM) is a method for documenting and analyzing the state or flow of a process. A value stream map, also called a flow chart, is a visual tool that displays all critical steps in a specific process from beginning to end and quantifies the time, materials, and information used at each step.[16]

There are two kinds of VSMs: current state and future state. The current-state VSM is used to determine what the process currently looks like, and the future-state VSM focuses on what the process will (ideally) look like after process improvements have been made. The current-state VSM must be created before the future-state VSM.

The VSM process requires input from everyone involved. Stakeholders must agree on an acceptable way of describing the current process taking place. Details are discussed and opportunities for improvement come into focus. These details are captured as opportunities to be evaluated when developing a future-state VSM. VSM allows the team to visualize the entire flow of the process and shows the linkage between the information gathered and material flow.[12] For example, a VSM can identify sources of waste in a process; this information will prove valuable when revising or recreating the process. Figure 13.6 provides a sample VSM illustrating the role of RDNs in the Nutrition Care Process.

FIGURE 13.6 Sample value stream map or flowchart illustrating the role of registered dietitians in the Nutrition Care Process

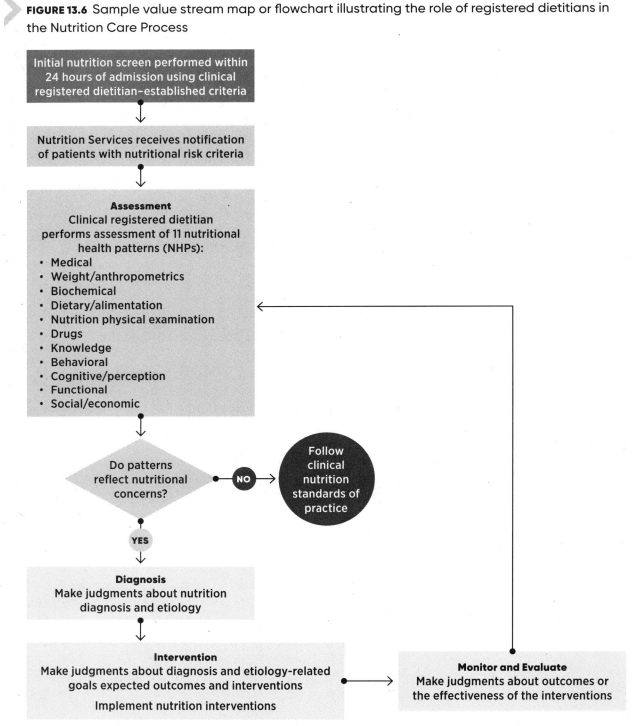

Reproduced with permission from Hakel-Smith N. Quality management and improvement. In: Grim J, Roberts S, eds. *The Clinical Nutrition Manager's Handbook*. Academy of Nutrition and Dietetics; 2014:111.

Affinity Diagram

The affinity diagram is a project management tool for organizing ideas and data. The name was devised by Jiro Kawakita in the 1960s and is sometimes referred to as the K-J method. The benefit of this tool is that it allows large numbers of ideas stemming from brainstorming to be sorted into groups, based on their commonalities.[18,19]

An affinity diagram is a great tool to use when starting to identify possible issues, challenges, or opportunities around an identified problem. For example, perhaps a foodservice department receives poor satisfaction scores on a recent survey; there could be many factors contributing to this (see Figure 13.7 for an example affinity diagram on this topic). In a brainstorming session, team members can take time to think about and write down all the possible reasons they feel food satisfaction scores might have declined. The ideas can then be grouped into categories. Some categories are likely to have more ideas than others, which can help a team know where to begin improving the process. The brainstorming process identifies the issues, and the affinity diagram helps sort these issues into categories.

The affinity diagram process follows these common steps:

1. Present the topic or define the problem clearly to the team.

2. Give the team index cards or sticky notes.

3. Ask the team to write an idea or issue on each card or sticky note.

4. Collect the ideas or issues and read them to the team as you post them on the wall.

5. Lead the team in sorting the ideas or issues into categories. If there are duplicates of an idea, group them together rather than tossing out the duplicates.

6. Lead the team in labeling each category of cards. You should end up with the ideas grouped together into categories.

7. To complete your affinity diagram, draw arrows between the categories you've identified, indicating all notable relationships (affinities) between them.

Once the affinity diagram is complete, the team should have a better understanding of the causes of the problem, which will guide their discussion of the most effective, targeted solutions.

FIGURE 13.7 Sample affinity diagram

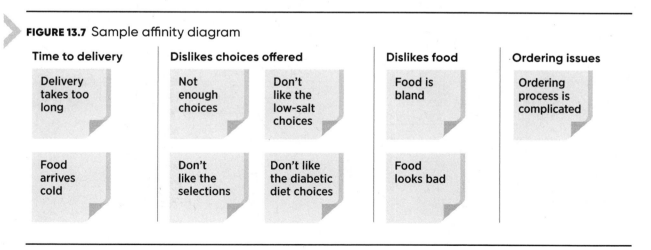

Fishbone Diagram

The fishbone diagram is also known as a cause-and-effect diagram or an Ishikawa diagram (after Kaoru Ishikawa who created the tool for quality control purposes). The fishbone diagram identifies many possible causes for a specific effect or problem. It can be used to structure a brainstorming session while at the same time sorting ideas into useful categories.[20]

The fishbone diagram process commonly follows these steps[20]:

1. Agree on a problem statement. Write the problem in the "head" of the fishbone.

2. Brainstorm the major categories of causes of the problem. If this is difficult, use generic headings such as Methods, Machines, People, Materials, Measurement, or Environment.

3. Write the categories as headers in the fishbone diagram. These categories should all relate to the primary problem.

4. Brainstorm all the possible causes of the problem under each category. For example, in our patient weight loss example, the problem is "average weight loss is up 10% in the geriatric population over the past 6 months." Ask, "Why does this happen?" As each idea is given, write it on a "bone" under the appropriate category header. Note that causes can be written in several places if they relate to several categories.

5. When the group runs out of ideas, focus attention on fleshing out places on the chart where ideas are few.

This process guides the team in discussing how to solve the issues contributing to the problem. As these issues are resolved, the problem identified should begin to improve.[20] Figure 13.8 shows an example of a fishbone diagram used to assess enteral feedings in the intensive care unit.

FIGURE 13.8 Sample fishbone (cause-and-effect) diagram

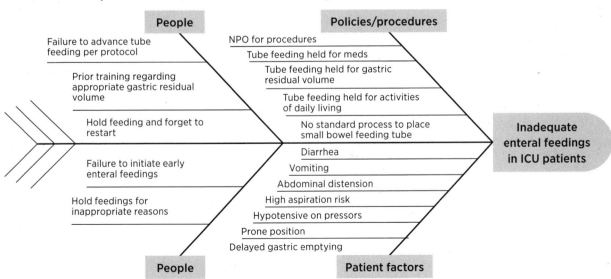

Abbreviations: NPO = nil per os (nothing by mouth) | ICU = intensive care unit

Reprinted with permission from Roberts S, Grim J. ICU Enteral Feedings. ABC Baylor Quality Improvement Presentation. Baylor Health Care System; 2009.

Five Whys Analysis

A Five Whys analysis is a tool you can use to explore cause-and-effect relationships underlying a particular problem. The goal is to determine the root causes of a problem by repeating the question "Why?" five (or more) times in response to explanations for a problem. This method was pioneered by Sakichi Toyoda to improve Toyota's automotive manufacturing processes and has since been adapted for use in many diverse settings. The Five Whys analysis can be very useful in tracking down an elusive root cause of a problem or when there may be multiple root causes.[21] For example, if the intensive care unit continues to have problems with the availability of enteral feeding formula on the unit, it may be due to insufficient storage availability on the unit, the frequency with which the stock levels are replenished, or even removal of unused formula. Asking the question "Why?" helps you zero in on different possibilities for a problem.

Not all problems have a single root cause. To uncover multiple root causes, the method must be repeated each time. The method provides no set rules about what lines of questions to explore or how long to continue the search for additional root causes. Thus, even when the method is closely followed, the outcome still depends upon the knowledge and persistence of the people involved.

The Stories From the Field box provides an example of the Five Whys process.

STORIES FROM THE FIELD: Wasted Tube Feeding Product

A foodservice department had a problem with expired tube feeding products on the shelf. This issue was costing the department more than $500 in waste each month. The team used the Five Whys tool as follows:

1. *Why* is there expired tube feeding product on the shelf?
   A: It is not used before the expired date.

2. *Why* is it not being used before the expiration date?
   A: Too much product is ordered.

3. *Why* is too much product ordered?
   A: Because the standard weekly order is five cases.

4. *Why* is the standard amount—five cases—ordered each week?
   A: Because that's what we've always done, and nobody checks inventory before placing the order.

5. *Why* is there not a process in place to check inventory prior to ordering new inventory?
   A: We don't know.

The team identified the root cause of the problem, the solution was clear and, in this case, simple: create a process for checking inventory prior to ordering new product.

Process Improvement Step 4: Implement a New or Changed Process

After identifying a problem, brainstorming, and assessing data, it is now time to make improvements to the process or create a new process. One way to do this is to go back to your current-state VSM and map out the new process using future-state VSM. The team can refer to the current-state VSM created during the baseline analysis phase and modify it as needed.

This is the team's chance to think big. What would the improved process look like in an ideal world? What staffing, resources, tools, and support would you need to drive the process to success? Imagine what is possible, what you *can* do, and what you might be able to do in that ideal world. Then, identify any barriers that threaten your ability to realize that ideal and consider opportunities that exist for overcoming them or working around them. Follow the steps discussed earlier in the process, but this time map out what the *new* process flow will look like. Brainstorming is again a useful process at this stage because it can generate innovative new ideas.

Once you map out a future state, your next step is to list all action items needed to implement the new process.[22] Create an implementation plan and a communication plan, revise your description of standard work, complete a mistake-proofing process, provide training in the new process, and run a pilot test, all before the official launch. Let's look at each step individually.

Implementation Plan

An implementation plan is a step-by-step action plan that outlines what tasks need to be completed to get to the future state. It outlines the who, what, and when of various tasks that need to be accomplished.[23] The question, "Who is going to do what, and when should it be completed?" helps guide the team through all the steps needed to implement the new process and keeps the team on task. When completing the plan, it is important to make deadlines realistic based on the resources you have available. This is a great time to set SMART (specific, measurable, achievable, relevant, and time bound) goals.

Communication Plan

The communication plan is similar to the implementation plan in that it outlines who, what, and when communication to stakeholders needs to occur.[24] To accomplish this, take the stakeholder analysis you developed at the beginning of the project and think about the best ways to communicate to each stakeholder group on the list. You will almost certainly need to communicate to different groups of people in different ways. The stakeholder analysis can also be used to determine the level of communication you need to provide to each stakeholder. People who will be deeply involved with the new process will need training on carrying it out efficiently and effectively. In contrast, people with little to no direct contact with the new process might simply need to be informed that the change will occur. *It is better to communicate too much than too little.* Also, just because you think you have communicated does not mean the stakeholder received the information. You should confirm that all stakeholders are aware of changes and the associated actions they need to take. If you identify a group of stakeholders as well as their needs and concerns and consider their input into the new process, you will have the most successful results.

Standard Work

Standard work (also known as standard operating procedures) should be used to encourage process standardization. Once a new process is established, standardize it by documenting the steps in a policy, protocol, or procedure. It can also be helpful to create graphics (like the ones discussed earlier in this chapter) to serve as visual guides. All of these will help reinforce the standard work.

Standardizing work will ensure that team members are clear about the work they need to do. There are many benefits to using standard work, including establishing consistency, maintaining efficiency, standardizing training, and establishing clear roles and responsibilities on teams. Ultimately, standard work ensures customer needs are met in a consistent way. Standard work should be clearly documented, so the process does not rely on one person or a few individuals, but rather enables others to follow the same process.

Unless standard work is properly documented, it lives only in the minds of the people who participated in the change process. Standard work is very effective in both training and monitoring new processes. As turnover occurs in an organization, new employees will be trained to do things in whatever way the person training the new employee does them. This may not always be the correct or most efficient way. Without standardization, processes will naturally change over time. Often in process improvement projects, the root cause of the problem is that the original process is not being followed as it was established.[25]

Mistake Proofing

Mistake proofing is the ideal way to assure standardizing. This technique makes it much more difficult, or even impossible, to make a mistake.[11,25,26] For example, when designing a new electronic form, setting up fields that must be filled in order to advance to the next field is a common form of mistake proofing. With "go/no-go" situations like this, you are assured all fields will be filled before the electronic form can be submitted. Whenever possible, build in an ability for the program to identify the designated value or range of values to be input in any given field. If anything other than the specific value or range of values is indicated—including an absence of any input at all—a message pops up prompting the user to add, verify, or adjust the information before continuing. In Microsoft Excel, the mistake-proofing function is called *data validation*. Mistake proofing limits the variation of acceptable responses, which is exactly what is needed in many (but not all) situations. In some cases, this type of electronic support is not available, and then it is critical to include clear, detailed instructions during the training process and in any training materials to reduce mistakes.

Training

Effective training on any new process is imperative. An effective training plan focuses on the direct needs of the audience and explains why the change is needed and how it will benefit the person being trained. The first thought many people have when asked to change is, "What's in it for me?" Anyone you are asking to comply with a process change should be provided with training that includes not only *how* to make the change, but *why* (for example, information about how the change will save them time, money, errors, effort, or other resources). It is best to have interactive training in which the employee can gain hands-on practice in the new skill under the supervision of a trainer. This type of training can reinforce buy-in among the people making the change, which in turn bolsters the likelihood the change will be implemented correctly and consistently and ultimately be successful. Effective training provides certainty to the employee, which increases satisfaction and improves morale in the workplace. It also leads to more positive attitudes toward the changes implemented.[27]

Pilot Test

A pilot test is a preliminary trial of a process improvement prior to full-scale implementation. A pilot test should be built into your timeline for launching the project. Pilot tests allow you to test the performance of solutions in a controlled environment to identify any adjustments that might be needed prior to rolling out the change to the full cadre of users.[28] One of the great things about piloting a solution is that it also provides timely feedback and decreases the risk of failure. Pilot testing is not always an option, as some projects require immediate implementation at full scale. For example, if a form is changed in the medical record, it may not be possible to pilot the form on one unit but not another unit; all units may need to start using the new form simultaneously. Although a pilot test is the optimal time to provide training as well as troubleshoot it, if you are unable to pilot test a process, all users should still be trained prior to launching the project.

Project Launch

Once a pilot test is complete (if applicable) and any changes to the process have been addressed, it is time to go live with the project improvement strategy. This is where the communication plan is key. Be sure you *over*communicate what changes have been made, why they have been made, and where users should turn for answers when questions inevitably arise. As you launch a project, assign team members involved with its development to assist in the implementation. Team members may not be actively participating in the new process; however, during the launch period, they should be monitoring how the process is going and what further changes might need to be made.

Process Improvement Step 5: Measure and Sustain the Success of the New Process

The fifth step of this process is maintenance, which involves keeping momentum high, sustaining the changes, and measuring the success of the new process.

You must continue to monitor outcomes to measure and sustain the success of any project. It is only by monitoring the results of your project over time that you will know whether the change has persisted or if employees have reverted to the earlier way of doing things. To determine how to monitor your project's success, start by asking yourself the following questions[29]:

> What measurable outcome or outcomes need to be monitored?

> How will you monitor the outcome or outcomes?

> Who will be responsible for tracking these data?

> How frequently will you monitor outcomes?

> How long will you continue to monitor outcomes (6 months, 12 months, 24 months, etc)?

> Who needs to be kept informed of the results?

> Who is responsible for keeping the process functioning properly?

> What will be done if the monitoring detects a condition that could create a defect or cause the output to fall outside of the target range?

> Where will your plan documentation, including the monitoring plan, reside?

Monitoring and sustaining success can be a challenge with many projects, but it is essential that you continue to require and reinforce standardization, accountability, and compliance with the new process. In time, especially without monitoring and reinforcing use of the new process, things often slip back to the old ways of doing things, or the new process gets interpreted and modified by individual users. Add to this the fact that every organization's staff changes over time. Your change process must include a plan for sustaining the new process through these and similar, predictable circumstances.

The data measured during the baseline problem analysis should be remeasured in this stage to determine whether the original problem has improved as a result of the interventions implemented. New processes and work throughout the project may inform new metrics that should be followed and reported, but at a minimum, the original baseline data metrics should be collected again and reassessed. One way to track these metrics is with a dashboard.

Dashboard

A dashboard is a system to track key performance indicators within an organization. Dashboards are designed to be simple to read and understand, providing quick indications of which things are going well and which are experiencing problems that need to be addressed. A dashboard should include short-term indicators to ensure milestones and outcome measures reflect whether goals are being met. A dashboard may include simple test documents, data spreadsheets, or sophisticated graphs. Data results are reported for multiple time periods to show trends over time and include benchmarks or goals to summarize performance. A dashboard needs to be easy to read and show the desired target outcomes of the improvement process.

There are several ways to display your data with a dashboard. Determine what type of dashboard you are creating and its purpose. For example, if you are implementing a change to the process of patient meal tray delivery, you would design a dashboard highlighting the key metrics, such as elapsed time between placing and receiving the order, patients' reported satisfaction with food temperature, and percentage of tray items consumed. These same data could be presented in a simple table or a sophisticated visual graphic, depending on the resources and expertise available. Establish the principal measures to include in the dashboard. What metrics are most important? Develop a routine plan (weekly, monthly, quarterly, etc) for data collection and reporting. Remember, your data are a living tool that will evolve over time—and so should your dashboard. If indicators are no longer useful, they may need to be removed or replaced with something more pertinent to your stakeholders.[30] Box 13.5 shows an example dashboard tracking completion of nutrition assessments.

BOX 13.5 Nutrition Assessment Completion Dashboard

Performance measure	Target	Quarter 1	Quarter 2	Quarter 3	Quarter 4
Percentage of nutrition assessments completed within 24 hours	>90%	78%	84%	89%	92%
Percentage of patients with completed admission weight	>90%	65%	72%	84%	89%

Recognize Your Team

Although you have completed the five steps of process improvement, you still have one important activity: recognizing your team for all the time, effort, and care they put into the project. Along with celebrating outcomes, don't forget to celebrate your team! There are countless ways to recognize a team's efforts, depending on your team and your budget. Some simple ideas include the following:

> sending a personalized, handwritten note of thanks to each team member;

> publishing recognition of the project and its successful implementation in a newsletter or on your organization's intranet site;

> posting a story board in a public area, such as the lobby, break room, or cafeteria;

> holding a final team meeting to review outcomes and recognize and celebrate with team members; and

> inviting your organization's leadership to join you in a meeting or small event recognizing the team's work.

If your budget allows, refreshments are always welcome and help an event feel celebratory.

Process Improvement Methodologies

Although there are many tools and methods for process improvement, all are designed to help us improve not only the speed of our work but also its quality while simultaneously meeting customers' needs. The methods discussed in this chapter follow the principles and key steps we have discussed: identifying and defining the problem, measuring current performance, assessing and determining how best to improve the process, implementing a new or changed process, and measuring and sustaining the success of the new process.

When selecting a methodology, first investigate if a standard one is utilized within your organization and, if not, familiarize yourself with a few alternatives and pick the one you think will work best. Two of the most widely used models are Plan, Do, Study, Act and Lean Six Sigma.

Plan, Do, Study, Act

Plan, do, study, act (PDSA) is one of the most widely recognized models for process improvement. The PDSA model continuously cycles through four phases for ongoing process refinement and improvement (see Figure 13.9).[6,29,31]

Plan In this first phase, time is taken to state the objectives of the project, determine necessary improvements, design a process change to achieve the improved objectives, and develop a plan to implement the change. It is important in this phase to identify what metrics will be used to determine whether objectives have been met. Tools that may be used in this phase include benchmarking, customer feedback (sometimes called voice of the customer or VOC), and stakeholder analysis.

Do In the second phase, changes are implemented on a small scale, such as a pilot project in several nursing units. Smaller-scale implementation allows time to identify early problems or unexpected challenges.

Study Once the new process is implemented, the third step is to gather and analyze the data to determine whether the changes were effective. The metrics identified in the plan phase of the project will help determine whether or not improvement has occurred. If the implementation led to successful results, you can move onto the next phase, but if the study indicates objectives were not met, going back to the plan phase to reevaluate the process will help determine what changes are needed.

Act If the study phase results determine that the changes were effective, the project can be implemented on a larger scale in the act phase. To monitor how well the process is working, remeasure the metrics identified at the beginning of the project.

FIGURE 13.9 The plan, do, study, act model for improvement

- Identify the current problem and determine root cause(s) using cause-and-effect theory.
- Formulate a plan to implement change.
- Agree on metrics to measure for success.

- Adopt process if working well.
- Adjust process if changes are needed.
- Abort project and begin work on new solutions if process not effective.

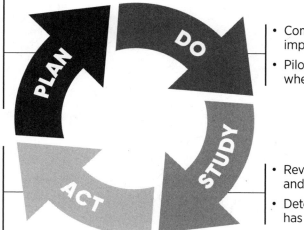

- Communicate and implement the plan.
- Pilot change(s) when possible.

- Review, measure, and analyze results.
- Determine if goal has been met.

Rapid-Cycle Improvement

The rapid-cycle improvement (RCI) model is an accelerated form of the PDSA method and is designed to improve a process in a short amount of time. It supports rapidly repeated, incremental improvements in a practice to optimize performance.[32] Ideas are trialed and evaluated for success. If they are not successful, a new plan is trialed and evaluated. This continues until the ideal process is identified. This process is often used when there are not a lot of resources or costs needed for implementation of the interventions that are trialed.

Lean Six Sigma

Lean Six Sigma, which is an offshoot of the original Six Sigma management model, has been used in health care since the early 2000s. Like its predecessor, Lean Six Sigma focuses on reducing eight different types of organizational waste (identified next).[11]

Lean Six Sigma consists of two different ways of making process improvements to reduce waste. "Lean" tools focus on reducing the time and number of steps it takes to deliver our service to the customer, and "Six Sigma" tools focus on delivering the best quality service possible. This model asserts that project selection is directly tied to business results, and the process of project selection focuses on internal and external customers as well as coworkers. Lean Six Sigma projects are managed by cross-functional teams in which members learn about processes in other departments; improvements made need to be acceptable to all areas. As in all models, projects and team leaders need to be supported by engaged leadership to be successful.[11]

Lean Six Sigma uses the define, measure, analyze, improve, control (DMAIC) roadmap as a tool for process improvement. In Box 13.6, these steps are defined for the identified problem of long wait times in a health care setting.[11,23]

BOX 13.6 Sample Define, Measure, Analyze, Improve, Control Roadmap[11,23]

Define	Patient wait times are too long
Measure	Gather data on actual wait times (registration times, laboratory times, provider times, checkout times)
Analyze	Determine key reasons for wait times (duplicate forms, unclear roles, too many handoffs)
Improve	Make process changes (eliminate duplicate forms, remove unnecessary steps, define responsibilities)
Control	Monitor to ensure shorter wait times (create and update a chart of improvement or results)

Eight Types of Waste

As mentioned earlier, Lean Six Sigma relies on removing as much waste as possible from processes while still meeting customers' needs. The eight types of waste defined in this model are as follows, and can be remembered more easily by recognizing the acronym DOWNTIME[33,34]:

> **Defects:** work containing errors, needing rework, or lacking something necessary

> **Overproduction:** producing more than the customer or patient needs right now

> **Waiting:** idle time created when material, information, people, or equipment is not ready

> **Nonutilized talent:** employees' skills not being fully appreciated or utilized

> **Transportation:** transport of patients, medications, supplies, or information that doesn't add value

> **Inventory:** keeping on hand more materials, medications, and products than are required

> **Motion:** movement of people, products, or supplies that does not add value

> **Excess processing:** extra effort or activities that add no value from the customer or patient's perspective; using complex solutions when you should be using simple ones

Using the DOWNTIME tool to evaluate a workflow or area of operation can identify and help to eliminate waste.[34]

Kaizen

Kaizen is a Japanese concept that, when applied to a business or organization, refers to a continuous effort to improve processes, services, and products. In Lean Six Sigma, *kaizen* is used to refer to a short-term project aimed at improving a particular process, usually involving a small group of people directly involved with the problem.[35]

5S

5S is also a tool of lean management. It is built around five Japanese words associated with a clean, safe, productive, and efficient workplace, which are the goals of 5S. In English, the words *sort*, *set* (set in order), *shine*, *standardize*, and *sustain* are used.[36] The idea behind this tool is similar to the adage of home decluttering: "a place for everything, and everything in its place." Consider an example of 5S in the diet office. A diet office was struggling when it went from using paper menus to electronic menus. Specifically, the team was worried about removing the inventory of paper menus "just in case" they needed to revert back to using them. The team got together and decided it was time to do something different. They first separated all the items that were needed for the new process from the old process. They then filed what was essential to save from the old process. Instead of piles of paper menus, one copy of each menu was saved. A few samples of the paper forms used for menu tallies, supplement use, and diet changes were also filed away. The diet office increased its open workspace and reduced unused materials in addition to encouraging team members to commit to the new electronic process.

Resources for Quality and Process Improvement

Quality management and process improvement are expanding, complex, and critically important in health care. Fortunately, there are many respected organizations that provide reliable information to support our work in the areas discussed below.

National Association for Healthcare Quality

Founded in 1976, the National Association for Healthcare Quality (NAHQ) is the only organization dedicated to health care quality professionals, defining the standard of excellence for the profession and equipping professionals and organizations across the continuum of health care to meet these standards. NAHQ offers the only accredited certification in health care quality, extensive educational programming, networking opportunities, and career resources to help members meet the challenges they face and demonstrate their value. This is an excellent organization where nutrition leaders can find guidance and tools for process improvement projects.[35]

National Quality Forum

Measures endorsed by the National Quality Forum (NQF) are considered the gold standard for health care measurement in the United States. Expert committees of various stakeholders (patients, providers, and payers) evaluate measures for NQF endorsement. The federal government and many private-sector entities use and trust NQF-endorsed measures above all others because of the rigor and consensus process behind them. NQF provides information, tools, events, and reports to help health care professionals make informed decisions and continuous changes in the field.[37]

Centers for Medicare & Medicaid Services

The Centers for Medicare & Medicaid Services (CMS) has developed a number of quality improvement initiatives, establishing standardized quality measures to evaluate and compare hospitals and other health care facilities. A portion of CMS reimbursements to facilities is based on how their performance meets this set of quality measures. A key component of this program is the the Hospital Consumer Assessment of Healthcare Providers and Systems (HCAHPS) survey, which measures patient experience of care. In 2017, CMS launched a comprehensive initiative (Meaningful Measures), which identifies priority areas for quality measurement and improvement with a goal of improving outcomes for patients, their families, and providers while also reducing burden on clinicians and providers.[38]

National Academy of Medicine

The National Academy of Medicine (NAM) is an independent, nonprofit, nongovernmental organization providing unbiased, authoritative advice to decision makers in health care and the public. NAM is driving quality by educating health care professionals on ways to improve their health care systems.[39]

The Joint Commission

The Joint Commission (TJC) is one of the key accreditation organizations for health care facilities. Operationalized by TJC in 1999, the ORYX Performance Measurement Initiative is a standardized set of core performance measures, including quality improvement efforts, used in the accreditation process to evaluate the quality of health care delivery at facilities.[40]

Agency for Healthcare Research and Quality

The mission of the Agency for Healthcare Research and Quality (AHRQ) is to produce evidence to make health care safer; higher quality; and more accessible, equitable, and affordable. The AHRQ is a department of the US Department of Health and Human Services (HHS) and offers health care professionals a variety of research-based tools and information to make health care safer in all settings.[17]

Summary

Quality assurance and process improvement are critically important activities in health care today. As a nutrition leader, you are in a position to contribute knowledge and become a change agent for improvement. This chapter reviewed some of the many tools available in identifying and designing process improvements in the work setting. Many large organizations have a preferred quality improvement method; if this is the case in your institution, the food and nutrition department should use the preferred methodology. Regardless of the specific tool or methodology used, what matters most is that you follow the principles reviewed in this discussion. As we have seen by learning about various models, tools, and approaches to process improvement, the fundamentals remain constant.

REFERENCES

1   Institute of Medicine (US) Committee on Quality of Healthcare in America. *Crossing the Quality Chasm: A New Health System for the 21st Century.* National Academies Press; 2001.

2   AHRQ Agency for Healthcare Research and Quality. The National Quality Strategy: Fact Sheet. US Department of Health and Human Services website. November 2016. Accessed March 17, 2022. www.ahrq.gov/workingforquality/about/nqs-fact-sheets/nqs-fact-sheet-0214.html#:~:text =The%20National%20Quality%20Strategy%20%28NQS%29%20was%20first%20published,U.S. %20Department%20of%20Health%20and%20Human%20Services%20%28HHS%29

3   Berwick DM, Nolan TW, Whittington J. The triple aim: care, health, and cost. *Health Aff.* 2008;27(3):759-769.

4   Smith C. Understanding the change management curve. Change Management website. April 10, 2014. Accessed June 1, 2020. https://change.walkme.com/understanding-the-change -management-curve

5   McLaughlin DB, Olson JR. *2017 Healthcare Operations Management.* 3rd ed. Health Administration Press; 2017.

6   Agency for Healthcare Research and Quality. Health Literacy Universal Precautions Tool Kit, 2nd Edition: Plan, Do, Study, Act (PDSA) Directions and Examples. Updated September 2020. Agency for Healthcare Research and Quality website. Accessed April 6, 2022. www.ahrq.gov/health -literacy/improve/precautions/tool2b.html

7   Foster J. Differentiating quality improvement and research activities. *Clin Nurse Spec.* 2013;27(1):10-13. doi:10.1097/NUR.0b013e3182776db5

8   Creasy T. Why do improvement projects in healthcare fail? Becker's Hospital Review website. Accessed April 2, 2022. www.beckershospitalreview.com/hospital-management-administration /why-do-improvement-projects-in-healthcare-fail.html

9   Brock M. QI: Getting Inside Quality Improvement Mindset. National Center for Quality Assurance website. January 13, 2016. Accessed April 2, 2022. www.ncqa.org/blog/qi-insidemindset/

10 Weick KE, Sutcliffe KM. *Managing the Unexpected: Sustained Performance in a Complex World.* 3rd ed. Jossey-Bass; 2015.

11 de Koning H, Verver JP, van den Heuvel J, Bisgaard S, Does RJ. Lean Six Sigma in healthcare. *J Healthc Qual.* 2006;28(2):4-11.

12 Chassin MR, Loeb JM. The ongoing quality improvement journey: next stop, high reliability. *Health Aff.* 2011;30(4):559-568.

13 Perla RJ, Provost LP, Murray SK. Sampling considerations in healthcare improvement. *Qual Manage Health Care.* 2014;23(4):268-279. doi:10.1097/QMH.0000000000000042

14 Institute for Healthcare Improvement. Run chart tool. Accessed April 1, 2022. Institute for Healthcare Improvement website. www.ihi.org/resources/Pages/Tools/RunChart.aspx

15 Institute for Healthcare Improvement. Pareto chart. Institute for Healthcare Improvement website. Accessed April 2, 2022. www.ihi.org/resources/Pages/Tools/ParetoDiagram.aspx ?PostAuthRed=/resources/_layouts/download.aspx?SourceURL=/resources/Knowledge %20Center%20Assets/Tools%20-%20ParetoChart_a8d425fd-ac16-4197-be1a-5c27d1d23fbe /QIToolkit_ParetoChart.pdf

16 Institute for Healthcare Improvement. Improvement stories. Institute for Healthcare Improvement website. Accessed April 2, 2022. www.ihi.org/resources/Pages /ImprovementStories/SuccessfulMeasurementForImprovement.aspx

17 Brainwriting. Agency for Healthcare Research and Quality website. Accessed April 9,2022. www.ahrq.gov/cpi/index.html

18 Institute for Healthcare Improvement. Idea generation tools: brainstorming, affinity grouping, and multivoting. Institute for Healthcare Improvement website. Accessed April 9, 2022. www.ihi .org/resources/Pages/Tools/BrainstormingAffinityGroupingandMultivoting.aspx?

19 Use of an affinity diagram as a brainstorming tool. Six Sigma website. March 22, 2017. Accessed April 9, 2022. www.6sigma.us/six-sigma-articles/affinity-diagram-as-brainstorming-tool

20 Best M, Neuhauser D. Kaoru Ishikawa: from fishbones to world peace. *Qual Safe Health Care.* 2008;17(2):150–152.

21 Serrat O. The Five Whys technique. In: Serrat O. *Knowledge Solutions: Tools, Methods, and Approaches to Drive Organizational Performance.* Springer; 2017:307–310.

22 Zidel TG. *Lean Done Right: Achieve and Maintain Reform in Your Healthcare Organization.* Health Administration Press; 2012.

23 American Society for Quality. The define, measure, analyze, improve, control (DMAIC) process. American Society for Quality. Accessed April 7, 2022. https://asq.org/quality-resources/dmaic

24 Agency for Healthcare Research and Quality. Ways to approach the quality improvement process. Agency for Healthcare Research and Quality website. Accessed April 7, 2022. www.ahrq.gov/cahps /quality-improvement/improvement-guide/4-approach-qi-process/index.html

25 Hagan P. Waste not, want not: leading the lean health-care journey at Seattle Children's Hospital. *Glob Bus Org Exc.* 2011;30(3):25–31. doi: 10.1002/joe.20375

26 Bredal F. Using communications strategies to accelerate quality improvement. Institute for Healthcare Improvement website. November 19, 2019. Accessed April 5, 2022. www.ihi.org /communities/blogs/using-communications-strategies-to-accelerate-quality-improvement

27 Courtney F. Change management: 3 reasons why training supports organizational change. eLearning Industry website. 2016. Accessed April 9, 2022. https://elearningindustry.com/change -management-3-reasons-training-supports-organizational-change

28 Institute for Healthcare Improvement. Science of improvement: implementing changes. Institute for Healthcare Improvemen websitet. Accessed April 9, 2022. www.ihi.org/resources/Pages /HowtoImprove/ScienceofImprovementImplementingChanges.aspx

29 Institute for Healthcare Improvement. Science of improvement: testing changes. Institute for Healthcare Improvement website. Accessed April 7, 2022. www.ihi.org/resources/Pages /HowtoImprove/ScienceofImprovementTestingChanges.aspx

30 Grout J. *Mistake-Proofing the Design of Health Care Processes.* Agency for Healthcare Research and Quality; May 2007. Accessed April 7, 2022. https://archive.ahrq.gov/professionals/quality -patient-safety/patient-safety-resources/resources/mistakeproof/mistakeproofing.pdf

31 Varkey P, Reller MK, Resar RK. 2007. Basics of quality improvement in health care. *Mayo Clin Proc.* 2007;82(6):735–739.

32 Brown P, Hare D. Rapid cycle improvement: controlling change. J Ark Med Soc. 2003 Apr;99(10):320–321.

33 Skhmot N. The 8 wastes of lean. The Lean Way website. August 5, 2017. Accessed June 5, 2020. https://theleanway.net/The-8-Wastes-of-Lean?msclkid=5af06545ba6311ecbd9b6fd1423acc46

34 8 wastes. GoLeanSixSigma.com website. Accessed April 9, 2022. https://goleansixsigma.com/8 -wastes

35 National Association for Healthcare Quality. About NAHQ. National Association for Healthcare Quality website. Accessed April 9, 2022. https://nahq.org/about-nahq

36 5S methodology explained. WhatIsSixSigma.net website. 2019. Accessed June 5, 2020. www .whatissixsigma.net/5s

37 National Quality Forum. NQF's work in quality measurement. 2017. National Quality Forum website. Accessed May 15, 2020. www.qualityforum.org/about_nqf/work_in_quality _measurement/#:~:text=Through%20our%20Measure%20Incubator%2C%20NQF,itself%20will %20not%20develop%20measures

38 Centers for Medicare & Medicaid Services. Electronic Clinical Quality Improvement resource center. CMS website. Accessed April 12, 2022. https://ecqi.healthit.gov

39 National Academy of Medicine. About the National Academy of Medicine. National Academy of Medicine website. Accessed April 9, 2022. https://nam.edu/about-the-nam

40 The Joint Commission. About The Joint Commission. Joint Commission website. Accessed June 22, 2020. www.jointcommission.org/AboutUs

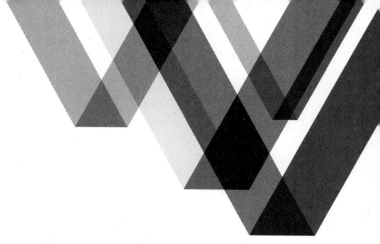

CHAPTER 14
Nutrition Informatics

Pamela Charney, PhD, MS, RDN, LDN, FAND

Introduction

This chapter addresses the important question of how nutrition managers can ensure their staff understand and use health care informatics and health care information technology (HIT) to provide appropriate and effective nutrition care for their patients. It provides an overview of the field of health informatics, explains why informatics is of increasing relevance today, describes some of the technologies that every registered dietitian nutritionist (RDN) should understand, and gives an overall picture of the informatics-related competencies required for safe, high-quality, effective nutrition care.

In health care today, virtually all information resources are computer based. Therefore, this chapter will focus on computer- and technology-based resources, including electronic health records (EHRs). However, a few caveats must be noted. First, information resources predate the "technology age" (many of us recall the days when the National Library of Medicine sent hard copies of *Index Medicus*, the forerunner of PubMed, to medical libraries every month). Second, health care informatics is *not* merely a synonym for HIT or EHRs. Think of nutrition informatics as encompassing what we know about nutrition and health and how we store, manage, evaluate, and share that information.

What Is Health Care Informatics?

In his fundamental theorem of informatics, Charles Friedman[1] describes "what informatics is and what it is not." Friedman posits that informatics is a tool clinicians can use to improve practice and "a person working in partnership with an information resource is 'better' than that same person unassisted."[1] Notably, this theorem does not equate informatics with technology alone. Instead, it focuses on two components: technology and the people who use it. When either component is ignored, mistakes are bound to happen. People can use technology incorrectly, but there is also ample evidence that technology can fail to meet the needs of clinicians in practice.[2-6] In sum, health informatics is the discipline that focuses on supporting health care professionals who need ready access to accurate information via secure and accessible technology platforms in order to optimize patient care and health outcomes.

According to the American Medical Informatics Association (AMIA), "health care informatics is focused on using data, information, and knowledge to improve human health and the delivery of health care services."[7] The health care informatician can be described as someone who creates and supports information resources that augment clinician reasoning and support provision of safe, effective care.[1] Health care informatics includes management of complex databases needed for research, integration of knowledge sources in health care, and evaluation of clinical systems and ensures seamless communication among providers, patients, and other stakeholders. Nutrition managers must understand and use health informatics principles and tools to ensure that the dietetics practitioners they manage have the skills and resources needed to thrive in an environment that is increasingly dependent on technology.

Data, Information, Knowledge, and Wisdom

Patient care generates tremendous amounts of data every day. Every laboratory test, vital sign, and anthropometric measurement is entered into the EHR as data. Data become useful only when they have been processed in ways that give them meaning. For example, the number 150 by itself has no meaning; it is only when we ascribe the term *lb* (pounds) that we know 150 lb is a measure of weight. When data have been given meaning, they become information. Figure 14.1 describes the data, information, knowledge, wisdom (DIKW) model. Using this model, it is possible to see data are generally meaningless. Once a description has been added to the data, information is created. When the information is used to do something, knowledge has been created. Finally, when knowledge is used to support actions that are in the best interest of the patient (or health care system), the result is wisdom that can be used to support future actions.

FIGURE 14.1 Data, information, knowledge, wisdom (DIKW) model

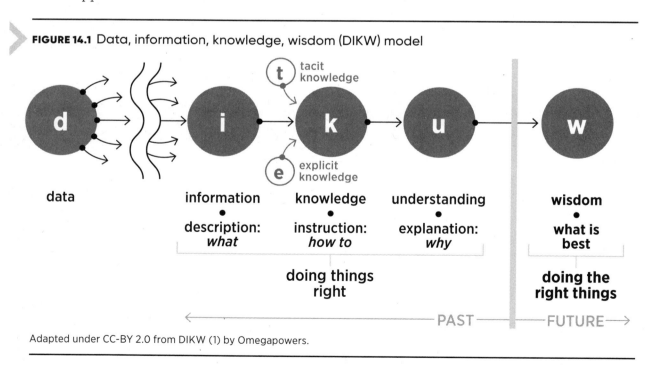

Adapted under CC-BY 2.0 from DIKW (1) by Omegapowers.

Informatics, Patient Safety, and Quality of Care

Patient safety and quality of care are the leading issues driving the health informatics movement. Have you ever had trouble reading a health care provider's handwriting in a paper-based medical record? Have you ever found mistakes made when patient data, such as height or weight, are written on a nutrition assessment form? Do clinicians sometimes forget to order vital components of a multipart feeding protocol? Each of these scenarios can be defined as a preventable medical error, and the appropriate use of HIT could help avert such mistakes.

Given that virtually all health care organizations are now using EHRs and other types of clinical information systems, you might feel that the types of errors described earlier would be a thing of the past. However, in some cases, the move to EHRs and other clinical systems resulted in the introduction of new types of errors. Use of tools such as *copy* and *paste* without adequate review of the data included results in mistakes being propagated throughout a patient's medical record. Poorly designed order sets still result in vital components being omitted or lost.[8] Inability to edit food allergy lists results in risk for potentially serious allergic reactions. Nutrition managers with a solid understanding of the strengths and weaknesses of HIT can play a vital role in preventing these new types of medical errors.

A preventable medical error occurs when a clinician inadvertently omits some component of care or makes a mistake in implementing care. Experts estimate that 180,000 people die every year in the United States as a result of preventable errors (the equivalent of three jumbo jet crashes every 2 days).[9] Unsurprisingly, these statistics have led to an outcry for improvements in the way health care is delivered in the United States, and many people and organizations have advocated for technological solutions. For example, a 2001 Institute of Medicine report, *Crossing the Quality Chasm*, concluded that preventable medical errors were a major problem in the United States health care system and suggested that improved use of HIT, including implementation of EHRs in all care settings, could help decrease the incidence of medical errors and improve patient safety.[10-12]

Meaningful Use of Electronic Health Records: A Brief History

Although many health care facilities have used HIT tools for decades, implementation of the EHR in all United States health care settings lagged far behind technology implementation in other areas of daily life. In 2009, the American Recovery and Reinvestment Act (ARRA) was signed into law. Part of this landmark legislation was the Health Information Technology for Economic and Clinical Health (HITECH) Act, which provided substantial funds to spur the implementation and use of technology in health care. One component of the legislation offered incentives to health care providers and organizations that demonstrated they were "meaningfully using" EHRs, and penalized those that did not meet meaningful use (MU) criteria.[13] In July 2010, final rules were released that described separate sets of criteria that providers and health care organizations had (and still have) to meet in order to qualify for financial incentives based on their MU of an EHR. MU initially was designed to include three stages, as follows:

> **Stage 1** was focused on adoption of EHRs and promotion of data sharing.

> **Stage 2** was designed to encourage care coordination and sharing of patient information in order to improve care.

> **Stage 3** was aimed at using EHRs and other health care technology to improve patient health outcomes.

To demonstrate MU, health care providers and facilities were required to show that they were using interoperable computer systems (ie, systems able to safely and accurately share information). As you can imagine, making sure systems are interoperable continues to be a huge task. One requirement of MU is that providers and hospitals must use certified EHRs. RDNs, particularly those in private practice, should be aware of this requirement, which does not apply specifically to the RDN but will apply to providers who refer to the RDN. In addition to ensuring that systems can "talk" to each other, many health care systems are still dealing with the need to transfer the vast amount of patient care information found in paper records to an electronic format. Also, as information is moved into an electronic format, it is necessary to determine how to make the information available only to individuals who are authorized to access it. Finally, in order to study health outcomes informatics, professionals with skills in data extraction and analysis are needed to retrieve the information to generate reports.

Meaningful Use: Where Are We Now?

In 2018, MU was revised and renamed promoting interoperability.[14] Since MU stages 1 and 2 are now complete, promoting interoperability is focused on stage 3 requirements. There are separate requirements for eligible providers and eligible hospitals. The 2019 requirements are of particular interest due to their inclusion of electronic prescribing (e-prescribing), supporting health information exchange, providing patients with access to their health information, and public health and clinical data exchange.[14] One component of this is the OpenNotes project (www.opennotes.org). OpenNotes has its roots in a movement that began in the 1970s to promote the practice of providing patients with all of the information related to their care. Beginning in April 2021, much of the information related to patient care must be made easily available and at no cost to patients. It is important that RDNs understand the implications of the OpenNotes requirements. Research is emerging that shows a positive impact on patients when notes are correct and easily understood.

Promoting Interoperability and Nutrition Care

At this time, RDNs are not identified as providers who must participate in promoting interoperability. However, if RDNs were to be included, those in ambulatory settings or private practice will be required to purchase, install, and use certified EHRs that can share information with all referring health care providers. Also, RDNs working in clinical settings will be included under the facility's requirements for demonstration of achievement of interoperability goals.

Requirements for promoting interoperability are designed to support the following five national pillars of health outcomes policy priorities[15]:

> improving the quality, safety, and efficiency of health care while reducing health disparities;

> engaging patients and their families in their health care;

> improving care coordination;

> improving population and public health; and

> ensuring adequate privacy and security for personal health records.

Each of these goals has implications for nutrition care. See Box 14.1 for examples of actions RDNs can take to support optimal national health outcomes.[15-17]

BOX 14.1 Five National Health Outcome Goals and the Role of the Registered Dietitian Nutritionist[15-17]

Health outcome goal	Suggested dietitian role
Improving the quality, safety, and efficiency of health care while reducing health disparities	Work with community leaders to identify "food deserts" that may impact nutritional health, and use information systems to connect the community to hospital systems in order to ensure access to a safe, adequate food supply.
Engaging patients and their families in their health care	Use health information technology to ensure patients and clients have ready access to information about diet and nutrition. Develop nutrition sections of personal health records.
Improving care coordination	Lead or participate as a member of a multidisciplinary medical home team.
Improving population and public health	Develop, implement, and evaluate community nutrition programs.
Ensuring adequate privacy and security for personal health records	Take steps to ensure patient and client information is protected. Share only information that is needed to accomplish safe patient care.

What Education, Training, and Skills Are Needed to Work in Nutrition Informatics?

As this chapter has emphasized, RDNs must become comfortable with and skilled in the use of health care technology to succeed in the current health care environment. In this endeavor, RDNs are not alone. Asan and colleagues[18] studied the perceptions of oncologists related to use of EHRs. Their results found several areas for improvement, including presentation of too much unnecessary information, inadequate flagging of abnormal test results, and increased workload required to document patient care. It is imperative that nutrition managers focus on usability and workflow for their staff, as other research found that EHR-related factors were associated with burnout in a group of advanced practice registered nurses.[19] Others noted a strong association between EHR use and burnout in a group of primary care providers, as well.[19,20]

What sort of education and training leads to success in health or nutrition informatics? This question is subject to ongoing debate. In the past, it was possible for the RDN to obtain positions in health care informatics or IT departments without formal training in the field, but these opportunities are rare now unless the RDN has extensive on-the-job experience. Today, most positions require advanced training in the form of baccalaureate or graduate degrees in health or biomedical informatics.

Recent efforts have been centered on creation of a new certification for health care informatics professionals through programs such as the one offered by the AMIA.[21]

Dietetics Education and Nutrition Informatics

In 2017, the Accreditation Council for Education in Nutrition and Dietetics (ACEND) adopted a new set of standards for dietetics education.[22] Core knowledge statements do not specifically include nutrition informatics. While a health care or nutrition informatics professional might see the potential to include informatics in each of the core knowledge statements, there is no requirement to do so. Therefore, it would be possible for students to complete the requirements specified in the verification statement without exposure to nutrition informatics.

Information technology (IT) is included in the standards for dietetic internship programs, but the concept is vaguely defined, giving program directors and preceptors great leeway in incorporating technology in dietetics education. The only competency for individuals training to become an RDN (Competency Registered Dietitian Nutritionist [CRDN]) that specifically mentions nutrition informatics does so in a very narrow way that misuses the terms "information" and "data" (CRDN 4.4: "Apply current nutrition informatics to develop, store, retrieve, and disseminate information and data").[23] Unfortunately, educators who have not been exposed to emerging technology may not understand the full range of tools available for nutrition care and may not require dietetics students to master technology or nutrition informatics beyond the use of word processing, spreadsheet, and presentation software. Most educators now include some exposure to the EHR as a data entry tool. Therefore, nutrition managers cannot assume RDNs who have completed training in the past few years have all the skills they need to function in today's technology-dependent health care setting. Instead, nutrition managers must evaluate the informatics and technology skills of staff and be ready to provide training as needed.

As RDNs debate how nutrition informatics will affect the dietetics profession, it can be helpful to look at developments and advances in related health care fields. Medical and nursing professional organizations have basic competency sets for physicians and nurses working in clinical practice along with advanced competencies for those specializing in health informatics.

Lessons From Medical Informatics

In 2008, AMIA's board of directors approved core content and training program requirements for physicians in clinical informatics. These requirements allow for the establishment of formal training programs for physicians at the fellow level or those who have completed medical education and residency training. Core content is divided into four major categories: informatics fundamentals, clinical decision making and care process improvement, health information systems, and leadership and management of change.[24] AMIA's application for approval by the American Board of Medical Specialties for formal establishment of clinical informatics as a medical subspecialty has been approved. Clinical informatics is also now recognized as a subspecialty under the American Board of Preventive Medicine.

Box 14.2 provides a broad overview of the knowledge required by physicians who plan to specialize in clinical informatics.[24] The first group of physicians was certified in 2011.

BOX 14.2 Core Content Areas for Physicians Practicing in Clinical Informatics[24]

» **Fundamentals:** Basic knowledge in clinical informatics

» **Clinical decision making and care process improvement:** Knowledge and skills that enable physician informaticists to participate in creation of systems and processes that support provision of effective, high-quality health care

» **Health information systems:** Knowledge and skills that support development, selection, implementation, and evaluation of clinical information systems

» **Leading and managing change:** Knowledge and skills that are needed to lead and manage changes associated with implementation of clinical information systems and to promote use of clinical systems from other health professionals

---

Lessons From Nursing Informatics

Nurses make up approximately half of the health care workforce and are major users of informatics tools in all care settings. As health care becomes increasingly dependent on technology to accomplish many patient care tasks, the need for basic knowledge and skill in nursing informatics has become evident. In 2007, Bond described nursing as a profession that lacked sufficient technology skills and divided nurses into the following three groups based on their attitudes toward IT[25]:

> **Engagers** were those nurses with experience using computers in work settings as well as to research evidence-based care resources.

> The **worried willing** were those who would use computers if they felt they had the skills needed to effectively do so.

> **Resisters** were those who did not want to use computers and thought computers interfered with effective care.

Interestingly, neither age nor experience necessarily correlates with competency in IT in the nursing profession. Although it is often assumed that older health professionals are less likely to possess computer skills, a survey of Australian nurses found that computer usage and skills were not associated with either age or length of nursing career. In the same survey, more than 92% of respondents reported that computer skills were essential for nursing practice. Only 2.9% stated that they avoided using computers whenever they could.[26]

Recognizing that educational programs may not be providing student nurses with the skills needed to thrive in a care environment heavily dependent on informatics, the Technology Informatics Guiding Education Reform (TIGER) Initiative was charged with developing solutions.[27] Informatics skills are now being incorporated into entry-level nursing education,[28] and the computer skills and informatics competencies proposed for undergraduate nursing programs may help nutrition managers assess the learning needs of current staff as well as new hires. These competencies include[29]:

> understanding computer basics (file and folder management, basic trouble-shooting);

> understanding and meeting information needs to support individual professional practice as well as patients' information needs; and

> being able to work in an environment that relies heavily on information and technology.

Developments in nursing informatics at more advanced levels could also provide models for nutrition informatics. Nurses can now achieve certification in informatics from several organizations,[30,31] and professional nursing organizations are developing competencies for nurses who specialize in informatics practice.[32,33] Furthermore, there are several accredited graduate-level programs in nursing informatics. Of particular interest to RDNs, some of these programs, such as the Clinical Informatics & Patient Centered Technology program at the University of Washington,[34] do not require nursing experience for entry.

American Medical Informatics Association Health Informatics Certification

Following creation of the medical informatics subspecialty for physicians, AMIA turned to investigation of knowledge and skills needed for safe, effective practice in health informatics. This practice analysis identified five domains of practice that included 74 tasks and 144 knowledge statements. The identified domains are discussed here.[35]

Domain 1: Foundational Knowledge Fundamental knowledge and skills that provide health informaticians with a common vocabulary, basic knowledge across all health informatics domains, and understanding of the environment in which they function.[35]

Domain 2: Enhancing Health Decision Making, Processes, and Outcomes Support and enhance decision making by clinicians, patients, and public health professionals; analyze existing health processes and identify ways that health data and health information systems (HIS) can enable improved outcomes; evaluate the impact of HIS on practice; pursue discovery and innovation in HIS and informatics practice.[35]

Domain 3: Health Information Systems Plan, develop or acquire, implement, maintain, and evaluate health information systems that are integrated with existing IT systems across the continuum of care, including clinical, consumer, and public health domains, while addressing privacy and safety considerations.[35]

Domain 4: Data Governance, Management, and Analytics Establish and maintain data governance structures, policies, and processes. Acquire and manage health-related data to ensure their quality and meaning across settings and to use them for analysis that supports individual and population health and drives innovation.[35]

Domain 5: Leadership, Professionalism, Strategy, and Transformation Build support and create alignment for informatics best practices; lead health informatics initiatives and innovation through collaboration and stakeholder engagement across organizations and systems.[35]

This new certification was offered for the first time in fall 2021. RDNs who have an advanced degree and meet criteria for time spent in health informatics practice are eligible to take the certification examination.

Electronic Health Record Systems: What They Are and What They Do

As noted earlier in this chapter, EHRs are only one component of the field of biomedical and health informatics. However, for many nutrition managers and the staff they manage, EHRs are the primary technology encountered in the workplace. Nutrition managers must understand the capabilities of the EHR to ensure information needed by dietetics practitioners and other providers is timely, accurate, and readily available.

The EHR is not simply a computerized replacement for the paper medical record. While early versions of the EHR included only transcribed versions of patient encounters and had limited functionality for data sharing or editing, such "flat" files are rapidly becoming a thing of the past. Current technology has expanded the scope of the EHR from a simple repository of clinical encounters for use in one setting to an interactive database containing information that can be accessed and utilized by clinicians in a variety of care settings. The ultimate goal in implementation of the EHR is to provide individuals with a repository of their personal health information that is accessible to authorized users regardless of the setting.

EHR systems vary depending on facility needs and budget. Older legacy systems often provide limited interoperability (information sharing between different departments or systems), whereas new systems purchased or licensed from commercial vendors generally offer seamless interface between departments and facilities. System interface is an important concept for dietetics practitioners to understand, as interoperability directly affects the efficiency and accuracy of clinical nutrition operations. For example, if a facility's foodservice department uses a commercial program to manage menus and inventory that is not interoperable with the EHR system, there will be no automated way for diet orders entered in the EHR to be correctly transmitted to the foodservice department.

Although the concept of an interface between systems might seem simple at first glance, health care providers must overcome major hurdles to ensure data are shared safely. Until recently, standards for data transmission were not available, and as a result, systems might not be able to send data to other systems in reliable ways. Current initiatives are focusing on developing data standards that will be used by all vendors that sell clinical information systems. However, even when all users agree on a data standard, clinicians will likely continue to encounter roadblocks to information sharing that need to be overcome. Therefore, nutrition managers must be wary when told that systems are "completely interoperable." In order to ensure information is transmitted appropriately, nutrition managers need to work closely with the IT department and EHR vendor to define the different types of data being sent.

To envision what is meant by standards for transmission or communication of data, it can be helpful to think about other standards that have become part of daily life. When you purchase an electrical appliance, you do not need to determine how electrical current will be supplied to the appliance. There is a standard that specifies which type of electrical outlet will be used in home construction and which type of plug will be used to connect appliances to electricity sources. At this time, there is no accepted data transmission standard comparable to the one used for electricity. However, the organization HL-7 (health level 7—the application level in standards) is developing and promoting communication standards for use in exchanging information in health care. Universal use of these standards should facilitate the smooth sharing of information both within and outside health care organizations.[36]

The following sections touch on some of the ways nutrition managers and their staff are involved in information sharing and the use of technology to transmit data.

Food and Nutrition Management Software Systems and the Electronic Health Record

Nutrition managers may be expected to take the lead in managing food and nutrition management software (FNMS) for a health care facility. A variety of FNMS systems are available to manage food production and management, clinical nutrition functions, or both. These systems are typically a small component of a facility's software needs. Therefore, the nutrition manager must act as a champion for FNMS systems and articulate departmental needs and capabilities during the early phases of any major facility software purchase or upgrade. Following are some of the key issues that should be considered when evaluating FNMS systems:

> Who will be responsible for database maintenance?

> Can the FNMS system interface with the facility's EHR? If so, what information will be shared between systems? If not, who will be responsible for ensuring information is entered into each system? Who will be responsible for maintaining the interface between the two systems?

> Can the system manage patient allergies and preferences?

> Can the software be customized to meet user needs?

Components of an Electronic Health Record

In addition to focusing on the interoperability of FNMS systems and EHR systems, nutrition managers should understand more generally how EHR systems can differ, both so they can use the facility's system correctly and so they can effectively explain the differences between systems to their staff. While all EHRs have the same capabilities, user experience will differ depending on the system and the purchasing contract between the system vendor and the organization. Newly hired staff might have experience in facilities using different systems with differing capabilities or their formal education about EHRs may have been limited in scope. The successful nutrition manager will help RDNs on staff understand that solutions that work in one care setting might not work in others due to differences in vendor contracts, system capabilities, and organizational behaviors.

Several vendors offer EHR products. Most of these systems provide a graphic user interface (GUI) with icons and buttons used to navigate through the system. This interface is sometimes referred to as the *front end* and will vary depending on facility needs and vendor design. All EHR systems also have a huge database of consolidated information regarding every patient's demographic profile, health insurance coverage, clinical data, and providers; this information is sometimes referred to as the *back end*.

Health care professionals responsible for evaluating EHR products can become overwhelmed with the complexity of systems offered. Vendors might offer products focused on one particular function in health care (eg, admissions, discharges, and transfers software; pharmacy software; or laboratory software) or products that purport to meet the needs of an entire facility or system. Federal standards provide guidance regarding which core functions must be included in the EHR system to meet interoperability requirements.[37] The core functions include (but are not limited to) the following:

> structured clinical documentation, which enables all providers to document the care provided in the system;

> computerized provider order entry (CPOE), which allows authorized providers to enter patient care orders directly into the system;

> documentation of patient demographics;

> retrieval of laboratory, procedure, and test reports;

> access to all provider clinical notes, past and present;

> clinical decision support systems (CDSSs), which provide alerts, reminders, and clinical practice guidelines as well as diagnostic support;

> medication management and tracking to include medication reconciliation;

> clinical flow sheets (vital signs, input and output records, etc); and

> problem list documentation.

Clinical Documentation

The transition from documenting patient care in a paper medical record to entering patient information into an EHR is incredibly complex. Although health care providers spend a good deal of time documenting patient care, some evidence indicates that much of this documentation is not read by others.[38] Thus, ideally, EHR documentation tools should be designed to ensure information documented by all providers is readily accessible to others in a format that can be easily interpreted and used. Information contained in the EHR must be accessible for several uses, including the following:

> billing

> regulatory compliance

> medicolegal action

> quality assurance

> teaching

> communication

Nutrition managers must be aware of all of these potential uses of information when developing documentation formats and screens for nutrition care. There are benefits and drawbacks associated with each documentation format.

One decision that must be made regarding documentation concerns the type of data (structured or unstructured) that can be entered into the EHR. Structured data entry allows discrete segments of information (eg, patient demographics, medical diagnoses, and laboratory and test results) to be saved and reused based on a predetermined format that defines where information is placed in a database. This type of data entry is often accomplished through the use of drop-down lists, menus of radio buttons, and other choice-limiting features. While structured data entry allows quick entry of information into the EHR database and supports extraction of information from the EHR, users are typically limited in the ways they are allowed to describe or document the care they provide. A poorly designed user interface for structured data entry may also lead to documentation errors.

Unstructured data (also called free-text data) is information that does not have special formatting applied to it in order to allow for searching or retrieval. A narrative description of a patient care encounter is an example of unstructured or free-text data. Natural language processing (NLP) is the area of clinical informatics that focuses on finding relevant information in free-text data. To illustrate the challenges involved in NLP, consider the word "lead." It might be present in an EHR in reference to an electrocardiogram lead, the heavy metal lead, or a lead role assumed by providers. NLP software must be able to properly evaluate each of these uses. Current technology does not allow efficient or accurate searching of free-text data in most EHR systems.

Clinicians often prefer the rich narrative capabilities of free-text documentation, whereas database managers and administrators prefer the ability to analyze and reuse information entered as structured data. Therefore, interface designers must carefully determine what information absolutely should be entered as structured data and what can be entered as free text. Nutrition managers should develop documentation formats that allow the entry of both types of data, as appropriate to the needs of clinicians and the facility.[37] Nutrition managers should detail how data will be used prior to requiring clinicians to use structured data entry formats that limit documentation of a patient encounter. Structured data that can be used to justify staffing and gain knowledge necessary to improve care processes include:

> measures of patient acuity (see Chapter 4),

> nutrition diagnoses,

> nutrition interventions, and

> monitoring and evaluation of patient response to nutrition interventions.

Use of structured data is facilitated by incorporation of standardized terminologies into the EHR. The Academy of Nutrition and Dietetics has developed the electronic Nutrition Care Process Terminology (eNCPT) to provide a mechanism to define and capture aspects of dietetics practice in standardized terms.[39] Nutrition managers should promote use of terms included in the eNCPT database to describe the work of dietetics in the steps of the Nutrition Care Process (NCP): nutrition assessment, nutrition diagnosis, nutrition intervention, and nutrition monitoring and evaluation. Using these terms allows for evaluation of the timeliness and effectiveness of nutrition care provided across care settings. The Stories From the Field box describes challenges facing a nutrition department attempting to incorporate clinical notes into the EHR.

STORIES FROM THE FIELD: Implementing an Electronic Health Record

Inpatient and outpatient clinical nutrition staff at a large academic medical center had been using their facility's electronic health record (EHR) for more than 10 years. Registered dietitian nutritionists (RDNs) were not included in initial EHR design; instead they were reassured that the design team would take nutrition care into account. The nutrition manager at the time was not aware of the importance of provider input into EHR design and told staff they would "get used to things" over time. Inpatient and outpatient RDNs used the same documentation format for their notes.

The design team determined (without conducting a workflow analysis, due to "time and money constraints") that RDNs should document using "flowsheets" that included mainly structured data entry. RDNs were told that data entered into the flowsheet would "flow" into an appropriately formatted nutrition progress note that could be easily read by other providers. The rationale given to clinical nutrition staff was that nursing preferred to use flowsheets, and nursing leaders determined that other allied health professionals should also use flowsheets to document care.

Shortly after the new system was implemented, RDN staff realized documentation was problematic for several reasons:

» Although the patient's height and weight were entered by the RDN at the beginning of documentation, this information did not flow to calculations of BMI or estimated nutrition requirements, thus requiring double data entry.

» RDNs were required to check off a series of data points for all patients. Radio buttons and check boxes were constructed using inpatient workflow and were not always applicable to each patient.

» RDNs were required to check boxes that documented exactly which educational handouts were given to patients. This flowed to the preformatted nutrition note. There was no plan to analyze these data, leading to unnecessary work for the RDN and a cluttered final note. While inpatient RDNs simply ignored this requirement, outpatient RDNs were required to document handouts provided. To date, none of these data have been used for analytics purposes.

» Data collection for nutrition focused physical examination was difficult to complete and was found in two different areas using two different formats. Information on oral examination was not included.

» The electronic Nutrition Care Process Terminology (eNCPT) was included but used drop-down menus that listed each diagnosis, etiology, and sign or symptom, leading to very long drop-down menus. This information was evaluated, and it revealed that busy RDNs tended to select the most convenient diagnosis instead of actually diagnosing the nutrition problem. In addition, only one diagnosis was allowed, so when a patient had more than one nutrition diagnosis, the RDN had to manually enter each as free text. Because this took more time, RDNs noted that many nutrition diagnoses were not documented.

It was thought that these problems may be due the following circumstances:

» Although much of nursing documentation works well as structured data entry fields, it is not known whether nutrition data works well as structured data.

» There are substantial differences between nursing and dietetics workflows.

» The flowsheet and nutrition note did not take RDNs' workflow into account, leading to several cognitive breaks during the documentation process when RDNs had to switch between using the flowsheet and entering free text. Each cognitive break interrupted the RDNs' thought process and required them to refocus, thus risking loss of time and clinical information.

The nutrition manager requested a formal workflow analysis for both inpatient and outpatient clinical nutrition settings. This resulted in separate documentation formats for each area of practice. Drop-down menus for nutrition diagnoses were streamlined and allowed for documentation of more than one nutrition diagnosis. The requirement for checking boxes for handouts was removed.

Computerized Provider Order Entry

Implementation of CPOE has been a major focus of the patient safety movement. Use of electronic systems for order entry ensures orders are timely, correct, and legible.[40] CPOE systems allow order entry by all providers who have order-writing authority, including those RDNs who are authorized by facility bylaws and licensure or scope of practice. While not without controversy, CPOE has been shown to be cost-effective and prevent medication errors.[41] For example, compared to a manual system, a CPOE system for parenteral nutrition (PN) orders in a pediatric hospital led to fewer errors in ordering and calculating PN solutions.[42]

Development of orders and order sets for use in CPOE is extremely complex work, and lack of attention to provider needs during development of CPOE systems may be a contributing factor to less-than-ideal rates of implementation. Poorly designed systems can also lead to increased time required for order entry, errors in data entry, and frustration with or rejection of systems. Therefore, to improve the acceptance, use, and efficacy of CPOE systems, providers must be involved in all steps of their development and implementation.

Implementation of CPOE can lead to dramatic changes in workflow for all involved.[43] System developers must be aware of the human aspects of CPOE implementation and take steps to ensure a smooth transition from paper to electronic order entry. When order sets are developed, they must include all necessary components of the order and be designed to minimize "click time" for the providers ordering diets or medications. During the development process, nutrition managers must carefully evaluate how diets and nutrition-related orders are entered in paper systems and translate this process to ensure the CPOE system is easy to use. For example, if the CPOE system forces the user to enter 10 different items before a complex diet can be ordered, providers will find the system to be less efficient than the previous practice of simply writing the desired order. When this happens, incorrect diet orders may be entered simply because busy providers do not have the time to spend trying to enter correct diet orders.

Clinical Decision Support Systems

A CDSS provides clinicians with guidelines, reminders, and alerts. Depending on the knowledge base associated with the system, information provided may range from simple reminders for appointments, preventive care, and follow-up to sophisticated diagnostic decision support.[44] Advanced CDSSs scan for patient characteristics that match information stored in the knowledge base[42] and provide sophisticated decision tools to aid clinicians in the diagnostic and therapeutic process. For example, a CDSS focused on nutrition support would identify patients receiving enteral nutrition (EN) or PN. The system would then provide clinicians caring for the patient with guidance in selecting feeding routes, formulas, and monitoring information. Providers initiating EN or PN would then be asked whether a nutrition support consult is needed. To encourage referrals to the nutrition support teams, the CDSS could make it easier for the provider to request the consult than to not request it.

Coding and Terminology

Standardized terminologies are now part of EHR databases, but they were used by health care providers long before the advent of electronic systems. The International Classification of Diseases (ICD) terminology has its modern origins in the 19th century, when it was used to facilitate reporting of mortality statistics.[43] Currently, health care providers in the United States use ICD clinical modifications (ICD-CM) to code medical diagnoses for billing purposes. While other developed nations began using ICD-10-CM in the 1990s, the US delayed implementation of ICD-10-CM until 2015. Because ICD was not originally intended to be used as a vehicle for billing, the use of ICD codes has been criticized for several reasons.[45,46] In many cases, multiple ICD codes could be used to identify a medical problem. In addition, ICD codes are often assigned before complete information is available, resulting in coding errors.[47] Attempts to better identify and study some medical conditions have resulted in the development of coding algorithms that can be used to improve accuracy in documenting diagnostic data.[48]

Other terminologies used in health care include Current Procedural Terminology (CPT); Systematized Nomenclature of Medicine Clinical Terms (SNOMED CT); Logical Observation Identifiers, Names, and Codes (LOINC); and the North American Nursing Diagnosis Association (NANDA) terminologies. As mentioned earlier, the eNCPT can be used specifically for standardized terms in nutrition care.

Support for Evidence-Based Practice

Evidence-based practice (EBP) in health care demands that the clinician use the best published scientific evidence combined with clinical experience and judgment to provide high-quality patient care.[49] EBP has been touted as a critical factor in improving the safety and quality of health care.[50,51] EHRs have the ability to provide clinicians with quick access to a wealth of information to support EBP. However, EBP resources are not always used at the point of care. Reasons for not using EBP resources include their lack of applicability, difficulty accessing the information, and users' lack of awareness of their value.[52,53] RDNs should ensure that EBP tools used in practice are accurate, up to date, and user friendly. Resources available for RDNs include the Academy of Nutrition and Dietetics Evidence Analysis Library, the Cochrane Library, and the American College of Physicians Journal Club. While these tools provide a readily available source of information that has presumably been reviewed and analyzed by experts in the field, they do not relieve the RDN from learning skills needed to find and analyze information.[54] Nutrition managers must ensure that EBP resources are easily accessible by staff at the point of care.

Privacy and Security

Use of technology in health care ensures that patient information is private and secure. When Congress enacted the Health Insurance Portability and Accountability Act (HIPAA) in 1996, the intent was to prevent abuse of information related to health insurance and to ensure that individuals had access to insurance coverage when changing jobs.[55] Administrative simplifications to HIPAA added more protection for patients regarding the electronic sharing of personal information.[56] HIPAA regulations can be complex and confusing; RDNs are urged to contact compliance specialists to ensure that appropriate information about patients and clients is shared only with those who have a need to know.[57]

Emerging Technologies: Smartphones, Data Analytics, and Collaborative Workspaces

No discussion of technology in health care is complete unless it addresses emerging (and sometimes already entrenched) trends in social networking, smartphone use, and electronic communication tools, such as wikis, blogs, and online collaboration software. It would be impossible to provide a detailed description of all these tools, particularly since they are constantly changing and evolving. Instead, the following sections briefly describe examples of some technologies that allow the rapid sharing of information. Dietetics practitioners should become familiar with technology tools and use critical thinking to determine which appropriately support application of the NCP.

Big Data and Health Care Data Analytics

The term *big data* refers to the tremendous amounts of data generated every day in health care. It wasn't so long ago that we measured health care data in terms of gigabytes. Current measures of data are done in exabytes; 1 exabyte is the equivalent of 1 billion gigabytes. Traditional analytic methods are unable to adequately examine the complex relationships between current data sources and types. The rapidly growing field of big data analytics uses newer techniques, tools, and skills for analyzing these data, including machine learning algorithms that allow for rapid analysis of terabytes of data.

To see how this can be done, imagine a public health professional who is responsible for allocating vaccination programs during flu season. To track outbreaks, data scientists might pull data from Twitter ("I'm home sick today—so achy I can't sit up"), Facebook posts, sales of cold and flu supplies from local pharmacies, and recent emergency room visits for a given set of signs or symptoms in order to predict when and where flu outbreaks might occur. Nutrition researchers might use big data to identify disease trends related to some aspect of nutritional health in communities with different socioeconomic characteristics.

Smartphones

Because smartphones have internet connectivity, they offer a wealth of tools, such as calendars, calculators, cameras, contact management databases, and thousands of mobile-based applications related to health care and nutrition.

Smartphone use has grown exponentially over the past decade. According to the Pew Research Center, in 2011 only about 35% of adults in the United States were smartphone users. By 2019, more than 80% of adults in the United States were using smartphones.[58] There are demographic differences in smartphone ownership, with 92% of American adults aged 30 to 49 years and 55% of those aged 65 years or older owning smartphones. There are no notable age differences when considering ownership of any type of cell phone. Therefore, because of the rapid increase in smartphone use among all age groups, RDNs should not immediately assume patient age is a factor when recommending nutrition and fitness smartphone apps.

Smartphones are small and easily portable for work, and they can provide a multitude of tools to facilitate patient care. However, the advantages of smartphones must be weighed against the potential risks associated with their use. Because these devices are small, they can be easily lost or stolen, which can put protected health information at risk. Nutrition managers who are contemplating use of (or are already using) these handy tools must be careful to ensure that any patient or client information is stored in an employer-approved, password-protected manner. Policies that provide clear guidance on proper security measures along with penalties for improper use of these tools must be developed and explained to staff. It would be advisable to check with security experts at the workplace to ensure that protected health information is kept safe and secure. Furthermore, when selecting mobile-based applications to use for reference, communication, and productivity, care must be taken to choose tools that are reliable, accurate, and compliant with standards and regulations.

It is also helpful for health care providers to understand how patients are using mobile-based applications to manage their health care. Smartphones are now widely used as tools to facilitate adherence to complex medical regimens.[59,60] In addition, patients are using their smartphones to track calories and exercise, find recipes, make shopping lists, and look for information on health, nutrition, and well-being. A newer use of smartphones in health care is in *gamification* or use of gaming tools and techniques to help engage patients in their care in order to improve health outcomes.[61] Researchers have recognized that people of all ages enjoy playing games, particularly if there is a good chance of winning. Gamification in health care combines the desire to win with positive reinforcement for desired behaviors.

Collaborative Workspaces

The user-generated encyclopedia Wikipedia (from the Hawaiian word for "quick") was the first successful collaborative workspace.[62] Wikipedia and other collaborative workspaces allow users to directly edit materials online, eliminating the need to download and share document files. Other collaborative workspaces include Google Docs and Microsoft Teams.

Wikipedia allows users to register for free accounts, which permit them to add content. Because Wikipedia users are not required to log in or register to edit content, concerns have been raised regarding the accuracy of the encyclopedia's articles. (Wikipedia has addressed this concern to some extent, but these efforts are mainly focused on preventing misinformation in biographies of living people.) Nevertheless, health-related content on Wikipedia seems to meet an acceptable level of accuracy.[62-65]

In dietetics, collaborative workspaces are becoming more popular because they allow users to create and edit pages while keeping a record of edits made. RDNs might use a collaborative workspace to create educational materials, coordinate meeting schedules and agendas, or maintain shared information in a central repository. A number of collaborative workspace tools are available, such as PBworks (http://pb works.com), which offers basic collaborative tools for free as well as several levels of paid support. In addition, RDNs may have access to employer-provided spaces, such as eRoom or network drives assigned to specified groups.

Summary

The past few decades have seen tremendous changes in the way health care professionals do their work, and the next few years will see even more changes as EHRs and other technology systems are implemented across all health care settings. Dietetics practitioners must therefore possess a strong framework for evaluating, implementing, and using technology to support practice in all care settings. Nutrition managers in particular should recognize the limits of their own knowledge and skills in nutrition and health care informatics; optimizing data entry in the EHR requires specific expertise in user-centered design and usability. This requires nutrition managers to develop a collaborative relationship with clinical informatics professionals in all care settings.

Health and nutrition informatics experts will be leaders in the efforts to develop and implement tools designed to improve patient care. Health informatics aims to turn information into knowledge and uses technology to support this objective. When used appropriately, technology helps the user and does not replace the critical thinking skills implicit in the NCP. Increasing numbers of dietetics professionals are seeking advanced training and skills in health informatics as well as tools that will support positive changes in how we work. However, unintended consequences can occur when the wrong technology is selected. It is therefore crucial that dietetics practitioners use the NCP to support decision making when identifying and using technology in the workplace.

REFERENCES

1   Friedman CP. A "fundamental theorem" of biomedical informatics. *J Am Med Inform Assoc.* 2009;16(2):169-170. doi:10.1197/jamia.M3092

2   Ash JS, Sittig DF, Poon EG, Guappone K, Campbell E, Dykstra RH. The extent and importance of unintended consequences related to computerized provider order entry. *J Am Med Inform Assoc.* 2007;14(4):415-423. doi:10.1197/jamia.M2373

3   Baron RJ, Fabens EL, Schiffman M, Wolf E. Electronic health records: just around the corner? Or over the cliff? *Ann Intern Med.* 2005;143(3):222-226. doi:10.7326/0003-4819-143-3-200508020 -00008

4   Fieschi M, Dufour JC, Staccini P, Gouvernet J, Bouhaddou O. Medical decision support systems: old dilemmas and new paradigms? *Methods Inf Med.* 2003;42(3):190-198.

5   Ford EW, Menachemi N, Peterson LT, Huerta TR. Resistance is futile: but it is slowing the pace of EHR adoption nonetheless. *J Am Med Inform Assoc.* 2009;16(3):274-281. doi:10.1197/jamia.M3042

6   Harrison MI, Koppel R, Bar-Lev S. Unintended consequences of information technologies in health care—an interactive sociotechnical analysis. *J Am Med Inform Assoc.* 2007;14:542-549. doi:10.1197/jamia.M2384

7   American Medical Informatics Association. Informatics: research and practice—what is informatics? AMIA website. Published 2019. Accessed December 19, 2019. www.amia.org/fact -sheets/what-informatics

8   Sarzynski E, Ensberg M, Parkinson A, Shahar K, Brooks K, Given C. Health information exchange of medication lists: hospital discharge to home healthcare. *Home Healthc Now.* 2019;37(1):33-35.

9   Anderson JG, Abrahamson K. Your health care may kill you: medical errors. *Stud Health Technol Inform.* 2017;234:13-17.

10 Institute of Medicine Committee on Quality of Healthcare in America. *Crossing the Quality Chasm: A New Health System for the 21st Century.* National Academies Press; 2001.

11 Office of the National Coordinator for Health Information Technology. About ONC. HealthIT.gov website. 2019. Accessed January 5, 2020. www.healthit.gov/topic/about-onc

12 Agency for Healthcare Research and Quality. Health information technology standards panel. 2020. Agency for Healthcare Research and Quality website. Accessed January 6, 2020. https://ushik.ahrq.gov/portals/hitsp/archive/?system=hitsp

13 Blumenthal D. Launching HITECH. *N Engl J Med*. 2010;362(5):382-385. doi:10.1056/NEJMp0912825

14 US Department of Health and Human Services. Promoting interoperability. Updated 2022. HHS website. Accessed May 14, 2022. www.cms.gov/Regulations-and-Guidance/Legislation/EHRIncentivePrograms

15 Centers for Disease Control and Prevention. Public health and promoting interoperability programs (formerly known as electronic health records meaningful use). Updated February 8, 2022. CDC website. Accessed May 14, 2022. www.cdc.gov/datainteroperability/index.html

16 Halamka JD. Making the most of meaningful use. *Health Aff*. 2010;29(4):596-600. doi:10.1377/hlthaff.2010.0232

17 Darmon N, Drewnowski A. Does social class predict diet quality? *Am J Clin Nutr*. 2008;87(5):1107-1117. doi:10.1093/ajcn/87.5.1107

18 Asan O, Nattinger AB, Gurses AP, Tyszka JT, Yen TWF. Oncologists' views regarding the role of electronic health records in care coordination. *JCO Clin Cancer Inform*. 2018;2:1-12. doi:10.1200/CCI.17.00118

19 Harris DA, Haskell J, Cooper E, Crouse N, Gardner R. Estimating the association between burnout and electronic health record-related stress among advanced practice registered nurses. *Appl Nurs Res*. 2018;43:36-41.

20 Gardner RL, Cooper E, Haskell J, et al. Physician stress and burnout: the impact of health information technology. *J Am Med Inform Assoc*. 2019;26(2):106-114. doi:10.1093/jamia/ocy145

21 American Medical Informatics Association. Become an AMIA certified health informatics professional. AMIA website. Accessed May 7, 2021. https://amia.org/amia-health-informatics-certification

22 Accreditation Council for Education in Nutrition and Dietetics. ACEND accreditation standards for nutrition and dietetics didactic programs (DPD). 2019. Updated January 26, 2018. eatrightPRO website. Accessed December 24, 2019. www.eatrightPRO.org/-/media/eatrightPRO-files/acend/about-program-accreditation/accreditation-standards/2017-standardsfordpdprograms.pdf?la=en&hash=18A1A38F32363415418B9E72E055AC98DD0438C0

23 Accreditation Council for Education in Nutrition and Dietetics. ACEND accreditation standards for nutrition and dietetics internship programs (DI). 2018. Updated January 26, 2018. eatrightPRO website. Accessed December 24, 2019. www.eatrightPRO.org/-/media/eatrightPRO-files/acend/about-program-accreditation/accreditation-standards/2017-standardsfordiprograms.pdf?la=en&hash=B1F08833AABC0FA8A6EBB7B76778A09BE7EDB667

24 American Board of Preventive Medicine. Clinical informatics content outline. 2019. American Board of Preventive Medicine website. Accessed January 5, 2020. www.theabpm.org/become-certified/exam-content/clinical-informatics-content-outline

25 Bond CS. Nurses' requirements for information technology: a challenge for educators. *Int J Nurs Stud*. 2007;44(7):1075-1078. doi:10.1016/j.ijnurstu.2007.01.009

26 Eley R, Soar J, Buikstra E, Fallon T, Hegney D. Attitudes of Australian nurses to information technology in the workplace: a national survey. *Comput Inform Nurs*. 2009;27(2):114-121. doi:10.1097/NCN.0b013e318197557e

27 Healthcare Information and Management Systems Society. TIGER initiative: an update. Updated 2022. Healthcare Information and Management Systems Society website. Accessed May 14, 2022. www.himss.org/what-we-do-initiatives/technology-informatics-guiding-education-reform-tiger

28 Thompson BW, Skiba DJ. Informatics in the nursing curriculum: a national survey of nursing informatics requirements in nursing curricula. *Nurs Educ Perspect*. 2008;29(5):312-321.

29 Bond CS, Procter PM. Prescription for nursing informatics in pre-registration nurse education. *Health Informatics J.* 2009;15(1):55-64. doi:10.1177/1460458208099868

30 Bakken S, Stone PW, Larson EL. A nursing informatics research agenda for 2008-2018: contextual influences and key components. *Nurs Outlook.* 2008;56(5):206-214. doi:10.1016/j.outlook.2008.06.007

31 American Nursing Informatics Association. Update on ANCC certification credentials. Updated March 2021. American Nursing Informatics Association website. Accessed May 15, 2022. www.ania.org/courses/ancc-update-2021

32 Hart MD. Informatics competency and development within the US nursing population workforce: a systematic literature review. *Comput Inform Nurs.* 2008;26(6):320-329. doi:10.1097/01.NCN.0000336462.94939.4c

33 Staggers N, Gassert CA, Curran C. A Delphi study to determine informatics competencies for nurses at four levels of practice. *Nurs Res.* 2002;51(6):383-390.

34 University of Washington. Online master of science in clinical informatics and patient-centered technologies. 2020. University of Washington website. Accessed January 7, 2020. https://clinical-informatics.uw.edu

35 Gadd CS, Steen EB, Caro CM, Greenberg S, Williamson JJ, Fridsma DB. Domains, tasks, and knowledge for health informatics practice: results of a practice analysis. *J Am Med Inform Assoc.* 2020;27(6):845-852. doi:10.1093/jamia/ocaa018

36 Health Level 7 International. HL7 home page. Health Level 7 International website. 2020. Accessed January 5, 2020. www.hl7.org

37 US Department of Health and Human Services. The Office of the National Coordinator for Health Information Technology. Updated 2022. HealthIT.gov websit.e Accessed May 14, 2022. www.healthit.gov

38 Hripcsak G, Vawdrey DK, Fred MR, Bostwick SB. Use of electronic clinical documentation: time spent and team interactions. *J Am Med Inform Assoc.* 2011;18(2):112-117. doi:10.1136/jamia.2010.008441

39 Academy of Nutrition and Dietetics. Electronic Nutrition Care Process Terminology (eNCPT). Accessed November 21, 2019. www.ncpro.org

40 Prgomet M, Li L, Niazkhani Z, Georgiou A, Westbrook JI. Impact of commercial computerized provider order entry (CPOE) and clinical decision support systems (CDSSs) on medication errors, length of stay, and mortality in intensive care units: a systematic review and meta-analysis. *J Am Med Inform Assoc.* 2017;24(2):413-422. doi:10.1093/jamia/ocw145

41 Roumeliotis N, Sniderman J, Adams-Webber T, et al. Effect of electronic prescribing strategies on medication error and harm in hospital: a systematic review and meta-analysis. *J Gen Intern Med.* 2019;34(10):2210-2223. doi:10.1007/s11606-019-05236-8

42 Lehmann CU, Conner KG, Cox JM. Preventing provider errors: online total parenteral nutrition calculator. *Pediatrics.* 2004;113(4):748-753. doi:10.1542/peds.113.4.748

43 Dougherty JA, Bonfiglio M. The future CPOE workflow: augmenting clinical decision support with pharmacist expertise. *Hosp Pharm.* 2019;54(3):149-152. doi:10.1177/0018578718791556

44 Loftus TJ, Tighe PJ, Filiberto AC, et al. Artificial intelligence and surgical decision-making. *JAMA Surg.* 2020;155(2):148-158. doi:10.1001/jamasurg.2019.4917

45 Cimino JJ. Review paper: coding systems in health care. *Methods Inf Med.* 1996;35(4-5):273-284.

46 McCarthy EP, Iezzoni LI, Davis RB, et al. Does clinical evidence support ICD-9-CM diagnosis coding of complications? *Med Care.* 2000;38(8):868-876. doi:10.1097/00005650-200008000-00010

47 O'Malley KJ, Cook KF, Price MD, Wildes KR, Hurdle JF, Ashton CM. Measuring diagnoses: ICD code accuracy. *Health Serv Res* 2005;40(5 Pt 2):1620-1639. doi:10.1111/j.1475-6773.2005.00444.x

48 Ginde AA, Blanc PG, Lieberman RM, Camargo CA Jr. Validation of ICD-9-CM coding algorithm for improved identification of hypoglycemia visits. *BMC Endocr Disord.* 2008;8(4). doi:10.1186/1472 -6823-8-4

49 Bordoni B. The benefits and limitations of evidence-based practice in osteopathy. *Cureus.* 2019;11(11):e6093. doi:10.7759/cureus.6093

50 Green LA, Seifert CM. Translation of research into practice: why we can't "just do it." *J Am Board Fam Pract.* 2005;18(6):541-545. doi:10.3122/jabfm.18.6.541

51 Miser WF. An introduction to evidence-based medicine. *Prim Care.* 2006;33(4):811-829. doi:10.1016 /j.pop.2006.10.001

52 Liang L. The gap between evidence and practice. *Health Aff.* 2007;26(2):w119-w121. doi:10.1377 /hlthaff.26.2.w119

53 Stewart WF, Shah NR, Selna MJ, Paulus RA, Walker JM. Bridging the inferential gap: the electronic health record and clinical evidence. *Health Aff.* 2007;26(2):w181-w191. doi:10.1377 /hlthaff.26.2.w181

54 Gooding B, Probst Y, Houston L, Neale E. Exploring perceptions, barriers and use of systematic reviews amongst nutrition professionals and nutrition students. *Nutr Diet.* 2020;77(1):151-159. doi:10 .1111/1747-0080.12598

55 Centers for Disease Control and Prevention. Health Insurance Portability and Accountability Act of 1996 (HIPAA). Updated September 14, 2018. CDC website. Accessed May 14, 2022. www.cdc .gov/phlp/publications/topic/hipaa.html

56 Chung K, Chung D, Joo Y. Overview of administrative simplification provisions of HIPAA. *J Med Syst.* 2006;30(1):51-55. doi:10.1007/s10916-006-7404-1

57 Choi YB, Capitan KE, Krause JS, Streeper MM. Challenges associated with privacy in health care industry: implementation of HIPAA and the security rules. *J Med Syst.* 2006;30(1):57-64. doi:10 .1007/s10916-006-7405-0

58 Pew Research Center. Mobile fact sheet. 2019. Pew Research Center website. Accessed December 26, 2019. www.pewresearch.org/internet/fact-sheet/mobile

59 Carroll AE, Marrero DG, Downs SM. The HealthPia GlucoPack diabetes phone: a usability study. *Diabetes Technol Ther.* 2007;9(2):158-164. doi:10.1089/dia.2006.0002

60 Marshall A, Medvedev O, Antonov A. Use of a smartphone for improved self-management of pulmonary rehabilitation. *Int J Telemed Appl.* 2008;2008:753064. doi:10.1155/2008/753064

61 Phillips EG, Nabhan C, Feinberg BA. The gamification of healthcare: emergence of the digital practitioner? *Am J Manag Care.* 2019;25(1):13-15.

62 Jemielniak D. Wikipedia: why is the common knowledge resource still neglected by academics? *Gigascience.* 2019;8(12):giz139. doi:10.1093/gigascience/giz139

63 Azzam A, Bresler D, Leon A, et al. Why medical schools should embrace Wikipedia: final-year medical student contributions to Wikipedia articles for academic credit at one school. *Acad Med.* 2017;92(2):194-200. doi:10.1097/ACM.0000000000001381

64 Weiner S, Horbacewicz J, Rasberry L, Bensinger-Brody Y. Improving the quality of consumer health information on Wikipedia: case series. *J Med Internet Res.* 2019;21(3):e12450.

65 Murray H, Walker M, Maggio L, Dawson J. Wikipedia medical page editing as a platform to teach evidence-based medicine. *BMJ Evid-Based Med.* 2018;23(suppl 1):A12–A13.

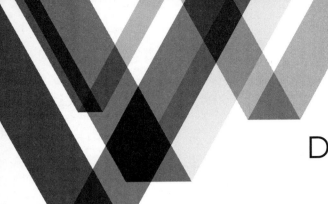

APPENDIX

Developing a Business Plan

Julie Grim, MPH, RDN, LD

Introduction

Whether you are an entrepreneur or are developing a new service, writing a business plan may give you the direction you need to make your new initiative a success. Business plans are often required for proposals for new services, especially if the initiative will require funding for staff, information technology, and so on. A business plan is also necessary if you wish to borrow money from a financial institution.[1]

Even when it is not a required part of an application, a business plan is an essential tool in moving your business forward. Benefits to creating a business plan include determining your target market, developing your organizational structure and financial plan, and establishing goals and strategies for your new business initiative.[1-4] Make sure the plan you create is specific, not vague. Your goal is to demonstrate how your business will solve a real problem or fill an actual need.[2,3]

Creating a business plan is not as difficult as you might think. There are a multitude of print, online, and software resources available, including free online templates to assist you in this process, and you can find advisors at Small Business Development Centers (SBDCs)[4] and business schools. In sum, a successful business plan[1-5]:

> presents a well-conceived idea,

> contains clear, concise writing,

> has a clear, logical structure,

> illustrates management's ability to make the business a success,

> communicates a practical approach,

> assigns tasks to people or departments and sets milestones and deadlines for tracking implementation, and

> shows profitability.

Sections of the Business Plan

There are many models for business plans, some of which are much more extensive and detailed than others. A discussion with your target audience to identify their priorities will help you determine the best model for your specific business plan. For the purposes of this chapter, our model will contain the following eight sections:

> Executive Summary
> Market Analysis
> Company or Department Description
> Organization and Management
> Marketing and Sales Management
> Service or Product Line
> Strategy and Implementation
> Financial Analysis

Section 1: Executive Summary

The executive summary—a succinct overview of the entire plan along with a history of your programs and services—is the first and most important section of your business plan. This section describes why you think your business ideas will succeed and tells the potential funder or decision maker where you want to take your new business or service. It is the first part of the business plan that your potential funder will see, and it will either grab their interest and make them want to keep reading or make them want to put the plan down and forget about it. Typical content in the executive summary includes the following[2,3]:

> your mission statement
> business start date (or projected start date)
> names of your management team and functions they perform
> number of employees on your team
> description of facilities
> products manufactured or services rendered
> summary of business growth, including financial or market highlights
> summary of future growth plans

The executive summary should be brief (one to two pages), with the details for each of these sections reserved for the body of your business plan. Although it appears first, write the executive summary last, after you have worked out all the details of your plan and are in the best position to write a succinct, effective summary of it.[2,3]

Section 2: Market Analysis

The market analysis illustrates your knowledge about the particular services or products your business will provide. It should also present general highlights and conclusions about any marketing research data you have collected. Imagine, for example, that your goal is to implement a series of fee-based, healthy cooking classes. Given this objective, the information you provide in this section might include:

> a summary of the type, length, and fee structure of current healthy cooking classes within your community;
> the market outlook for this type of training, such as attendance numbers at competitor's classes and the prevalence of chronic disease in your community;

> the amount of time required to prepare your classes for implementation;

> a summary about the competition (who else provides this type of education, what they charge if they charge, and why your offerings are superior); and

> information about why this type of education is particularly timely (eg, note relevant trends regarding increased interest in home cooking, culinary nutrition programs, and functional medicine).

You may find that the data you collected for your original exploratory analysis are sufficient to write the market analysis section, or you may need to expand your information base. Make sure your competitive analysis is thorough, and do not limit your analysis to programs involving RDNs. The analysis should identify your competitors by product line or service as well as by market segment, assess their strengths and weaknesses, evaluate how important your target market is to your competitors, and point out any barriers that may hinder you in entering the market.[3] Other specific details of your marketing research studies can be included in an appendix to your business plan, rather than in the marketing analysis section.

As part of the market analysis, you also need to define the levels of your pricing; your gross margin levels; and any institutional discount structures that apply to your business, such as discounts for volume or bulk orders, prompt payment, or patients paying cash. If relevant to your plan, gather information about how your primary payers reimburse for services, as these data can help you determine the length of billable time allowed for initial and follow-up visits. The following components should be included in the market analysis, as well:

> resources for finding information related to your target market,

> media you will use to reach your target audience,

> the purchasing cycle of your potential customers (eg, January tends to be the busiest month for weight management programs, and December tends to be the slowest; August through November may be very busy months because patients who have met their insurance deductibles will request appointments before the end of the year),

> trends and potential changes that could impact your primary target market, and

> notable characteristics of your secondary markets (ie, customers other than those to whom a product was originally offered, such as hospital employees or visitors who buy cookbooks designed and priced for patients).

The final area to evaluate as you complete your market analysis is regulatory issues. Be sure to capture data about current customer or governmental regulatory requirements as well as any anticipated changes in the future.

If your business plan involves any type of initiative to generate revenue from insurance reimbursement, be sure to address all issues related to reimbursement with individuals in your finance department or your billing or payment advisor. You should also determine whether regulations related to the Health Insurance Portability and Accountability Act (HIPAA) are relevant to your plan and be prepared to ensure compliance.

Section 3: Company or Department Description

The company or department description outlines your management structure, other services you provide, how long you have provided specific services, and other general information about operations. A brief description of the start-up plan for your new revenue-generating opportunity should also be provided in this section.

Section 4: Organization and Management

The organization and management section should include a broad picture of how all the different parts of your business fit together, such as your department's organizational structure and the qualifications and roles of you and your team. The length of this section will vary depending on the size and complexity of your department or company.

Section 5: Marketing and Sales Management

The marketing and sales management section describes your market penetration strategy, strategies for growing your business, and communications strategies as well as the methods you will use to evaluate the effectiveness of your marketing plan. When determining what tools to use to reach potential customers, marketing experts recommend a combination of the following promotions: advertising, public relations, personal selling, social media, and printed materials (such as brochures, catalogs, and flyers). In your plan, you may want to include sample copies of your actual or proposed marketing brochures and flyers, or screenshots from your website.[2]

Finally, remember that providing an outstanding service is fundamental to growing your business. Positive word of mouth is gold, from a marketing standpoint.[6]

Section 6: Service or Product Line

In this section, describe in detail the product or service your business offers. Be sure to emphasize the benefits customers receive from your product or service, how it differs from the competition's offerings, and the specific need it fills for your target customers. In addition, provide information about the current developmental stage of your product or service (eg, concept, pilot program, or completed program). Also describe how the product or service will be sold, any anticipated copyright or patent filings, and any plans for future product or service lines.

Section 7: Strategy and Implementation

Specificity is critical in the strategy and implementation section of your business plan. Identify management responsibilities, establish and communicate concrete goals, lay out the anticipated timelines for tasks, and provide budgets. Make sure your strategy includes how you plan to track results.

Section 8: Financial Analysis

A financially sound business plan should include at least the following financial projections:

> a break-even analysis that shows income and expense estimates for a year or more;

> a profit-and-loss forecast (pro forma) that shows a formal, monthly projection of your business's net income for at least the first year of operation (pro forma analyses are more refined than break-even analyses);

> a start-up estimate of the initial financial investment needed to launch the business (for example, if you are starting an outpatient medical nutrition therapy program, you might include estimated costs for educational materials and laptops, brochures, salaries, expanded liability insurance, and expanded telephone lines); and

> a cash-flow projection that identifies how much cash you anticipate will be coming in during each month vs each month's anticipated expenditures—this analysis helps you plan for adequate funding during months when the cash coming in is likely to be less than the cost of doing business.

Be sure that sales revenue, gross profit, and net income all feature prominently in this section of the business plan.

As you create your financial projections, do not underestimate possible expenses, and be conservative about your revenue expectations, especially if your revenue is based on insurance reimbursement. Remember that your staff will not generate revenue during every hour of the workday. Your projections must include realistic assessments of the time required for nonrevenue-producing activities and how much time is left for revenue generation. When in doubt, be less optimistic. This conservatism will make it easier for you to defend your projections. Your finance department, accountant, and the Small Business Administration (SBA) can help. If you are just starting out, your financial analysis will be based on projected costs and income.

Sample Business Plan

Executive Summary

Mercy Medical Center has operated an outpatient nutrition counseling department for the past 2 years. During this time, we have averaged 75 individual patient visits per month and achieved a monthly net profit of 15%. The mission of the Nutrition Counseling Center at Mercy Medical Center is to partner with our clients through nutrition consultation to enable them to maximize their health and wellness through healthy eating.

Our goal is to expand our services to include video and audio medical nutrition therapy (MNT) for individuals and groups in addition to our present face-to-face program. Analysis of the present market indicates high demand for these services and strong potential for profitability.

The benefits of this new service delivery model include:

> patient convenience,

> ease of access,

> expanded service area,

> increased physician satisfaction (physicians at our outlying hospitals will now have an accessible resource for their patients),

> increased patient satisfaction, and

> revenue generation.

The program will be housed in the clinical nutrition department and use a part-time registered dietitian nutritionist (RDN) to provide telehealth services and market the program in conjunction with the clinical nutrition manager (CNM). Part-time RDN hours will be flexed to accommodate changes in patient volume. Market analysis indicates high demand for this service and strong potential for profitability. Frequent requests from physicians and patients for this service indicate a solid customer base. We would like to begin offering these services effective January 10, 2021.

The initial service provided will be audio and video individual nutrition counseling. There is the potential to expand services to include audio and video group visits using the health care system's secure platform and communication portal for the following potential audiences: prenatal nutrition, diabetes prevention, and bariatric nutrition classes. Marketing materials, social media messaging, and an implementation plan have been developed.

We estimate that the start-up cost for equipment and staff training will be $9,500.00. Based on reimbursement history for outpatient MNT services at Mercy Medical Center, the new program is expected to recover initial start-up investment cost and reach profitability by July 2021 and continue to generate revenue on an ongoing basis.

Market Analysis

Mercy Medical Center has 670 employees and 309 active physicians on staff. In the surrounding area, four main hospitals offer outpatient nutrition counseling services to the community and at least five commercial businesses offer weight-loss nutrition services, but no other facilities offer telehealth for nutrition counseling.

According to reports from the Centers for Disease Control and Prevention (CDC), telehealth utilization increased as much as 154% in late March 2020 compared to the same period in 2019.[1] Although usage has since leveled off somewhat, it is clear telehealth is now a key part of health care delivery. According to a Healthcare Information and Management Systems Society (HIMSS) webinar presented in late November 2021, 90% of more than 700 survey respondents plan to increase (or continue to increase) telehealth access, and most organizations expect telehealth volume to increase post pandemic by an average of 53%.[2]

During the past year, we have received approximately four requests per week for video nutrition counseling from physician's offices and patients alike, indicating a clear need for and interest in this service. In addition, Dr Ofosu, Dr Shah, Dr Smith, and other providers have asked repeatedly for this service to be made available to their patients.

Following are drafts of (1) an updated outpatient nutrition counseling services brochure featuring telehealth services and (2) draft updated language for our website's home page.

Department Description

The Mercy Medical Center Clinical Nutrition Department is composed of Sally Hall, CNM; five RDNs; and a part-time diet clerk who also serves as an administrative assistant. Present services include inpatient MNT, outpatient MNT, and community nutrition education. Measured by volume, the top three inpatient diagnoses are cardiovascular disease, gastrointestinal disease, and diabetes. A part-time RDN will be added to provide telehealth MNT services; this RDN will work flexible hours based on patient volume. Sally Hall will partner with the outpatient RDN to market and manage the outpatient services.

Organization and Management

The Mercy Medical Center CNM is proposing to hire a part-time RDN. Part-time RDN staff hours will be increased as telehealth appointment volume grows to ensure there is corresponding revenue to cover costs and no increase in net costs. The two outpatient RDNs will provide cross-coverage and adjust workload based on the volume of face-to-face vs virtual appointments scheduled.

An additional consultation office on the third floor has been secured to meet patient privacy and HIPAA guidelines. Standardized charge codes are already in place to enable MNT billing in 15-minute increments. A computer, printer, and two monitors will be needed to maximize clinician effectiveness and enhance the patient experience. A desk or workstation will also be needed. The anticipated start date of telehealth nutrition services is January 10, 2021.

The new part-time RDN will require approximately 40 hours of training, which includes orientation to the hospital, MNT billing and coding, electronic health record (EHR) and patient portal, use of the hospital's virtual visit software, and virtual presentation training with the hospital media department.

Service or Product Line

Medical Nutrition Therapy (MNT) Individualized nutrition counseling that, in most cases, includes a 1-hour initial consultation with an RDN. The RDN reviews the patient's medical history and partners with the patient to identify nutrition and health goals and develop a personalized eating plan. In addition, supplemental materials, such as a list of websites, recipes, and tips for success, will be provided. Follow-up appointments, generally lasting 30 minutes, will be scheduled at the end of each session. Various counseling techniques, such as motivational interviewing, will be used. Patient outcomes are tracked and shared with the referring provider.

Strategy and Implementation

1. Billing, electronic registration, consent for service, and insurance verification and payment and receipt processes developed and approved by Finance and Admissions Department: September 30, 2020
2. Recruiting for part-time RDN begins: October 1, 2020

3. MNT content for EHR and for patient portal built by Information Technology: October 15, 2020

4. Educational materials uploaded to patient portal: November 1, 2020

5. Office equipment and computer purchase and installation: November 1, 2020

6. Office staff and current outpatient RDN training: November 15, 2020

7. Marketing materials, website, social media, and voice mail updated: December 1, 2020

8. Physician and community marketing campaign begins: December 1, 2020

9. New, part-time RDN hired (target date): December 1, 2020

10. New, part-time RDN training and practice with simulated patients: December 15, 2020

11. Scheduling for telehealth patients begins: December 20, 2020

12. Telehealth service begins: January 10, 2021

Financial Analysis

A review of reimbursement for MNT Current Procedural Terminology (CPT) codes for the past fiscal year indicates an average reimbursement of 60% of charges. The top five payers were contacted to confirm reimbursement policies for telehealth services. The payers contacted confirmed that their reimbursement in dollars and allowable reimbursement was the same for telehealth as for face-to-face consultations. Financial services verified that this had been the experience with other departments (eg, Medicine, Psychiatry) utilizing telehealth.

See financial data summarized in Table 1 (2021 estimated charges and revenue), Table 2 (2021 estimated net income), and Table 3 (telehealth pro forma) on pages 322 and 323.

Financial Summary

The addition of the telehealth initiative in the Nutrition Counseling Center is projected to break even within 6 months of implementation (July 2021) and generate $9,052.00 in net income during the first year of operation. The pro forma projects stable revenue and decreased expenses in year 2, and a doubling of both volume and net revenue in year 3, with progressive increases in net income each year. While Centers for Medicare & Medicaid Services rule changes in regard to telehealth are ongoing, continued expansions in Medicare reimbursement indicate favorable reimbursement for MNT. We will work closely with the financial services and reimbursement departments to monitor reimbursement rules and adjust financial projections if necessary.

TABLE 1 Calendar Year 2021 Estimated Charges and Revenue

Month	Patients/ month	Patient charge/ hour	Gross revenue	Net revenue
January	30	$240	$7,200	$4,320
February	40	$240	$9,600	$5,760
March	42	$240	$10,080	$6,048
April	42	$240	$10,080	$6,048
May	42	$240	$10,080	$6,048
June	42	$240	$10,080	$6,048
July	42	$240	$10,080	$6,048
August	42	$240	$10,080	$6,048
September	42	$240	$10,080	$6,048
October	42	$240	$10,080	$6,048
November	42	$240	$10,080	$6,048
December	35	$240	$8,400	$5,040

Start-up costs	
RDN training salary and benefit cost for 40 hours/week	$1,500.00
IT/computer/printer/monitors/ telephone	$5,000.00
Workstation	$1,000.00
Marketing/Web development	$2,000.00
Total start-up cost	$9,500.00

Ongoing costs (monthly)	
RDN salary and benefits at 20 hours/ week at $39,000/year	$3,250.00
Web subscriptions and continuing education	$100.00
0.2 FTE allocated administrative assistant time	$800.00
Office supplies	$50.00
Marketing	$50.00
Total monthly ongoing costs for year 1	$4,250.00

Abbreviations: FTE = full time equivalent | IT = information technology | RDN = registered dietitian nutritionist

TABLE 2 Calendar Year 2021 Estimated Net Income

Month	Gross revenue	Reimbursement/ net revenue	Cost	Monthly net income	Year to date net income
January	$7,200.00	$4,320.00	$13,750.00[a]	($9,430.00)	($9,430.00)
February	$9,600.00	$5,760.00	$4,250.00	$1,510.00	($7,920.00)
March	$10,080.00	$6,048.00	$4,250.00	$1,798.00	($6,122.00)
April	$10,080.00	$6,048.00	$4,250.00	$1,798.00	($4,324.00)
May	$10,080.00	$6,048.00	$4,250.00	$1,798.00	($2,526.00)
June	$10,080.00	$6,048.00	$4,250.00	$1,798.00	($728.00)
July	$10,080.00	$6,048.00	$4,250.00	$1,798.00	$1,070.00
August	$.10,080.00	$6,048.00	$4,250.00	$1,798.00	$2,868.00
September	$10,080.00	$6,048.00	$4,250.00	$1,798.00	$4,666.00
October	$10,080.00	$6,048.00	$4,250.00	$1,798.00	$6,464.00
November	$10,080.00	$6,048.00	$4,250.00	$1,798.00	$8,262.00
December	$8,400.00	$5,040.00	$4,250.00	$790.00	$9,052.00

[a] January includes start-up costs.

TABLE 3 Telehealth Pro Forma

Expenses	Explanation	2021	2022	2023
Clinician salary and benefits	Part-time RDN	$39,000.00	$40,170.00	$82,750.00
Administrative support salary and benefits	0.2 FTE allocation for scheduling and patient portal assistance	$9,600.00	$9,888.00	$10,184.00
IT	Computer, monitors, printer, phone	$5,000.00		
Clinical training	Onboarding	$1,500.00		
Office furniture	Work station	$1,000.00		
Subscriptions and continuing education		$1,200.00	$1,200.00	$1,500.00
Marketing	Brochures, business cards	$600.00	$600.00	$600.00
Website	Maintenance/enhancements	$2,000.00		
Office supplies		$600.00	$600.00	$600.00
	Total expenses	$60,500.00	$52,458.00	$95,634.00
Revenue				
	MNT visit revenue	$69,552.00	$73,030.00	$146,059.00
	Total revenue	$69,552.00	$73,030.00	$146,059.00
	Net income	$9,052.00	$20,572.00	$50,425.00

Abbreviations: FTE = full time equivalent | IT = information technology | MNT = medical nutrition therapy | RDN = registered dietitian nutritionist

References

1   Centers for Disease Control and Prevention. Trends in telehealth usage. CDC website. 2020. Accessed November 30, 2020. www.cdc.gov

2   Havasy R. Consumer perspectives on telehealth and virtual healthcare survey highlights. Health Information and Management Systems Society website. 2020. Accessed November 30, 2020. www .himss.org/resources/consumer-perspectives-telehealth-and-virtual-healthcare-survey-highlights

REFERENCES

1   Silver A, Stollman L. *Making Nutrition Your Business: Building a Successful Private Practice.* 2nd ed. Academy of Nutrition and Dietetics; 2018.

2   Pakroo P. *Small Business Start-Up Kit: A Step-by-Step Legal Guide.* 11th ed. NOLO; 2020.

3   Bangs DH Jr. *Business Plans Made Easy.* 3rd ed. Entrepreneur Press; 2005.

4   US Small Business Administration. Write your business plan. US Small Business Administration website. Accessed April 22, 2020. www.sba.gov/business-guide/plan-your- business/write -your-business-plan

5   Do you need a business plan? PowerHomeBiz.com website. 2013. Accessed April 27, 2020. www.powerhomebiz.com/starting-a-business/business-planning/need-a-business-plan.htm

6   Gross M, Ostrowski C. Getting started in private practice: a checklist to your entrepreneurial path. *J Am Diet Assoc.* 2008;108(1):21–24. doi:10.1016/j.jada.2007.11.007

CONTINUING PROFESSIONAL EDUCATION

This edition of *Effective Leadership & Management in Nutrition & Dietetics* offers readers 10 hours of Continuing Professional Education (CPE) credit valid through December 31, 2025. Readers may earn credit by completing the interactive online quiz at:

https://publications.webauthor.com/educational_leadership

INDEX

Note: Page numbers followed by *f* refer to figures; page numbers followed by *t* refer to tables; and page numbers followed by *b* refer to boxes

productivity benchmarks, 82–83, 83*t*

staffing mix, 74–75

staffing models, 69–70

time study outcomes, 86–88

CMS. *See* Centers for Medicare & Medicaid Services (CMS)

CNMs. *See* clinical nutrition managers (CNMs)

CNSC. *See* Certified Nutrition Support Clinician (CNSC)

coaching for performance

coaching session, 18

effective coaching blueprint, 18

GROW model, 19

high performers, 19

low performers, 19

middle performers, 19

Code of Federal Regulations (CFR), 188

common mistakes in leaders

effective delegation, 14

effective feedback, 14

failing to develop trust, 13

hiring mistakes, 14

performance issues, 13

set expectations, 14

set goals, 14

communication

active listening, 4–5

situation, background, assessment, recommendation (SBAR), 6–7, 6*b*

speaking with clarity, 5–6

writing clearly, 7–8

competency-based education approach, 78

computerized provider order entry (CPOE), 303, 306

Conditions for Coverage (CfC), 189

Conditions of Participation (CoP), 189

CPOE. *See* computerized provider order entry (CPOE)

CPT. *See* Current Procedural Terminology (CPT)

cultural competency, 49

cultural humility, 40, 46*b*, 49–50

culture, 46*b*

Current Procedural Terminology (CPT), 93, 307

D

data, information, knowledge, and wisdom (DIKW), 294, 294*f*

define, measure, analyze, improve, control (DMAIC) roadmap, 288, 288*b*

Definition of Terms document, 75

Dietary Guidelines Advisory Committee, 51, 52

dietetics education

American medical informatics association health informatics certification, 300–301

medical informatics, 298–299, 299*b*

nursing informatics, 299–300

dietetics leadership taxonomy, 27*f*

dietitian

career ladder activities, 144*b*

lead role, 145

DIKW. *See* data, information, knowledge, and wisdom (DIKW)

diversity, 46*b*

diversity, inclusion, and cultural humility, 237

DNV Healthcare, Inc. (DNV), 190

doctor of medicine (MD), 194

doctor of osteopathic medicine (DO), 194

dominant culture, 46*b*

dominant-culture bias, 51

E

EBP. *See* evidence-based practice (EBP)

EEO. *See* Equal Employment Opportunity (EEO) laws

electronic health record systems (EHRs), 293

challenges, 305

clinical decision support systems (CDSS), 306

clinical documentation, 303–304

coding and terminology, 307

components of, 302–308

computerized provider order entry (CPOE), 306

description of, 301–302

evidence-based practice (EBP), 307

food and nutrition management software (FNMS), 302

functions, 303

graphic user interface (GUI), 302

implementation, 305

privacy and security, 307–308

structured data, 304

unstructured data, 304

electronic Nutrition Care Process Terminology (eNCPT), 304, 305, 307

employee absenteeism, 108

employee bulletin board, 114

employee engagement

communication and, 108

increasing, 107

measurement, 106–107

employee recognition, 109

eNCPT. *See* electronic Nutrition Care Process Terminology (eNCPT)

enteral nutrition (EN), 306
Equal Employment Opportunity (EEO)
    laws, 220
equity, 46b
ethics and leadership
    autonomy, 39
    justice, 40
    non-maleficence, 39
    professionalism, 39
evidence-based practice (EBP), 247, 307
exchange leadership theory, 2
extrinsic rewards, 30

F

facilitation, 38
Fair Labor Standards Act (FLSA), 239–
    240
Family and Medical Leave Act (FMLA),
    240
federal regulation of health care
    facilities
    Centers for Medicare & Medicaid
        Services (CMS), 188–189
    CMS State Operations Manual
        (SOM), 190–191
    Code of Federal Regulations (CFR),
        188
    deeming authority and
        accrediting organizations, 190
    governmental entities vs. survey
        agencies, 188f
financial management, 185, 186f
FLSA. See Fair Labor Standards Act
    (FLSA)
FMLA. See Family and Medical Leave
    Act (FMLA)
FNCE. See Food and Nutrition
    Conference and Expo (FNCE)
FNMS. See food and nutrition
    management software (FNMS)
Food and Nutrition Conference and
    Expo (FNCE), 122
food and nutrition management
    software (FNMS), 302
FoodCorps, 57, 58b
foodservice management
    benchmarking, 112
    company culture, 115–117
    dashboards, 112, 113t
    effective training programs, 111b
    elements of communication, 105
    employee empowerment, 115
    employee engagement, 106–108
    employee onboarding, 109–111
    human resources challenges,
        108–109
    interdepartmental
        communication, 106

key performance indicators (KPIs),
    112
management training, 112
optimized scheduling, 113–114
recognition, 115
training new employees, 111
two-way communication, 105–106

G

graphic user interface (GUI), 302
GROW model, 19, 30

H

HAC. See hospital-acquired conditions
    (HAC)
HAPUs. See hospital-acquired pressure
    ulcers (HAPUs)
Health and Human Services (HHS), 264
health care information technology
    (HIT)
    big data, 308
    collaborative workspaces, 309
    data, information, knowledge, and
        wisdom (DIKW), 294, 294f
    description, 293–294
    dietetics education, 298–301
    education and training, 297–298
    interoperability and nutrition care,
        296–297, 297b
    meaningful use of EHR, 295–296
    smartphones, 308–309
health care quality
    Agency for Healthcare Research
        and Quality (AHRQ), 290
    Centers for Medicare & Medicaid
        Services (CMS), 290
    change management. See change
        management, health care
    common metrics, 272
    dimensions of, 264
    The Joint Commission (TJC), 290
    National Academy of Medicine
        (NAM), 290
    National Association for
        Healthcare Quality (NAHQ),
        289
    National Quality Forum (NQF),
        289
    National Quality Strategy, 264–
        266
    quality assurance, 267
    quality improvement, 265, 267
Health Information Portability and
    Accountability Act (HIPAA), 231, 307
HHS. See Health and Human Services
    (HHS)